An Illustrated Guide to Pediatric Surgery

Ahmed H. Al-Salem

An Illustrated Guide to Pediatric Surgery

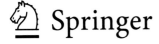

Ahmed H. Al-Salem
Pediatric Surgery Department
Maternity and Children Hospital
Dammam
Saudi Arabia

ISBN 978-3-319-06664-6   ISBN 978-3-319-06665-3 (eBook)
DOI 10.1007/978-3-319-06665-3
Springer Cham Heidelberg New York Dordrecht London

Library of Congress Control Number: 2014945252

© Springer International Publishing Switzerland 2014
This work is subject to copyright. All rights are reserved by the Publisher, whether the whole or part of the material is concerned, specifically the rights of translation, reprinting, reuse of illustrations, recitation, broadcasting, reproduction on microfilms or in any other physical way, and transmission or information storage and retrieval, electronic adaptation, computer software, or by similar or dissimilar methodology now known or hereafter developed. Exempted from this legal reservation are brief excerpts in connection with reviews or scholarly analysis or material supplied specifically for the purpose of being entered and executed on a computer system, for exclusive use by the purchaser of the work. Duplication of this publication or parts thereof is permitted only under the provisions of the Copyright Law of the Publisher's location, in its current version, and permission for use must always be obtained from Springer. Permissions for use may be obtained through RightsLink at the Copyright Clearance Center. Violations are liable to prosecution under the respective Copyright Law.
The use of general descriptive names, registered names, trademarks, service marks, etc. in this publication does not imply, even in the absence of a specific statement, that such names are exempt from the relevant protective laws and regulations and therefore free for general use.
While the advice and information in this book are believed to be true and accurate at the date of publication, neither the authors nor the editors nor the publisher can accept any legal responsibility for any errors or omissions that may be made. The publisher makes no warranty, express or implied, with respect to the material contained herein.

Printed on acid-free paper

Springer is part of Springer Science+Business Media (www.springer.com)

Preface

Pediatric surgery is a rapidly growing specialty. There are several textbooks on pediatric surgery but most of them are big and reference text books. Over more than 20 years of experience in the field of pediatric surgery and pediatric urology, I decided to write this book on pediatric surgery. This is different than any of the already written text books. It is actually a well-illustrated, easy to read and quick reference book. It is written in a simple way, point by point, and should be useful to consultant pediatric surgeons, fellows, specialists, residents, and nurses as well as pediatricians and neonatologists. The book covers most areas in pediatric surgery and pediatric urology with emphasis on the most important points relevant to the patient's management including clinical, operative, radiological, and hand drawn illustrations.

Ahmed H. Al-Salem

Acknowledgements

I would like to express my special thanks of gratitude to my family who supported me all these years as well as all my patients and their families.

Secondly, I would also like to thank all my friends who helped me a lot in finishing this project. A special thanks to Dr. Mohammed Ramadan for his support and help with the drawings.

Contents

1 Intravenous Fluids, Blood, and Blood Products 1
   Neonates (CC/kg/day) 1
   Infants (CC/kg/day) 2
      Electrolytes 2
   Replacement Solutions 3
   Blood and Blood Products Transfusion 4

2 Nutrition and Caloric Requirements for Infants and Children 5
   Nutrition Requirements 5
   Caloric Requirements 6
      Carbohydrates 6
      Fat 6
      Protein 6
      Electrolytes 7
      Vitamins and trace elements 7

3 Venous Access in Infants and Children 9
   Indications for Central Venous Access 9
   Types of Vascular Access 9
      Peripherally Inserted Central Catheter 9
      Central Venous Tunnelled Catheter 10
      Implantable Ports (Port-A-cath) 10
      Intraosseous Infusion 11
      Sites for Long-term Central Venous Access in Infants and Children ... 11
   Types of Catheters 12
      Catheter Care 13
   Complications of Central Venous Access 13
      Sepsis 13
      Catheter Occlusion and Malfunction 14
      Technical Complications 14
      Treatment of Catheter Occlusion 14
   Recommended Reading 14

4	**Abdominal Wall Hernias and Hydroceles**	15
	Inguinal Hernias	15
	Hydroceles	26
	Recommended Reading	27

5	**Lymphangiomas**	29
	Introduction	29
	Classification	30
	Lymphangioma Circumscriptum	33
	Cavernous Lymphangiomas	33
	Cystic Hygroma	33
	Sites of Lymphangiomas	34
	Treatment	34
	Recommended Reading	35

6	**Hemangiomas**	37
	Introduction	37
	Complications	37
	Treatment	39
	Treatment Options	39
	Prognosis	43
	Hepatic Hemangiomas	45
	Recommended Reading	45

7	**Branchial Cysts, Sinuses, and Fistulae**	47
	Introduction	47
	Embryology	47
	Types	48
	Clinical Features	49
	Investigations	50
	Treatment	50
	Recommended Reading	51

8	**Sternomastoid Tumor of Infancy and Torticollis**	53
	Introduction	53
	Etiology	53
	Diagnosis	54
	Management	54
	Recommended Reading	55

9	**Infantile Fibromatosis and Myofibromatosis**	57
	Introduction	57
	Histopathology	58
	Clinical Features	58
	Treatment:	60
	Prognosis	61
	Recommended Reading	61

Contents   xi

10 Thyroglossal Cyst ... 63
Introduction ... 63
Embryology ... 63
Sites ... 63
Clinical Features ... 64
Treatment ... 64
Recommended Reading ... 66

11 Undescended Testes (Cryptorchidism) ... 67
Introduction ... 67
Embryology ... 67
Etiology ... 69
Diagnosis ... 69
Treatment ... 70
Prognosis ... 71
    Fertility ... 71
    Testicular Cancer ... 72
Recommended Reading ... 72

12 Varicocele ... 73
Introduction ... 73
Clinical Features ... 73
Classification ... 73
Etiology ... 74
Diagnosis ... 74
Treatment ... 75
Recommended Reading ... 76

13 Acute Scrotum ... 77
Introduction ... 77
Treatment ... 81
    Intermittent Testicular Torsion ... 82
    Torsion of the Testicular Appendix ... 82
    Epididymitis and Epididmoorchitis ... 82
    Idiopathic Scrotal Edema ... 84
Other Causes of Acute Scrotum ... 85
    Scrotal Trauma ... 85
    Henoch–Schönlein Purpura ... 85
    Inguinal Hernia ... 86
    Hydrocele ... 87
    Varicocele ... 87
Recommended Reading ... 87

14 Esophageal Atresia and/or Tracheoesophageal Fistula ... 89
Introduction ... 89
Embryology ... 89
Anatomy ... 89
Clinical Features ... 90
Diagnosis ... 90

	Associated Anomalies	92
	Treatment	94
	Prognosis and Outcome	95
	Recommended Reading	98

15 H-type Tracheoesophageal Fistula — 101
	Introduction	101
	Etiology	101
	Presentation and Diagnosis	101
	Treatment	103
	Recommended Reading	103

16 Congenital Esophageal Stenosis — 105
	Introduction	105
	Incidence	105
	Classification	105
	Clinical Features	106
	Diagnosis	106
	Treatment	107
	Recommended Reading	108

17 Achalasia — 109
	Introduction	109
	Incidence	109
	Etiology	109
	Clinical Features	109
	Diagnosis	110
	Treatment	110
	Recommended Reading	113

18 Infantile Hypertrophic Pyloric Stenosis — 115
	Introduction	115
	Epidemiology and Etiology	115
	Pathophysiology	116
	Signs and Symptoms	116
	Diagnosis	117
	Treatment	117
	Recommended Reading	120

19 Congenital Gastric Outlet Obstruction (Pyloric and Antral Atresia and Web) — 121
	Introduction	121
	Anatomy	121
	Associated Anomalies	122
	Presentation	122
	Clinical Examination	123
	Investigation	123
	Management	124
	Prognosis	126
	Recommended Reading	126

20 Gastric Volvolus ... 127
Introduction ... 127
Classification ... 127
Treatment ... 130
Recommended Reading ... 131

21 Congenital Duodenal Obstruction ... 133
Introduction ... 133
Anatomy ... 133
Presentation ... 133
Examination ... 134
Associated Anomalies ... 134
Diagnosis ... 134
Preoperative Preparation ... 135
Operative Management ... 135
Postoperative Care ... 137
Complications ... 138
Recommended Reading ... 138

22 Neonatal Intestinal Obstruction ... 139
Introduction ... 139
Differential Diagnosis ... 139
Presentation ... 139
Examination ... 141
Investigations ... 141
Imaging Studies ... 142
Contrast Studies ... 145
    Important Things to Remember While Doing the Contrast Study ... 146
Treatment ... 147

23 Congenital Intestinal Stenosis and Atresia ... 149
Jejunoileal Stenosis and Atresia ... 149
    Introduction ... 149
Etiology ... 149
Classification ... 150
    Pathophysiology ... 153
    Clinical Features ... 154
    Diagnosis ... 155
    Treatment ... 157
    Outcome and Prognosis ... 161
Atresia and Stenosis of the Colon ... 162
    Introduction ... 162
    Etiology ... 162
    Associated Anomalies ... 163
    Clinical Features ... 163
    Classification ... 163
    Investigations ... 164
    Management ... 164
Recommended Reading ... 165

24 Intussusception ... 167
Introduction ... 167
Etiology ... 167
Types of Intussusceptions According to Etiology ... 167
Types of Intussusception According to Site ... 168
Symptoms and Signs ... 168
Diagnosis ... 169
Management ... 170
Recommended Reading ... 172

25 Intestinal Malrotation ... 173
Introduction ... 173
Embryology ... 173
Clinical Features ... 175
Investigations ... 177
Management ... 178
Complications ... 180
Recommended Reading ... 180

26 Meckel's Diverticulum ... 181
Introduction ... 181
Embryology ... 182
Symptoms ... 183
Volvolus ... 184
Diagnosis ... 186
Treatment ... 187
Recommended Reading ... 188

27 Meconium Ileus ... 189
Introduction ... 189
Etiology ... 189
Clinical Presentation ... 190
Differential Diagnosis ... 190
Investigations ... 191
Treatment and Outcome ... 191
Recommended Reading ... 194

28 Meconium Plug Syndrome ... 195
Introduction ... 195
Etiology ... 195
Associated Conditions ... 195
Clinical Features ... 196
Differential Diagnosis ... 196
Diagnosis, Treatment, and Outcome ... 196
Recommended Reading ... 197

29 Small Left Colon Syndrome ... 199
Introduction ... 199
Etiology ... 199

Contents

Clinical Features	200
Investigations	201
Treatment	201
Recommended Reading	202

30 Congenital Rectal Stenosis and Atresia ... 203
Introduction	203
Classification	203
Clinical Features	204
Diagnosis	204
Treatment	205
Recommended Reading	207

31 Necrotizing Enterocolitis ... 209
Introduction	209
Incidence	209
Etiology	209
Clinical Features	210
Diagnosis	212
Treatment	214
Indications for Surgery	215
Long-term Complications	217
Recommended Reading	217

32 Hirschsprung's Disease (Congenital Aganglionic Megacolon) ... 219
Introduction	219
Incidence	219
Pathophysiology	219
Etiology	220
Symptoms and Signs	220
Enterocolitis	222
Associated Anomalies	222
Diagnosis	223
Treatment	225
Laparoscopic Approach to the Surgical Treatment of Hirschsprung's Disease	226
Transanal Pull-through	226
Anorectal Myomectomy	227
Long-segment Hirschsprung's Disease	227
Neuronal Intestinal Dysplasia	228
Complications and Outcome	228
Recommended Reading	229

33 Congenital Segmental Dilatation of the Intestines ... 231
Introduction	231
Etiology	231
Sites	233
Diagnosis	234
Recommended Reading	235

34 Megacystis Microcolon Intestinal Hypoperistalsis Syndrome 237
Introduction 237
Etiology 237
Clinical Features 239
Treatment 240
Recommended Reading 240

35 Perianal Abscess and Fistula-in-Ano 241
Introduction 241
Classification 241
Etiology 242
Clinical features 244
Treatment 244
Recommended Reading 245

36 Gastroschisis 247
Introduction 247
Etiology 247
Diagnosis 248
Examination 248
Associated Anomalies 249
Management and Outcome 249
Recommended Reading 252

37 Omphalocele 253
Introduction 253
Etiology 253
Diagnosis 254
Associated Anomalies 255
Management and Outcome 256
Surgical Management 257
Hernia of the Umbilical Cord 259
Recommended Reading 259

38 The Spleen 261
Introduction 261
Embryology 261
    Functions of the Spleen 261
    Other Functions of the Spleen 262
    Splenectomy is Associated with 262
Pathological Conditions of the Spleen 262
    Splenomegaly 262
    Massive Splenomegaly 263
    Splenic Rupture 264
    Splenosis 264
    Accessory Spleen 264
    Asplenia (Congenital Absence of Spleen) 265
    Hepatolienal Fusion 265
    Polysplenia 265

Contents   xvii

    Splenogonadal Fusion 266
    Splenorenal Fusion 266
    Wandering Spleen 266
    Splenic Cysts 267
    Splenic Abscess 268
    Massive Splenic Infarction 268
    Congestive Splenomegaly 270
    Immunizations and Splenectomy 270
    Partial Splenectomy 270
  Recommended Reading 271

39 Splenogonadal Fusion 273
  Introduction 273
  Classification 273
  Etiology 274
  Clinical Features 274
    Associated Anomalies 274
  Treatment 275
  Recommended Reading 275

40 Cholelithiasis and Choledocholithiasis 277
  Introduction 277
  Etiology 278
  Complications 279
  Investigations 279
  Treatment 280
  Recommended Reading 281

41 Choledochal Cyst 283
  Introduction 283
  Etiology 283
  Classification 283
  Clinical Features 285
  Diagnosis 285
  Treatment 286
  Recommended Reading 289

42 Biliary Atresia 291
  Introduction 291
  Etiology 291
  Classification 292
  Associated Anomalies 293
  Clinical Features 293
  Differential Diagnosis 294
  Investigations 294
  Treatment 295
  Postoperative Care 296
    Postoperative Complications and Outcome 296
  Recommended Reading 297

43 Pancreatitis and Pancreatic Pseudocyst in Children ... 299
Introduction ... 299
Etiology ... 299
Acute Pancreatitis ... 300
    Clinical Features ... 300
    Diagnosis ... 301
    Medical Management ... 302
    Surgical Management ... 302
Pancreatic Pseudocyst ... 303
    Clinical Features ... 303
    Diagnosis ... 304
    Treatment ... 305
Recommended Reading ... 307

44 Congenital Pancreatic Cysts ... 309
Introduction ... 309
Embryology ... 310
Clinical Features ... 310
Diagnosis ... 311
Treatment ... 312
Recommended Reading ... 313

45 Intestinal Polyps and Polyposis Syndromes ... 315
Introduction ... 315
Classification ... 316
    Juvenile Polyps ... 316
    Familial Juvenile Polyposis Syndrome ... 318
    Peutz–Jeghers Syndrome ... 319
    Familial Adenomatous Polyposis ... 320
    Gardner Syndrome ... 321
    Turcot Syndrome ... 322
    MYH-associated Polyposis ... 323
    Cowden Syndrome ... 323
    Bannayan–Zonana Syndrome ... 324
    Cronkhite–Canada Syndrome ... 325
    Hereditary-mixed Polyposis Syndrome ... 326
    Gorlin Syndrome ... 326
    Lymphoid Polyposis ... 326
    Ruvalcaba–Myhre–Smith Syndrome ... 327
Recommended Reading ... 327

46 Congenital Diaphragmatic Hernia ... 329
Introduction ... 329
Embryology ... 333
Pathophysiology ... 335
Clinical Features ... 335
Associated Anomalies ... 336
Diagnosis and Management ... 337
    Surgical Repair ... 341
Long-Term Outcomes and Prognosis ... 342
Recommended Reading ... 344

47 Eventration of the Diaphragm ... 345
Introduction ... 345
Classification ... 346
Pathophysiology ... 347
Clinical Features ... 347
Diagnosis ... 347
Treatment ... 348
Recommended Reading ... 349

48 Morgagni's Hernia ... 351
Introduction ... 351
Presentation ... 352
Associated Anomalies ... 353
Diagnosis ... 353
Management ... 355
Recommended Reading ... 356

49 Congenital Paraesophageal Hernia ... 357
Introduction ... 357
Etiology ... 357
Classification ... 358
    Sliding Hiatal Hernia ... 358
    Paraesophageal Hernia ... 359
Clinical Features ... 359
Treatment ... 359
Recommended Reading ... 363

50 Congenital Lobar Emphysema ... 365
Introduction ... 365
Sites ... 365
Pathogenesis ... 366
Associated Malformations ... 367
Clinical Features ... 367
Diagnosis ... 367
Treatment and Outcome ... 370
Recommended Reading ... 372

51 Congenital Cystic Adenomatoid Malformation ... 373
Introduction ... 373
Classification ... 373
Presentation ... 376
Differential Diagnosis ... 377
Investigations ... 377
Treatment and Outcome ... 380
Recommended Reading ... 383

52 Bronchogenic Cyst ... 385
Introduction ... 385
Embryology ... 385
Sites and Pathology of Bronchogenic Cysts ... 386
Clinical Presentation ... 388

Investigations	389
Treatment	391
Recommended Reading	392

53 Pulmonary Sequestration ... 393
Introduction	393
Embryology	394
Classification	395
Intralobar Sequestration	395
Extralobar Sequestration (Figs. 53.2 and 53.3):	395
Diagnosis	396
Ultrasonography	396
Chest Radiography	397
Chest Computed Tomography	397
Arteriography	398
Magnetic Resonance Imaging	398
Treatment	398
Recommended Reading	399

54 Anorectal Malformations ... 401
Introduction	401
Associated Anomalies	401
Clinical Features	402
Investigations	403
Classification	406
Treatment	406
Diagnosis and Early Treatment	407
Postoperative Functional Disorders	415
Prognosis	415
Recommended Reading	416

55 Cloacal Anomalies ... 417
Introduction	417
Clinical Features	417
Associated Anomalies	419
Investigations	420
Classification	421
Management	421
Recommended Reading	424

56 Cloacal Extrophy ... 425
Introduction	425
Embryology	425
Associated Anomalies	427
Clinical Features and Management	427
Recommended Reading	430

57 Hepatoblastoma ... 431
Introduction	431
Etiology	431
Clinical Features	432

Contents xxi

    Investigations 432
    Staging 434
    Pathology 435
    Histological Classification of Hepatoblastoma 437
    Treatment and Prognosis 438
    Recommended Reading 440

58 Hodgkin's and Non-Hodgkin's Lymphoma 443
    Introduction 443
    Classification 443
    Staging 444
    Clinical Features 445
    Etiology 446
    Diagnosis 446
    Treatment 447
    Recommended Reading 450

59 Neuroblastoma 451
    Introduction 451
    Sites of Origin 452
    Etiology 452
    Clinical Features 452
    Investigations and Diagnosis 454
    Staging 456
    Treatment and Outcome 457
    Recommended Reading 460

60 Ovarian Cysts and Tumors 461
    Introduction 461
        Germ Cell Tumors 461
        Ovarian Teratoma 462
        Malignant Germ Cell Tumor 463
        Benign Cystic Teratomas (Dermoid Cysts) 463
        Dysgerminoma 464
        Rhabdomyosarcoma 464
        Ovarian Carcinomas 465
        Ovarian Cysts 465
    Recommended Reading 468

61 Pediatric Liver Tumors 469
    Introduction 469
    Investigations 469
    Classification 470
        Benign Tumors 470
        Malignant Tumors 470
        Hepatic Hemangiomas 470
        Mesenchymal Hamartomas 472
        Focal Nodular Hyperplasia and Hepatic Adenomas 473
        Hepatocellular Carcinoma 475
        Hepatic Metastases 476
    Recommended Reading 478

62	**Renal Tumors: Wilms Tumor (Nephroblastoma)**	479
	Introduction	479
	Epidemiology	479
	Clinical Features	479
	Investigations	481
	Pathology	482
	Treatment	485
	Prognosis	486
	Clear Cell Sarcoma of the Kidney	486
	Malignant Rhabdoid Tumor of the Kidney	487
	Mesoblastic Nephroma	489
	Recommended Reading	490
63	**Teratoma**	491
	Introduction	491
	Sacrococcygeal Teratomas	492
	Treatment	494
	Ovarian Teratoma	496
	Mature Teratoma	497
	Immature Teratoma	497
	Monodermal Teratoma	498
	Staging of Malignant Teratoma	498
	Complications	499
	Presentations	499
	Treatment	499
	Testicular Teratoma	500
	Mediastinal Teratoma	500
	Intraperitoneal Teratoma	500
	Cervical Teratoma	501
	Recommended Reading	503
64	**Testicular Tumors**	505
	Introduction	505
	Sertoli Cell Tumors	506
	Leydig Cell Tumors	506
	Juvenile Granulosa Cell Tumors	506
	Gonadoblastoma	507
	Paratesticular Tumors	507
	Clinical Features and Investigations	507
	Classification	508
	Staging	509
	Treatment	510
	Recommended Reading	511
65	**Thyroid Tumors**	513
	Introduction	513
	Classification	513
	Clinical Features	514
	Diagnosis	515

Contents

Staging	516
Treatment	516
Prognosis	517
Recommended Reading	517

66 Disorders of Sex Development ... 519
Introduction ... 519
Embryology ... 520
Classification ... 523
Etiology ... 524
Pathophysiology ... 526
Evaluation of a Newborn with DSD ... 526
Management of Patients with DSD ... 530
The More Common Causes of DSD ... 530
Sex Assignment and Therapy ... 537
    CAH ... 537
Recommended Reading ... 539

67 Persistent Müllerian Duct Syndrome ... 541
Introduction ... 541
Embryology ... 541
Clinical Features ... 541
Management ... 542
Follow-Up ... 543
Recommended Reading ... 544

68 Hypospadias ... 545
Introduction ... 545
Embryology ... 546
Classification ... 548
Etiology ... 549
Associated Anomalies ... 550
Treatment ... 551
Postoperative Complications ... 553
Recommended Reading ... 557

69 Pelviureteric Junction Obstruction ... 559
Introduction ... 559
Etiology ... 560
Clinical Features ... 561
Investigations ... 561
Treatment ... 563
Recommended Reading ... 566

70 Posterior Urethral Valve ... 569
Introduction ... 569
Clinical Features ... 570
Classification ... 570
    Glassberg's Classification of Ureters ... 571

Investigations	571
Secondary effects of PUV:	572
Pathophysiology	574
Management	575
Medical Management	577
Prognosis	578
Recommended Reading	579

71 Vesicoureteral Reflux — 581
Introduction	581
Etiology	582
Classification	583
Pathophysiology	584
Clinical Features	585
Investigations and Diagnosis	585
Treatment	586
Recommended Reading	590

72 The Exstrophy–Epispadias Complex — 591
Introduction	591
Embryology	591
Clinical Features	592
Isolated Epispadias	594
Introduction	594
Embryology	594
Classification	594
Classic Bladder Exstrophy	595
Introduction	595
Management	596
Recommended Reading	599

Index 601

Chapter 1
Intravenous Fluids, Blood, and Blood Products

Intravenous fluids and electrolyte requirements are variable and depend on the patient age and gestation, as outlined in this chapter.

Neonates (CC/kg/day)

- 10 % dextrose in water (D10W)
  - Day 1: 60–75.
  - Day 2: 75–85.
  - Day 3: 100.
- Electrolytes
  - Day1: D10W alone—except in major surgery or for those with abdominal wall defects.
  - Day 2: Na, 2–3 meq/kg/day.
  - Day 3: K, 2 meq/kg/day.
- For the first 24 h, supplemental sodium, potassium, and chloride are not usually required. Starting at 24 h, assuming that urine production is adequate, the infant needs 1–2 mEq/kg/d of potassium and 1–3 mEq/kg/d of sodium.
- Hyponatremia is defined as a serum sodium level of < 130 mEq/L. This is not a cause for concern until the serum sodium has dropped to < 125 mEq/L.
- Hypernatremia is defined as a serum sodium level > 150 mEq/L. This is not a cause for concern until the serum sodium level has risen to > 155 mEq/L.
- Hypokalemia is defined as a serum potassium level of < 3.5 mEq/L. Unless the patient is receiving digoxin therapy, hypokalemia is rarely a cause for concern until the serum potassium level is < 3.0 mEq/L. Severe hypokalemia can produce cardiac arrhythmias, ileus, and lethargy.
- Hyperkalemia is defined as a serum potassium level of > 6 mEq/L measured in a nonhemolyzed specimen. Hyperkalemia is more serious than hypokalemia, especially when serum potassium levels exceed 6.5 mEq/L or if there are electrocardiographic changes.
- Hypercalcemia is rarely observed in neonates; it is defined as a total serum calcium concentration of > 11 mg/dL or an ionized serum calcium concentration of > 5 mg/dL (1.25 mmol/L).
- Hypocalcemia is more common and is defined as a total serum calcium concentration of < 7 mg/dL or an ionized serum calcium concentration of < 4 mg/dL (1 mmol/L).

Table 1.1 Amount of fluid by weight

Weight (kg)	Amount of fluid, D/W 5% ¼ NS
1–10	100 CC/kg/day (4 CC/kg/h)
10–20	1000 CC + 50 CC/kg/day for wt > 10 kg (2 CC/kg/h)
>20	1500 CC + CC/kg/h for wt > 20 kg (1 CC/kg/h)

Table 1.2 Volume of maintenance fluid by body weight

Weight (kg)	Volume of maintenance fluid (CC/kg)
1–10	100
11–20	1000 + 50 (over 10 kg)
>20	1500 + 20 (over 20 kg)

Infants (CC/kg/day)

Tables 1.1 and 1.2 show the amount of fluid required by infants.

Electrolytes

Na 2–3 meq/100 CC.
K   2 meq/100 CC.

Commercially available saline solutions and their sodium concentrations are outlined as follows:

- Normal saline (0.9% NaCl/L): 154 mEq Na^+/L.
- One-half normal saline (0.45% NaCl/L): 77 mEq Na^+/L.
- One-third normal saline (0.33% NaCl/L): 57 mEq Na^+/L.
- One-quarter normal saline (0.2% NaCl/L): 34 mEq Na^+/L.
- Ringer's lactate: 130 mEq Na^+/L (contains 4 mEq K^+, 109 mEq Cl^-, 28 mEq bicarb equivalent all/ Liter, and 3 mg/dl of Ca^{++}).
- A guide for fluid maintenance therapy for term infants and older children is as follows:

    – Newborn:

    ○ Day 1: D10W infused at a rate of 50–60 mL/kg/d.
    ○ Day 2: D10W with 0.2% NaCl infused at a rate of 100 mL/kg/d.
    ○ After day 7: D5W with 0.45% NaCl or D10W with 0.45% NaCl infused at a rate of 100–150 mL/kg/d.

    – Child infusion rates:

    ○ 0–10 kg: 100 mL/kg/d (4 mL/kg/h).
    ○ 10–20 kg: 1000 mL/d + 50 mL/kg/d (40 mL/h + 2 mL/kg/h).
    ○ <20 kg: 1500 mL/d + 25 mL/kg/d (60 mL/h + 1 mL/kg/h).

- Maintenance fluid calculations in infants and children are as follows:

    – Hourly calculation:

    ○ 1–10 kg: 4 mL/kg/h.
    ○ 11–20 kg: 40 mL/h + 2 mL/kg/h.
    ○ >20 kg: 60 mL/h + 1 mL/h.

Table 1.3 Composition of body fluids

Body or IV fluid	Na⁺	K⁺	Cl⁻	HCO₃⁻
Gastric	70	5–15	120	0
Pancreas	140	5	50–100	100
Bile	130	5	100	40
Ileostomy	130	15–20	120	25–30
Diarrhea	50	35	40	50
RL solution	130	4	109	28
0.9% NaCL	154	0	154	0
0.45% NaCL	77	0	77	

- Daily calculation:
  - 1–10 kg: 100 mL/kg/d.
  - 11–20 kg: 1000 mL/d + 50 mL/kg/d.
  - >20 kg: 1500 mL/d + 20 mL/kg/d.

Replacement Solutions

The composition of body fluids is outlined in Table 1.3.

- Gastric losses: D5% 1/4 NS with 20 meq KCL/L.
  Replace losses cc by cc every 4 h.
- Duodenal and pancreatic losses: Replace with normal saline or Ringer lactate with 20 meq KCl/L.
  Replaces losses cc by cc every 4 h.
- Colonic loss (diarrhea): Replace with Ringer lactate.
- Dehydration:
  - For 5% dehydration, add 50 cc/kg/day.
  - For 10% dehydration, add 100 cc/kg/day.
  - For 15% dehydration, add 150 cc/kg/day.
  - Mild-to-moderate dehydration is corrected with D5 + 1/2 NS + 20 meq/L KCL.
  - Severe dehydration is corrected with normal saline or Ringer lactate.
- Normal urine output:
  1. Infants and toddlers: 2–3 m/kg/h.
  2. Preschool and young school-age children: 2–1 mL/kg/h.
  3. School-age adolescents: 0.5–1 mL/kg/h.
- Minimum urine output:
  Oliguria, a common fluid problem, is defined as a urine output of < 1 mL/kg/h.
  1. Infants and young children: 1 mL/kg/h.
  2. School-age adolescents >30 kg: 0.5 ml/kg/h.

Blood and Blood Products Transfusion

Blood and blood product transfusions can be given using the following formulas:

- Packed red blood cells: 3 × weight (kg) × (desired hemoglobin (Hb)—actual Hb).
- Whole blood: 6 × weight (kg) × (desired Hb—actual Hb).
- Fresh frozen plasma (FFP):
    - For volume expansion: 10–20 mL/kg given over ½–1 h.
    - For clotting factors replacement: 10 mL/kg.
- Platelets: 10 cc/kg.

Chapter 2
Nutrition and Caloric Requirements for Infants and Children

Nutrition Requirements

- Nutrient requirements for infants and children include the following:
  - Energy (measured as cal/kg/d)
  - Carbohydrates
  - Water
  - Minerals and trace elements
  - Protein
  - Vitamins
  - Fat

- The ideal energy ratio provides:
  - 65 % of the energy as carbohydrates
  - 35 % as lipids

- Most infants need 100–120 cal/kg/d for adequate growth. Some need up to 160–180 cal/kg/d.
- The primary goal in total parenteral nutrition (TPN) is to provide energy and nutrients in sufficient quantities to allow normal growth and development.
- The maximum dextrose concentration that can be delivered safely through a peripheral vein is 12.5 %.
- A 15–20 % dextrose concentration can be used in the presence of central venous line.
- At least 3 % of the total energy should be supplied as essential fatty acids. This can be accomplished by providing a fat emulsion (e.g., Intralipid, Liposyn), 0.5 g/kg/day, 3 times per week.
- Fat emulsions provide about 37.8–42 kJ/g.
- Parenteral fat emulsion is usually provided as a 20 % lipid emulsion made from soybeans (e.g., Intralipid).
- Intralipid is a concentrated source of energy with a caloric density of 8.4 kJ/mL (for 20 % Intralipid).
- Lipids play a primary role in supporting gluconeogenesis in parenterally fed preterm infants.
- Most practitioners start with 0.5–1.5 g/kg/d on the first day and increase steadily to 3–3.5 g/kg/d.
  - Term infants need 1.8–2.2 g/kg/d along with adequate nonprotein energy for growth.
  - Preterm very low birth weight (VLBW) infants need 3–3.5 g/kg/d along with adequate nonprotein energy for growth.
  - Once protein intake has been started, calcium and phosphorous should be added to TPN.
  - Calcium and phosphorous need to be concurrently administered for proper accretion.

- Take care to ensure that solubility is not exceeded; if this happens, calcium and phosphorous may spontaneously precipitate.
- Supplemental magnesium should be added to TPN once protein has been added.

Caloric Requirements

- Carbohydrates: 45%
- Lipids: 40%
- Proteins: 15%

  - 0–1 years→90–120 kcal/kg/day
  - 1–7 years→75–90 kcal/kg/day
  - 7–12 years→60–75 kcal/kg/day
  - 12–18 years→30–60 kcal/kg/day

Carbohydrates

The caloric density of carbohydrates in a solution is 3.4 kcal/g glucose.

D10%W solution has 10 g glucose/100 mL and provides (10 gm × 3.4 kcal/g) 100 mL = 0.34 kcal/ml. (D12.5% can be given through a peripheral line and D20% should be given through a central line.)

Fat

- Fat is used as an energy source and to provide essential fatty acids (linoleic and linoleic acid).
- The caloric density of fat in a solution is 9 kcal/g.
- 20% intralipids (20 g fat/100 ml fluid) solution has a caloric density of 2 kcal/ml.

Guidelines for infusion of 20% intralipids (g/kg/day) are provided in Table 2.1.

- Monitor the effect of infusion by measuring the serum triglyceride level. The goal is <200 mg%.
- Caution should be used in infusing fat emulsion in premature infants with pulmonary insufficiency, liver failure, jaundice, and coagulation disorders.

Protein

- The amino acid compositions for neonates, children, and adult TPN differ as there are some amino acids that are essential during the early phases of life.
- Protein requirements for growth and repair are age dependent.
- Protein requirement (q/kg/day):

  - Premature-term neonate 0–1 month 3.0–3.5
  - Infant (1–12 months) 2.5–3.0
  - Children 1.5–2.5
  - Adolescents 1.0–1.5

Caloric Requirements

Table 2.1 Guidelines for infusion of 20% intralipids (g/kg/day)

Initial	0.5	1	1
Increase daily by	0.25	0.5	0.5
Maximum dose	3	4	2

- The total calories to nitrogen ratio of the TPN formulation has a great impact on the optimal utilization of the carbohydrate calories and potentially on the incidence of TPN-associated liver disease.
- Ideally, it ranges from 150 to 180:1.

Electrolytes

Na^+	3–4 mmol/kg/day.
K^+	2–3 mmol/kg/day.
Ca^+	0.5–1.5 mmol/kg/day.
Mg^+	0.5 mmol/kg/day.
Cl^-	3–4 mmol/kg/day.
Phosphate	0.5 mmol/kg/day.

Vitamins and trace elements

- Vitamins A, D, E, and K are fat soluble.
- Vitamins B-1, B-2, B-6, B-12, C, biotin, niacin, pantothenate, and folic acid are water soluble.
- Vitamin supplementation should be started as soon as protein is added to TPN.
- Trace elements: zinc, copper, and chromium.

Chapter 3
Venous Access in Infants and Children

Infants and children, especially those with cancer, require long-term treatment. Venous access is necessary to administer intravenous drugs of chemotherapy, antibiotics, and total parenteral nutrition (TPN) or blood products. For this purpose, central lines are placed through a peripheral vein or central vein. These lines generally stay for longer duration and patients can move around with them.

Indications for Central Venous Access

- Peripheral access is not accessible.
- TPN.
- Chemotherapy.
- Exchange blood transfusion.
- Monitoring of central venous pressure.
- Haemodialysis.

Types of Vascular Access

- Peripheral percutaneous venous cannulation
- Peripherally inserted central line (PICC)
- Intraosseous infusion
- Percutaneous central venous access (Figs. 3.1 and 3.2)
- Peripheral venous cut-down
- Open central venous access:
  - Open central venous tunnelled catheters
  - Totally implantable venous access (Port-a-cath)

Peripherally Inserted Central Catheter

The simplest, safest, and most reliable vascular access is PICC (Fig. 3.1).

- These catheters are inserted through a peripheral vein and advanced into the heart.
- They require local anaesthesia.

Fig. 3.1 A clinical photograph showing a peripherally inserted central catheter (PICC)

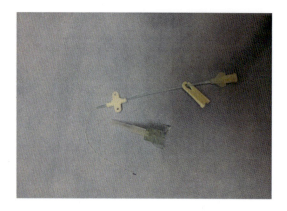

Fig. 3.2 Diagrammatic representation of a tunnelled double lumen central line. Note the proper position of the tip of the catheter in the superior vena cava

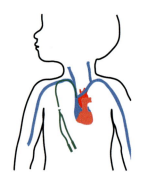

- They are easy to insert.
- They can be done at bedside.

Central Venous Tunnelled Catheter

- Centrally inserted tunnelled catheters are one of the most used options (Figs. 3.2 and 3.3).
- It can be single lumen or double lumen.
- It is inserted under anaesthesia through a big vein in the neck.
- Advantage is it can be inserted in any age group.
- It can be kept for longer duration until the treatment is over.

Implantable Ports (Port-A-cath)

Implantable ports are one of the best-suited options for children (Figs. 3.4, 3.5, and 3.6). They are:

- Used primarily in oncology patients for the administration of chemotherapy, nutritional therapy, blood, and blood products
- Associated with less infectious complications
- Require less care (no dressing or heparin flushing between use) and are out of site
- Do not interfere with patient activities

Types of Vascular Access

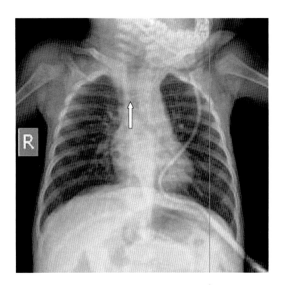

Fig. 3.3 A chest X-ray showing a tunnelled central line. Note the position of the tip of the catheter at the junction of the brachiocephalic vein and the internal jugular vein

- Cosmetically better and permit bathing and swimming
- Require general anaesthesia to insert and remove
- Require a special needle (Huber needle)
- Discomfort during port access which can be decreased with Emla cream
- Limited life span of the diaphragm

Intraosseous Infusion

Intraosseous infusion is illustrated in Fig. 3.7.

- A useful technique to establish intravascular access in emergency situations
- Should be used for less than 1 day and removed as soon as venous access is established
- Sites for intraosseous infusion:
    - Proximal tibia (1–3 cm below the tibial tuberosity on the flat anteromedial surface of the tibia).
    - After 5 years of age: Distal tibia (2–3 cm above the medial malleolus) or distal femur (On the flat anterior surface about 3 cm above the external condyle).
- Substances that can be given intraosseously: red blood cells (RBCs), fluids, antibiotics, anticonvulsants, muscle relaxants, inotropes, calcium, HCO_3, dexamethasone, glucose, and vasoactive drugs
- Hypertonic solutions are not to be given

Sites for Long-term Central Venous Access in Infants and Children

- External jugular vein
- Facial vein
- Internal jugular vein
- Subclavian vein
- Long saphenous vein

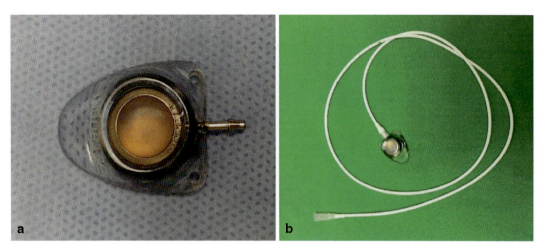

Fig. 3.4 a A photograph showing the single port. **b** The already connected port. There are also double ports. The length of the catheter to be used is determined intra-operatively and using fluoroscopy to determine the proper position of the catheter

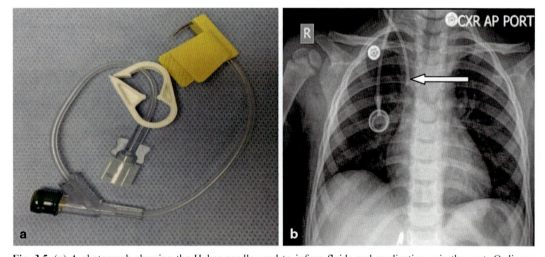

Fig. 3.5 (**a**) A photograph showing the Huber needle used to infuse fluids and medications via the port. Ordinary needles should not be used and a chest X-ray (**b**) showing the Port-A-cath. Note the position of the tip of the catheter in the superior vena cava

Types of Catheters

In the past, relatively stiff and thrombogenic polyvinyl catheters were used. Currently, more flexible inert catheters are used:

- Broviac
- Hickman

- They are made up of radio-opaque soft silicone with a Dacron cuff.
- The percutaneous subclavian approach is facilitated by a peel-away sheath.

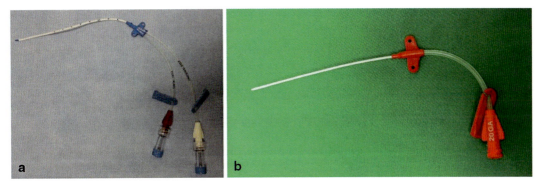

Fig. 3.6 a and **b**, Two types of percutaneously inserted *central lines*

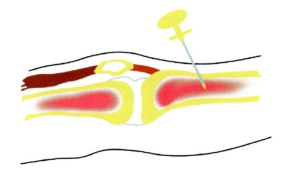

Fig. 3.7 Diagrammatic representation of intraosseous infusion

Catheter Care

- Flushing:
  - Done with heparinized solution (hepsal)
  - Should be done once daily or after administration of fluid or medications through the catheter
  - Neonates and infants up to 6 months of age: 3 mL of heparinized saline (10 units/mL)
  - Children more than 6 months old: 5 mL of heparinized saline (10 units/mL)
- Dressing:
  - Initially, every 2–3 days or sooner if they become soiled or moist and later every week
  - Should be done under aseptic technique
  - Transparent or dry gauze dressing can be used

Complications of Central Venous Access

Sepsis

- It is the most common and serious complication.
- Catheter-related bacterial infection can be successfully treated in the majority without catheter removal.
- The catheter has to be removed if sepsis cannot be controlled.

Catheter Occlusion and Malfunction

This complication can be caused by a number of factors:

- A thrombus within the lumen of the catheter or a fibrin sheath around the catheter end due to TPN ingredients or chemotherapeutic agents
- Malposition of the catheter tip against the vessel wall
- Catheter tip within a small branch vessel
- Thrombosis or stenosis in the native vein

Technical Complications

- Pneumothorax
- Haemothorax
- Hydromediastinum
- Subclavian artery puncture and haematoma
- Thoracic duct injury
- Brachial plexus injury and Horner's syndrome
- Catheter fracture and embolism
- Air embolism
- Catheter malposition
- Carotid artery injury

Treatment of Catheter Occlusion

- Streptokinase: (125,000 IU/mL). Use 10,000–15,000 IU. Fill the catheter and leave it for 2 h. Aspirate and flush with heparinized saline. Repeat 2 × if required.
- Urokinase: (5000 IU/mL). Instil 1 mL into the catheter, wait for 5 min, and withdraw and then flush with heparinized saline. Repeat if necessary.

Recommended Reading

Bagwell CE, Salzberg AM, Sonnino RE, et al. Potentially lethal complications of ventral venous catheter placement. J Pediatr Surg. 2000;35(5):709–13.

Chiang VW, Baskin MN. Uses and complications of central venous catheters inserted in a pediatric emergency department. Pediatr Emerg Care. 2000;16(4):230–2.

Smith R, Davis N, Bouamra O, Lecky F. The utilisation of intraosseous infusion in the resuscitation of paediatric major trauma patients. Injury. 2005;36(9):1034–8.

Stovroff M, Teague WG. Intravenous access in infants and children. Pediatr Clin North Am. 1998;45(6):1373–93.

Chapter 4
Abdominal Wall Hernias and Hydroceles

An abdominal wall hernia is a protrusion of the abdominal-cavity contents, usually intestines, through an opening or area of weakness in the abdominal wall. Abdominal wall hernias are very common and usually named for the area in which they occur.

Inguinal Hernias

- Inguinal hernias are by far the most common (up to 75–80 %) of all abdominal hernias in both boys and girls and appear as a protrusion of abdominal-cavity contents through the inguinal region or into the scrotum (Fig. 4.1).
- They are commonly seen in approximately 3–5 % of full-term infants.
- Inguinal hernias are three times more common in premature infants (hernias are found in as many as 30 % of prematurely born babies).
- These hernias appear more frequently in boys than in girls (the male to female ratio is 10:1).
- Girls however present more with bilateral inguinal hernias than boys.
- Inguinal hernias are more common on the right side (60 % of the time) and in some cases it is located on the left side or can be bilateral.
- Inguinal hernias are further divided into:
  - The more common indirect inguinal hernia in which the hernia enters through the internal inguinal ring (caused by failure of embryonic closure of the processus vaginalis).
  - The direct inguinal hernia type, where the hernia contents pass through a weak spot in the back wall of the inguinal canal which is formed by the transversalis fascia.
- Indirect inguinal hernias appear lateral to the inferior epigastric vessels while direct inguinal hernias occur medial to the inferior epigastric vessels.
- About 50 % of inguinal hernias are present clinically in the first year of life, especially in the first 6 months.
- There is a familial tendency for inguinal hernia.
- The incidence of inguinal hernias is higher in those infants with:
  1. Increased intra-abdominal pressure (Fig. 4.2)
  2. Undescended testis
  3. Congenital heart disease
  4. Cystic fibrosis
  5. Connective tissue disorders
  6. Bladder exstrophy
  7. Testicular feminization syndrome
  8. Intersex disorders

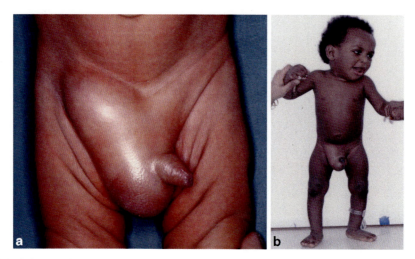

Fig. 4.1 Clinical photographs (**a** and **b**) of a large inguinoscrotal hernia

Fig. 4.2 Intraoperative photograph showing right-sided inguinal containing a ventriculo-peritoneal shunt

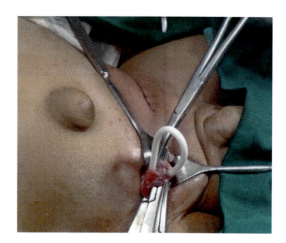

- Inguinal hernia also occurs more commonly in patients with chromosomal disorders, microdeletion disorders, and single gene disorders.
- A chromosomal study should be done if testicular feminization syndrome is suspected. The possibility of testicular feminization syndrome must be kept in mind in females who present with bilateral inguinal hernia.
- Inguinal hernias are classified into:
  - Reducible hernia: one in which the hernia contents can be pushed back into the abdomen by putting manual pressure to it.
  - Irreducible hernia: one in which the hernia contents cannot be pushed back into the abdomen by applying manual pressure.
- Irreducible inguinal hernias are considered an emergency and if it fails to be reduced after sedation then an emergency herniotomy should be done (Fig. 4.3).
- Obstructed inguinal hernia: a hernia in which the lumen of the herniated part of intestine is obstructed but the blood supply is intact.

Fig. 4.3 A clinical photograph showing an irreducible right inguinal hernia

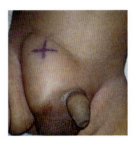

- Incarcerated inguinal hernia: a hernia in which adhesions develop between the wall of hernial sac and the intestines preventing it from being reduced.
- Incarceration occurs in about 12 % of infants and young children with an inguinal hernia, often during the first 6 months of life.
- The rate of incarceration decreases to 1 % at 8 years of age.
- Immediate surgery is indicated for the incarcerated hernia that is manually irreducible (Fig. 4.4).
- Strangulated inguinal hernia: A hernia that is irreducible and in which the blood supply of the herniated intestines is compromised leading to ischemia. Infarction of the small bowel, testis, or ovary may result (Figs. 4.5 and 4.6).
- Infants 6 months of age and younger who have inguinal hernias have a much higher risk of strangulation than older children.
- The content of an inguinal hernial sac is commonly small intestines but may also contain ovary, testes, Meckel's diverticulum, appendix, and urinary bladder.
- Amyand's hernia: an inguinal hernia in which the content of the hernial sac is the vermiform appendix.
- Littre's hernia: an inguinal hernia in which the content of the hernial sac contains a Meckel's diverticulum. It is named after the French anatomist Alexis Littré (1658–1726).
- Busse's hernia: an inguinal hernia in which the testicle is within the hernia sac.
- Richter's hernia: a hernia in which only one side of the wall of the bowel is trapped into the hernial sac, which can result in bowel strangulation leading to perforation through ischemia without causing bowel obstruction. It is named after the German surgeon August Gottlieb Richter (1742–1812).
- Sliding hernia: occurs when the herniated organ forms part of the hernia sac. The colon and the urinary bladder are the commonest to be involved in a sliding hernia.
- Pantaloon hernia (saddle bag hernia): This is a combined direct and indirect inguinal hernia, when the hernial sac protrudes on either side of the inferior epigastric vessels.
- Maydl's hernia: This is seen when two adjacent loops of small intestines are within a hernial sac with a tight neck. The intervening portion of bowel within the abdomen is deprived of its blood supply and eventually becomes necrotic.
- Surgical repair of inguinal hernia shortly after diagnosis is recommended for all patients, including premature infants. This is to avoid complications such as strangulation.
- There is controversy about whether the contralateral groin should be explored. Today, most surgeons do not routinely perform a contralateral exploration unless a contralateral inguinal hernia or patent processus vaginalis can be demonstrated either by preoperative ultrasonography or by intraoperative laparoscopy.
- A hernia develops in the other side of the groin in about 30 % of children who have had hernia surgery. This is more so if the initial hernia was on the left side.
- Complications of inguinal hernia repair include:
    - Wound infection
    - Hematoma

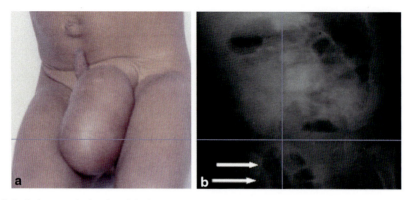

Fig. 4.4 a Clinical photograph showing right incarcerated inguinal hernia containing bowel loops. **b** Abdominal x-ray showing bowel loops in an incarcerated right inguinal hernia

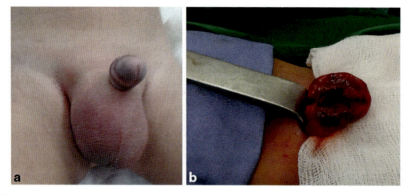

Fig. 4.5 a Clinical photograph showing *right* strangulated inguinal hernia. **b** Intraoperative photograph showing an ischemic bowel loop in an irreducible strangulated inguinal hernia

Fig. 4.6 Intraoperative photograph showing a necrotic ovary in an irreducible strangulated *left* inguinal hernia

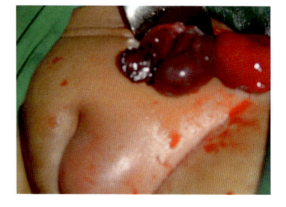

- Scrotal edema
- Ascent of testis
- Testicular atrophy
- Recurrence

- Laparoscopic inguinal hernia repair has become an alternative to the conventional open herniotomy. This procedure is safe, reproducible, and technically easy for experienced laparoscopic surgeons. It also does not impair testicular perfusion. The main advantages of laparoscopic inguinal hernia repair over conventional herniotomy are:

  - Less postoperative pain
  - Earlier postoperative recovery
  - Better wound cosmesis
  - The ability to detect and simultaneously repair contralateral patent processus vaginalis.

Umbilical *Hernia*:

- An umbilical hernia results from imperfect closure or weakness of the umbilical ring (Fig. 4.7).
- These hernias are common in infants and young children and make up roughly 5–10% of all primary hernias.
- Umbilical hernias are about 10 times more common in blacks than in whites.
- They are more common in low birth weight infants.
- The sex incidence is equal.
- Umbilical hernias often resolve spontaneously (Fig. 4.8).
- Most umbilical hernias are sporadic and occur as isolated findings in otherwise healthy infants. They may appear in children with increased intra-abdominal pressure as in those with ventriculoperitoneal shunt (Fig. 4.9).
- Umbilical hernias occur with increased frequency in patients with:

  - Down's syndrome, trisomy 13, trisomy 18, congenital hypothyroidism, Beckwith–Wiedemann syndrome, mucopolysaccharidosis, and cirrhosis of the liver with ascites.

- Complications, such as incarceration of intestine or omentum, strangulation, perforation of the intestine, and rupture with evisceration, are rare in children with umbilical hernia.
- Most umbilical hernias resolve spontaneously, usually within the first year of life (Fig. 4.10).
- Rarely, surgery may become necessary:

  - If the hernia becomes incarcerated or strangulated
  - If the hernia increases in size after the first year of life
  - If the hernia persists beyond the age of 2 years

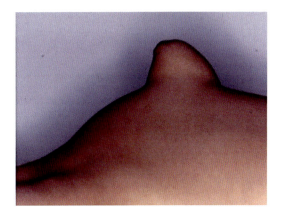

Fig. 4.7 A clinical photograph showing an umbilical hernia

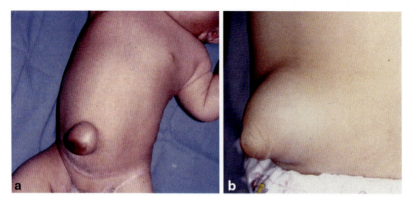

Fig. 4.8 Clinical photograph (**a** and **b**) showing umbilical hernias that may resolve spontaneously

Fig. 4.9 A clinical photograph showing an umbilical hernia in a child with ventriculoperitoneal shunt causing an increase in intra-abdominal pressure

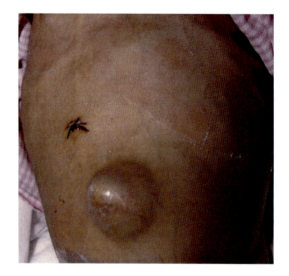

Fig. 4.10 A clinical photograph showing an umbilical hernia that is getting smaller in size

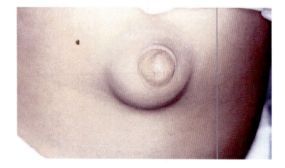

- Repair at the age of 2 years is advocated when the fascial defect is greater than 1.5 cm in diameter.
- For umbilical hernias with larger fascial defects, repair at a much earlier age is recommended.
- Of umbilical hernias not repaired in childhood, 10% persist into adulthood.

Paraumbilical hernia:

- Unlike an umbilical hernia, a paraumbilical hernia does not protrude through the umbilical area. Rather, it protrudes just above or below the umbilicus.
- The male-to-female ratio is about 1:5.
- The condition is more common in whites and obese children.
- The hernia contents include: omentum, small bowel, and large bowel.
- A paraumbilical hernia poses the risk of incarceration and strangulation.
- A paraumbilical hernia does not close spontaneously.
- Elective herniorrhaphy is advisable because of the recognized risk of complications.

Epigastric hernia:

- An epigastric hernia results from an intrinsic defect in the interstices of the decussating fibers of the linea alba.
- The hernia protrudes in the midline through the linea alba between the xyphoid and the umbilicus.
- It usually consists of extraperitoneal fat and, occasionally, a peritoneal sac that may contain abdominal viscera.
- Epigastric hernias account for 0.35–1.5% of all abdominal wall hernias.
- The condition is more common in males.
- The peak incidence is between 20 and 50 years of age and rarely seen in children.
- Although usually asymptomatic, an epigastric hernia may present with upper abdominal pain and dyspepsia.
- Epigastric hernia has to be differentiated from subcutaneous lipoma, fibroma, and neurofibroma.
- Incarceration and strangulation are rare but potential complications.
- Early surgical repair is advocated.

Femoral Hernia:

- Femoral hernias occur just below the inguinal ligament, when abdominal contents pass through a weak area at the posterior wall of the femoral canal.
- The femoral canal is located below the inguinal ligament on the lateral aspect of the pubic tubercle. It is bounded by the inguinal ligament anteriorly, pectineal ligament posteriorly, lacunar ligament medially, and the femoral vein laterally. It normally contains a few lymphatics, loose areolar tissue, and occasionally a lymph node called Cloquet's node. The function of this canal appears to be to allow the femoral vein to expand when necessary to accommodate increased venous return from the leg during periods of activity.
- In the pediatric age group, femoral hernia is considered congenital. This is supported by its occurrence in infants and twins. Previous inguinal herniotomy has been incriminated as an etiological factor for femoral hernia in children. This however is not well supported and in most cases the diagnosis of femoral hernia was missed initially (Fig. 4.11).
- They can be hard to distinguish from inguinal hernia; however, they generally appear more rounded, and, in contrast to inguinal hernias, there is a strong female preponderance in femoral hernias. This is because of the wider bone structure of the female pelvis.
- Femoral hernias are a relatively uncommon type, accounting for only 3% of all hernias. Femoral hernias are more common in adults than in children.
- Femoral hernias are rare in the pediatric age group. They form about 0.4–1.1% of all groin hernias.
- Femoral hernias are commonly seen in the 5–10-years age group, and unlike adults there is a similar sex incidence, and 58% are seen on the right side, 29% on the left side, and bilateral in 13%.

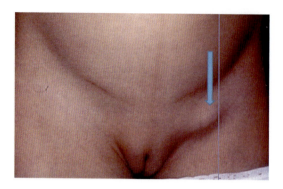

Fig. 4.11 Clinical photograph of a female child with femoral hernia. Note its location below the inguinal ligament. Note also the scars of previous bilateral herniotomy

- Cooper's hernia: a femoral hernia with two sacs, the first being in the femoral canal and the second passing through a defect in the superficial fascia and appearing almost immediately beneath the skin.
- Strangulation can happen in all hernias but is more common in femoral and inguinal hernias due to their narrow "necks." The incidence of strangulation in femoral hernias is high. A 15–20 % incidence of incarceration or strangulation among children with femoral hernias calls for early diagnosis and repair.

Lumbar Hernia:

- Congenital lumbar hernias are rare abdominal wall hernias in infants and children (Fig. 4.12).
- Approximately 10 % of all lumbar hernias are congenital and the majority are unilateral (Fig. 4.13).
- Lumbar hernias are divided into three types depending on the site:
  1. Superior: occur through the superior lumbar triangle (Grynfelt-Lesshaft triangle).
  2. Inferior: occur through the inferior lumbar triangle (Petit triangle).
  3. Combined.
     - Petit's hernia: A hernia through Petit's triangle (inferior lumbar triangle). It is named after the French surgeon Jean Louis Petit (1674–1750).
     - Grynfeltt's hernia: A hernia through Grynfeltt-Lesshaft triangle (superior lumbar triangle). It is named after physician Joseph Grynfelt (1840–1913).
- Acquired lumbar hernias are much more common and seen following surgery, infection, or trauma.
- Congenital lumbar hernias are associated with:

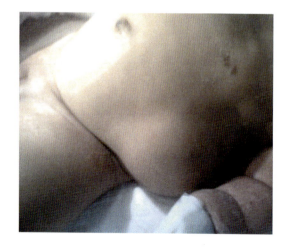

Fig. 4.12 Clinical photograph of a child with *left* lumbar hernia

Inguinal Hernias

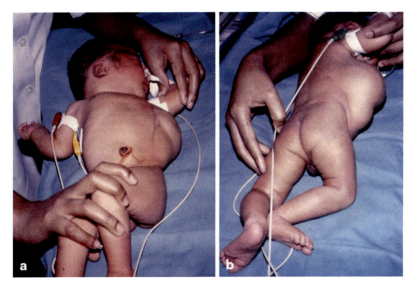

Fig. 4.13 a and **b** Clinical photographs of a newborn with a very large *left* side lumbar hernia

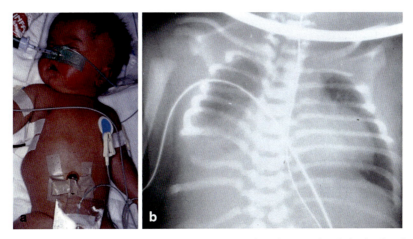

Fig. 4.14 Clinical photograph of a newborn with lumbocostovertebral syndrome and *right* lumbar hernia (**a**) and chest X-ray showing features of the lumbocostovertebral syndrome (hemivertebrae and absence of ribs) (**b**)

- Lumbocostovertebral syndrome (hemivertebrae, congenital absence of ribs, anterior myelominigocele, and hypoplasia of anterior abdominal wall presenting as congenital lumbar hernia; Fig. 4.14)–Anorectal malformations
- Hydrocephalus
- Congenital diaphragmatic hernia
- Caudal regression syndrome
- Pelvi-ureteric junction obstruction
- Cloacal extrophy
- Absent kidney
- Meningomyelocele

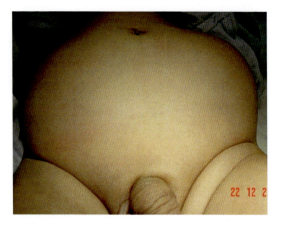

Fig. 4.15 Clinical photograph of a child with bilateral spigelian hernia

- In the majority of cases, congenital lumbar hernia is repaired primarily. This, however, is not always possible and sometimes in large defects prosthetic materials are required for the repair.

Spigelian hernia

- Spigelian hernia is rare and exceedingly so in infants and children (Fig. 4.15).
- It is commonly seen in adult females between the ages of 40 and 70 years, but only 3 % of all spigelian hernias are seen in children.
- Typically, spigelian hernia occurs through the spigelian fascia at the level of the semicircular line of Douglas where it is thinnest and usually lies deep to the external oblique aponeurosis (Fig. 4.16).
- Because of this, it is sometime difficult to localize the hernia if the sac is empty, and in situations where the diagnosis is not clear, ultrasonography is accurate in localizing the hernial defect (Fig. 4.17).
- It is also advisable to mark the site of the hernia preoperatively to obviate the difficulties in sometimes localizing the hernial defect intraoperatively.
- In children, spigelian hernia is more common in males, and although in the majority the hernia is congenital, traumatic as well as postoperative spigelian hernias have been reported.
- Associated anomalies are common with spigelian hernia and a 35 % incidence of associated anomalies has been reported.
- These include:
  - Inguinal hernia, umbilical hernia, congenital diaphragmatic hernia, meningomyelocele, neuroblastoma, cleft palate, clubfoot, micrognathia, and undescended testes (Fig. 4.18).
- Of interest was the finding of associated undescended testes in 28 % of male children with spigelian hernias which may have an etiological relationship.
- A variety of organs have been reported in the hernial sac which include small and large intestines, stomach, ovary, gallbladder, Meckel's diverticulum, and testes.
- Irreducibility and strangulation are common in spigelian hernia and because of this early diagnosis and treatment are advocated.

Incisional Hernia:

- An incisional hernia occurs when the defect is the result of an incompletely healed surgical wound (Fig. 4.19a).
- This type of hernia may develop many years after surgery (Fig. 4.19b).
- When these hernias occur in median laparotomy incisions in the linea alba, they are called ventral hernias.
- These can be the most frustrating and difficult hernias to treat.

Inguinal Hernias

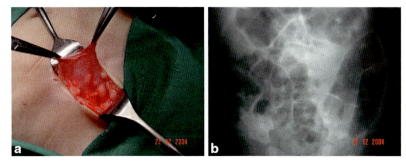

Fig. 4.16 a Intraoperative photograph showing the hernial sac of a spigelian hernia. **b** Abdominal radiograph showing the colon herniating into the spigelian hernia on the *left* side

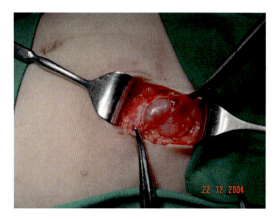

Fig. 4.17 Intraoperative photograph showing the colon herniating into a spigelian hernia

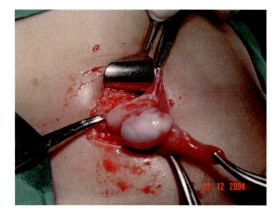

Fig. 4.18 Intraoperative photograph showing spigelian hernia with undescended testes. The presence of spigelian hernia may be a contributing factor for the development of undescended testes

Other rare abdominal wall hernias:

- Obturator hernia: a hernia through the obturator canal.
- Perineal hernia: A perineal hernia protrudes through the muscles and fascia of the perineal floor. It may be primary but usually is acquired following perineal prostatectomy, abdominoperineal resection of the rectum, or pelvic exenteration.

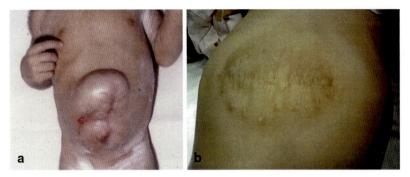

Fig. 4.19 Clinical photographs showing incisional hernia following repair of a large omphalocele (**a**) and an incisional hernia that developed several years following laparotomy as a neonate (**b**)

- Sciatic hernia: A hernia in the greater sciatic foramen most commonly presents as an uncomfortable mass in the gluteal area. Bowel obstruction may also occur. This type of hernia is a rare cause of sciatic neuralgia.
- Velpeau hernia: a hernia in the groin in front of the femoral blood vessels.

Hydroceles

- A hydrocele is a collection of fluid in the scrotum around the testicle. It is characterized by the following:
    - A narrow spermatic cord felt above the swelling.
    - It transilluminates.
    - It does not empty on squeezing.
- Hydroceles are not harmful to the testicles in any way.
- They do not cause discomfort.
- They are sometimes present at birth or may develop later.
- They can occur on one or both sides of the scrotum.
- The fluid typically makes the scrotum look large (Fig. 4.20).
- Hydroceles usually disappear on their own and no treatment is needed.

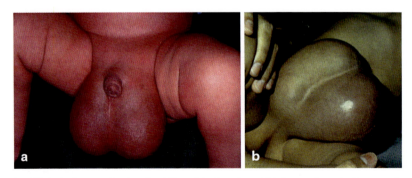

Fig. 4.20 a and **b** Clinical photographs showing bilateral hydroceles which is very large in the second one

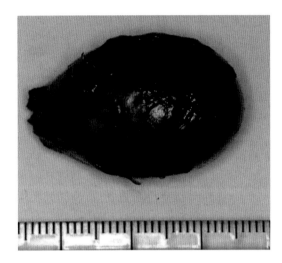

Fig. 4.21 Clinical photograph of a large encysted hydrocele after complete excision

- Surgery is indicated:
  - If the hydrocele has not disappeared by age 1 year.
  - If it becomes very large.
  - If it appears later after the age of 2 years (Fig. 4.21).
- Rarely, a hernia and hydrocele may occur together. Hydroceles need to be treated surgically if there is a hernia in addition to the hydrocele.
- Hydroceles need to be treated surgically when they develop as a complication of ventriculoperitoneal shunts. In these cases, both sides should be repaired and the communication to the peritoneal cavity should be closed with nonabsorbable sutures to avoid recurrence.
- Encysted hydrocele of the cord:
  - This is a loculated fluid collection along the spermatic cord, separated from and located above the testicle and the epididymis.
  - It usually resolves spontaneously.
  - Surgery is indicated only if they are large or appear after the age of 1 year (Fig. 4.21).
- Hydrocele of the canal of Nuck
  - The inguinal canal in the female transmits the round ligament and sometimes a finger-like extension of the peritoneum resembling the processus vaginalis in the male.
  - Accumulation of fluid may occur in this in the same manner as encysted hydrocele of the cord is formed in the male. It is then called hydrocele of the canal of Nuck.
  - They may also develop as a complication of ventriculoperitoneal shunts.

Recommended Reading

Kapur P, Caty MG, Glick PL. Pediatric hernias and hydroceles. *Pediatr Clin North Am*. 1998;45(4):773–89.

Lyngdoh TS, Mahalik S, Naredi B, Samujh R, Khanna S. Lumbocostovertebral syndrome with associated VACTERL anomaly. J Pediatr Surg. 2010;45(9):e15–7.

Chapter 5
Lymphangiomas

Introduction

- Lymphangiomas are rare congenital malformations of the lymphatic system, commonly seen in the head and neck.
- The lymphangiomas are uncommon lesions and their exact incidence is not known.
- Lymphangiomas can occur at any age and may involve any part of the body, but 90 % occur in children less than 2 years of age and involve the head and neck.
- Congenital lymphangiomas are often associated with chromosomal abnormalities such as Turner syndrome, although they can also exist in isolation.
- Treatment includes:
    - Aspiration
    - Surgical excision
    - Laser and radiofrequency ablation
    - Sclerotherapy
- Lymphangiomas are rare, accounting for 4 % of all vascular tumors in children and approximately 25 % of all benign vascular tumors in children.
- Although lymphangiomas can become evident at any age, 50 % are seen at birth and 90 % of lymphangiomas are evident by 2 years of age.
- Features of lymphangiomas:
    - Benign and commonly asymptomatic
    - Sometimes cause pressure and life threatening complications, especially massive lesions involving the neck and mediastinum in newborn infants
    - Cause a diagnostic confusion as a result of sudden enlargement following hemorrhage or infection
- Most lymphangiomas which are benign developmental malformations of the lymphatic system occur in the head and neck with the cervical region being the commonest site (Figs. 5.1, 5.2, and 5.3).
- Lymphangiomas can however appear at any age.
- This is specially so at sites other than the head and neck including the abdomen and mediastinum where they can attain a large size before being apparent clinically.
- Sometimes, they can attain a large size as a result of infection or hemorrhage. This can cause pressure symptoms or life-threatening complications at sites like the mediastinum (Figs. 5.3, 5.4, 5.5, 5.6, and 5.7).

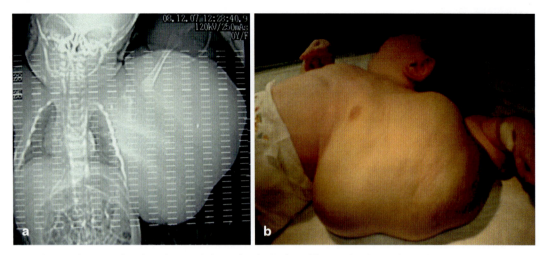

Fig. 5.1 a Plain X-ray showing a large soft tissue density in the axillary region in a patient with large cystic hygroma. **b** Clinical photograph of the same patient in showing a large axillary cystic hygroma extending downwards

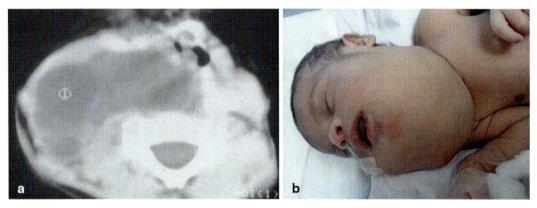

Fig. 5.2 a CT scan showing a large cervical lymphangioma. **b** clinical photograph showing a very large cervical lymphangioma

- An important observation is the sudden appearance of cervical lymphangioma as a result of bleeding. This causes diagnostic confusion and the final diagnosis is confirmed only intraoperatively and by histology.
- The possibility of lymphangioma should always be considered in children with sudden appearance of a cervical swelling.

Classification

- Lymphangiomas have traditionally been classified into three subtypes:
  - Capillary.
  - Cavernous lymphangiomas.
  - Cystic hygroma.
  - A fourth subtype the hemangiolymphangioma is also recognized.

Classification

Fig. 5.3 Clinical photograph showing a large cervical lymphangioma in an older child

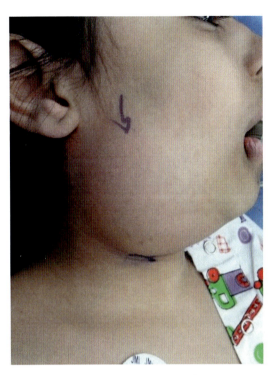

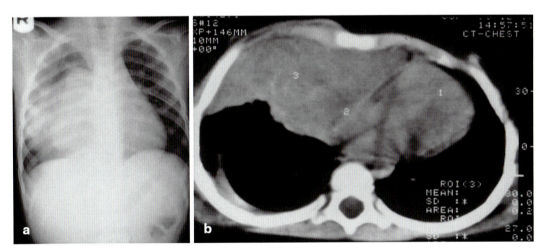

Fig. 5.4. a Chest ray showing a soft-tissue density in the right side of the chest and **b** CT scan of the chest for the same patient showing a large intrathoracic lymphangioma

- This classification is based on their microscopic characteristics.
- Capillary lymphangiomas are composed of small, capillary-sized lymphatic vessels and are characteristically located in the epidermis.
- Cavernous lymphangiomas are composed of dilated lymphatic channels and characteristically invade surrounding tissues.
- Cystic hygromas are large, macrocystic lymphangiomas filled with a straw-colored, protein-rich fluid.
- Hemangiolymphangiomas are lymphangiomas with a vascular component.

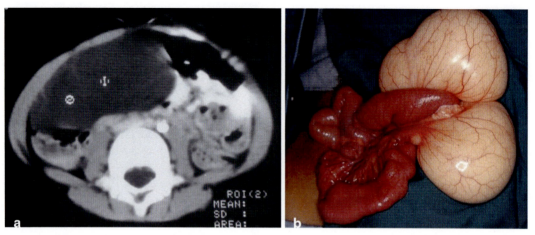

Fig. 5.5 a CT scan of the abdomen showing a large intra-abdominal lymphangioma and **b** intraoperative photograph showing a large mesenteric lymphangioma

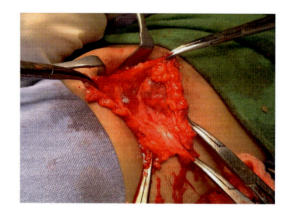

Fig. 5.6 Intra-operative photograph showing a macrocystic lymphangioma arising from the abdominal wall

- Lymphangiomas may also be classified according to the size of their cysts into (see Fig. 5.7):
  - Microcystic
  - Macrocystic
  - Mixed
- Microcystic lymphangiomas are composed of cysts, each of which measures less than 2 cm^3 in volume.
- Macrocystic lymphangiomas contain cysts measuring more than 2 cm^3 in volume.
- Mixed lymphangiomas: Lymphangiomas of the mixed type contain both microcystic and macrocystic components.
- Kennedy classified lymphangiomas into five groups:

  1. Superficial cutaneous lymphangioma (lymphangioma simplex and lymphangioma circumscriptum)
  2. Cavernous lymphangioma
  3. Cystic hygroma
  4. Diffuse system lymphangioma
  5. Mixed lymphangioma

Classification

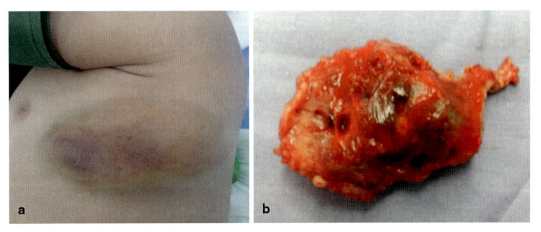

Fig. 5.7 **a** A clinical photograph showing lymphangioma of the chest wall. Note the spontaneous bleeding into the lymphangioma and **b** a clinical photograph of the resected lymphangioma. Note the bleeding inside the lymphangioma

Lymphangioma Circumscriptum

- It is a microcystic lymphatic malformation which resembles clusters of small blisters ranging in color from pink to dark red.
- They are benign and do not require treatment.
- May be removed surgically for cosmetic reasons.

Cavernous Lymphangiomas

- They are generally present at birth, but may appear at a later age.
- They appear deep under the skin, typically on the neck, tongue, and lips.
- Vary widely in size, ranging from as small as a centimeter in diameter to several centimeters wide.
- In some cases, they may affect an entire extremity such as a hand or foot.
- Although they are usually painless, the patient may feel mild pain when pressure is exerted on the area.

Cystic Hygroma

- They are similar to cavernous lymphangiomas.
- Cystic lymphangiomas usually have a softer consistency than cavernous lymphangiomas.
- They usually appear on the neck (75%), arm pit, or groin areas.
- Cystic lymphangioma that emerges during the first two trimesters of pregnancy is associated with genetic disorders such as Noonan syndrome and trisomies 13, 18, and 21.
- Chromosomal aneuploidy such as Turner syndrome or Down syndrome were found in 40% of patients with cystic hygroma.
- Cystic hygroma causes deep subcutaneous cystic swelling, usually in the axilla, base of the neck, or groin, and is typically noticed soon after birth.
- If the lesions are drained, they rapidly fill back up with fluid.
- The lesions will grow and increase to a larger size if they are not completely removed in surgery.

Fig. 5.8 A clinical photograph of a large lymphangioma arising in the upper thigh. There was spontaneous bleeding inside the lymphangioma

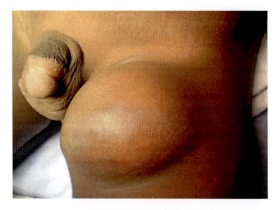

Fig. 5.9 A clinical photograph showing lymphangioma arising from the tongue

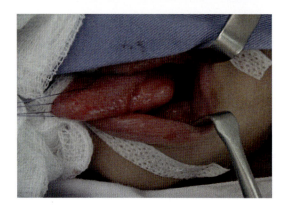

Sites of Lymphangiomas

- Lymphangiomas occur at any site in the body but:
  - They are most commonly seen in the head and neck area.
  - They can been seen rarely at other sites including:
    - The groin, axilla, mediastinum, mesentery, scrotum, spleen, retroperitoneium, chest wall, abdominal wall, tongue, and bones (Figs. 5.8, 5.9, and 5.10).
- Although rare, lymphangioma should be considered in the differential diagnosis of children presenting with cystic swellings at these unusual sites.

Treatment

- The treatment of lymphangiomas continues to be a challenge.
- Although spontaneous regression of lymphangiomas has been reported, it is however rare.
- It may be reasonable to treat small asymptomatic lymphangiomas expectantly.
- The treatment of lymphangiomas is early surgery as this is technically easier before further invasion of normal tissue and/or scarring secondary to infection has occurred. This however needs to be a complete radical resection, as with an incomplete resection, one faces the danger of a recurrence with a tendency to invasive growth.

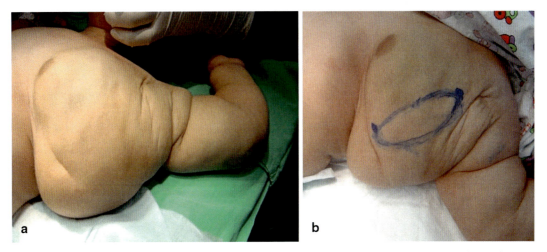

Fig. 5.10 Clinical photographs of a large cystic hygroma before (**a**) and after (**b**) sclerotherapy with bleomycin. Note the marked reduction in size

- The least invasive and most effective form of treatment is sclerotherapy.
- A sclerosing agent, such as 1 or 3 % sodium tetradecyl sulfate, doxycycline, bleomycin, or ethanol, may be directly injected into the lymphangioma.
- All sclerosing agents work by ablating the endothelial cells of the lymphangioma.
- Although surgical excision has been considered to be the treatment of choice by most surgeons, sclerotherapy with OK-432 (produced from the low virulent strain of type 3, group A Streptocccus pyogenes) and bleomycin has gained popularity during recent years (Fig. 5.10).
- OK-432 is safe and effective in the treatment of lymphangiomas and can be the first choice of treatment of lymphangiomas.
- Macrocystic lymphangiomas respond almost universally to OK-432 injections, whereas patients with microcystic lesions generally do not respond and should not therefore be injected with OK-432.
- They also advised against using this form of therapy for lesions outside the head and neck and for lymphangiomas surrounding the airways.
- Surgery is the treatment of choice for lymphangiomas but sclerotherapy has a place in the treatment of lesions where there is risk of damaging surrounding structures as well as to obviate the poor cosmetic results.
- Sclerotherapy can also be used as an adjunctive therapy in the treatment of wide spread and incompletely excised lymphangiomas.
- Treatment for cystic hygroma is surgical removal of the abnormal tissue; however, complete removal may be impossible. Cystic hygroma can also be treated with OK432 (Picibanil).

Recommended Reading

Marchese C, Savin E, Dragone E, et al. Cystic hygroma: prenatal diagnosis and genetic counseling. *Prenat Diagn.* 1985;5(3):221–7.

Okazaki T, Iwatani S, Yanai T, et al. Treatment of lymphangioma in children: our experience of 128 cases. *J Pediatr Surg.* 2007;42(2):386–9.

Chapter 6
Hemangiomas

Introduction

- The word "hemangioma" comes from the Greek *haema-* (αἷμα), "blood"; *angeio* (αγγείο), "vessel"; and *-oma* (-ωμα), "tumor."
- A hemangioma is a benign and usually a self-involuting tumor characterized by increased number of normal or abnormal blood vessels.
- Hemangioma is the most common tumor in infants.
- It usually appears during the first weeks of life and generally resolves by 10 years of age.
- Most infantile hemangiomas undergo rapid initial proliferation, with a subsequent plateau in infants aged about 9–10 months; finally, they become involuted.
- The involution phase extends from 1 year until 5–7 years of age.
- Hemangiomas are the most common childhood tumors, occurring in approximately 10 % of Caucasians and are less prevalent in other ethnicities.
- Hemangiomas are more common in females who are three to five times as likely to have hemangiomas as males.
- Approximately 80–85 % of hemangiomas are located on the face and neck, with the next most prevalent location being the liver. Hemangiomas however can affect any part of the body (Figs. 6.1, 6.2, 6.3, and 6.4).
- The cause of hemangioma is currently unknown; however, several studies have suggested the importance of estrogen in hemangioma proliferation.
- Most hemangiomas are easily diagnosed without any additional diagnostic tests. Deeper hemangiomas or questionable superficial lesions, however, may require imaging studies to confirm the diagnosis and to evaluate their extent. Ultrasound (US) and magnetic resonance imaging (MRI) are valuable in their assessment.

Complications

- The vast majority of hemangiomas are benign tumors and not associated with complications.
- Hemangiomas may however cause several complications:
    1. It can cause ulceration (Figs. 6.5 and 6.6).
    2. It can cause bleeding.

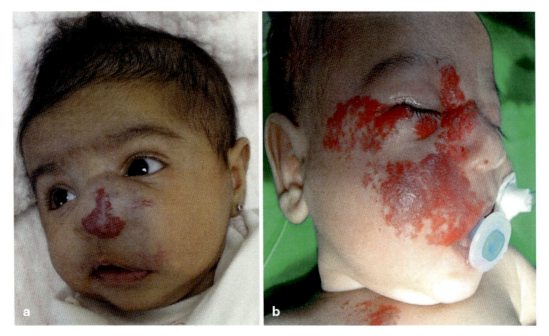

Fig. 6.1 a and **b** Clinical photographs showing extensive facial hemangiomas

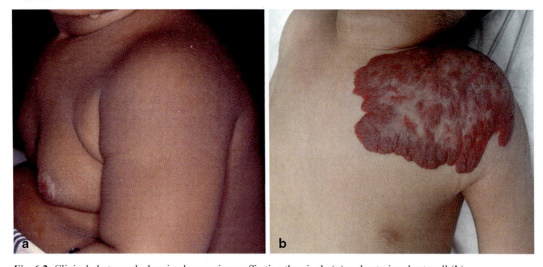

Fig. 6.2 Clinical photograph showing hemangioma affecting the nipple (**a**) and anterior chest wall (**b**)

3. If a hemangioma develops in the larynx, breathing can be compromised.
4. A hemangioma can grow and block one of the eyes, causing an occlusion amblyopia (Fig. 6.7).
5. Very rarely, extremely large hemangiomas can cause high-output cardiac failure due to the amount of blood that must be pumped to all the hemangiomas blood vessels.
6. Hemangiomas adjacent to bone can also cause erosion of the bone.
7. Psychosocial complications might occur to the patient and family from large hemangiomas on the face (Fig. 6.8).

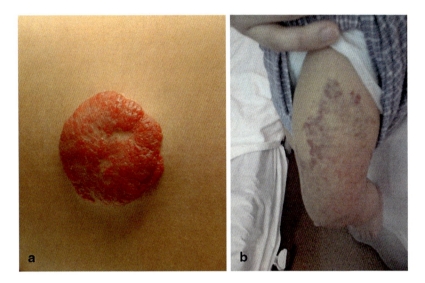

Fig. 6.3 Clinical photographs showing hemangioma at the back (**a**) and lower limb (**b**)

8. Children with large segmental hemangiomas of the head and neck can be associated with a disorder called PHACES syndrome (posterior fossa malformations, hemangiomas, arterial anomalies, cardiac defects, eye abnormalities, sternal cleft and supraumbilical raphe syndrome).
9. Rarely, large hemangiomas may cause Kasabach–Merritt syndrome (thrombocytopenia and hemangioma).

Treatment

- In general, most hemangiomas disappear without treatment, leaving minimal or no visible marks.
- Large hemangiomas can leave visible skin changes secondary to severe stretching of the skin or damage to surface texture.
- There are however hemangiomas which need treatment. When hemangiomas interfere with vision, breathing, or threaten significant cosmetic injury (facial lesions and in particular, nose and lips), they are usually treated.
- Whether to treat a hemangioma or not is determined by:
  1. The age of the patient
  2. Size of the hemangioma
  3. Location of the hemangioma
  4. How rapidly the hemangioma is growing
- Hemangiomas located in areas that can threaten health (airway or liver) or normal development (ear canal or on the eye) and those hemangiomas that are potentially disfiguring (face) are treated more quickly and aggressively than hemangiomas that pose less of a risk.

Treatment Options

- Observation: All hemangiomas should be watched closely for rapid growth and complications.
- Oral systemic corticosteroids:
  - The oral steroids are used to control or stop the growth of the hemangioma.

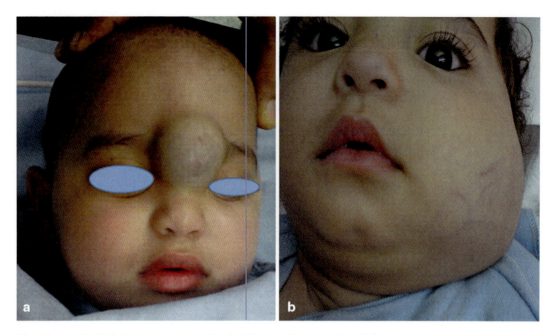

Fig. 6.4 a and **b** Clinical photographs showing facial hemangiomas causing disfigurement

Fig. 6.5 Clinical photograph showing an ulcerating hemangioma of the hand

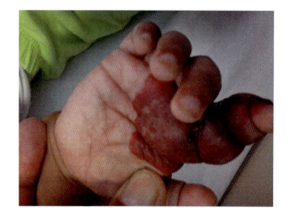

- They are only used during the growth period and in most cases do not usually shrink the hemagioma but slow its growth.
- Side effects include:
  ◦ Irritability, gastrointestinal upset, immunosuppression, hypertension, and growth retardation
- The duration of treatment ranges from a few weeks to many months, depending on the child's age, the indications for treatment, and the growth characteristics of the hemangioma.
• Corticosteroids can also be injected directly into the hemangioma and are effective for small, localized hemangiomas on the skin.
• Topical steroids also have been found to be effective in controlling the growth of small superficial hemangiomas, particularly on the eyelid and around the mouth.

Treatment

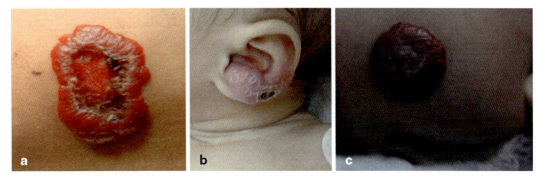

Fig. 6.6 a–c Clinical photographs showing ulcerating hemangiomas

Fig. 6.7 A clinical photograph showing hemangioma involving the lower eye lid. Further growth of the hemangioma may lead to lockage of the eye

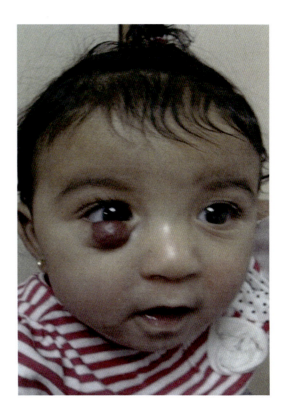

- Sclerotherapy:
    - Bleomycin is effective in the treatment of hemangiomas.
    - The effect however is variable ranging from total disappearance to only shrinkage of the hemangioma but the main effect is that it stops the growth of the hemangioma.
    - One of the side effects of bleomycin is the development of skin pigmentations at sites far away from the hemangioma.
    - The cause of this is not known. To avoid these pigmentations, metal contact to the skin should be avoided during injection (Figs. 6.9 and 6.10).

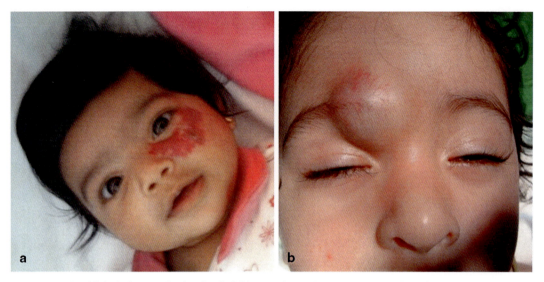

Fig. 6.8 a and **b** Clinical photographs showing facial hemangiomas that may cause psychosocial complications

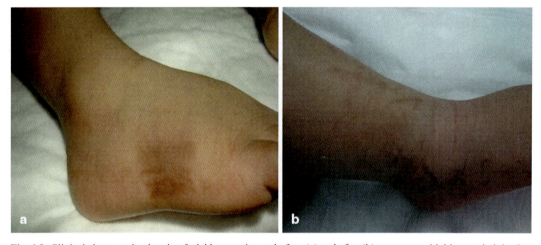

Fig. 6.9 Clinical photographs showing facial hemangiomas before (**a**) and after (**b**) treatment with bleomycin injection

- Surgical excision:
  - This is a reasonable option in selected cases.
  - This is particularly so if there was delay in commencing treatment and structural changes have become irreversible.
  - Surgery may also be necessary to correct distortion of facial features, again in the case of inadequate or failed early medical intervention.
- Laser therapy:
  - The flash-lamp pulsed dye laser is effective for superficial hemangiomas but has no impact on deeper or thicker hemangiomas.
  - It is also effective in treating ulcerated hemagiomas.
  - Continuous-wave lasers such as the argon, neodymium: yttrium-aluminium-garnet, and potassium titanyl phosphate have also been used but have a greater risk of scarring.

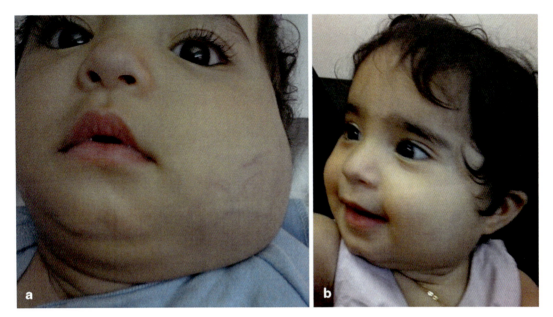

Fig. 6.10 a and **b** Clinical photographs showing pigmentations as a complication of bleomycin injection

- Interferon alpha:
  - It has been used successfully in treating life-theatening hemagiomas that have failed to respond to oral corticosteroid therapy.
  - Common side effects include irritability, neutropenia, and liver enzyme abnormalities.
- Embolization: has been rarely used in the treatment of hemangiomas.
- Vincristine: has been used successfully to treat hemangiomas that threaten to affect a vital function.
- Propranolol:
  - This is also effective in treating hemangiomas but must be used with caution because it can cause a drop in blood sugar and a drop in blood pressure or heart rate.
  - Propranolol can be given in combination with corticosteroids (Figs. 6.11 and 6.12).

Prognosis

Hemangiomas go through three stages of development:

1. The proliferation stage:
   - The hemangioma grows very quickly.
   - This stage can last up to 12 months.
2. The rest stage:
   - There is very little change in the hemangioma's appearance.
   - This usually lasts until the infant is 1–2 years old.

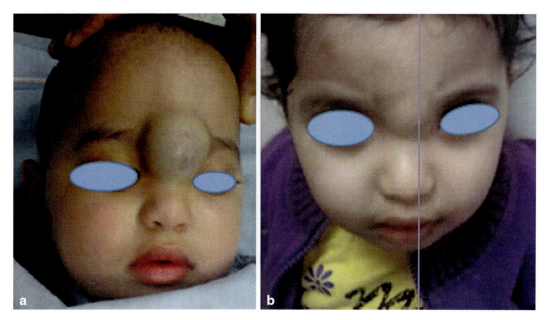

Fig. 6.11 Clinical photograph showing facial hemangioma before (**a**) and after (**b**) treatment with a combination of propranolol and corticosteroids

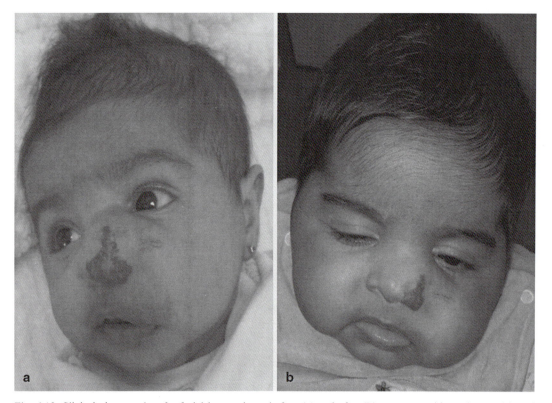

Fig. 6.12 Clinical photographs of a facial hemangioma before (**a**) and after (**b**) treatment with corticosteroids and propranolol and injection with bleomycin

3. The involution stage:
   - The hemangioma begins to diminish in size.
   - Fifty percent of lesions will have disappeared by 5 years of age and the vast majority will have gone by 10 years of age.

Hepatic Hemangiomas

- Hepatic hemangiomas are not rare and are thought to be present in as many as 7 % of healthy people.
- Hemangiomas are four to six times more common in females than in males.
- Hepatic hemangiomas usually are small in size measuring only a quarter inch in diameter, but they can be several inches in diameter or even larger.
- The vast majority of hepatic hemangiomas are asymptomatic.
- Most hepatic hemangiomas are discovered incidentally most commonly with ultrasound imaging or CT scan of the abdomen.
- Very large hemangiomas can cause symptoms. Pain, nausea, or enlargement of the liver can occur.
- Rarely, hepatic hemangioma can cause the Kasabach–Merritt syndrome.
- Rarely, larger hemangiomas can rupture, causing severe pain and bleeding into the abdomen that may be severe or even life threatening.
- When a hemangioma is suspected, the diagnosis can be confirmed using scintigraphy, CT scan, or MRI.
- In general, a biopsy of suspected hemangiomas is avoided because of their benign nature and the potential risk of bleeding from the biopsy.
- The vast majority of hepatic hemangiomas require no treatment. If a hepatic hemangioma is large, especially if it is causing symptoms, surgical removal is an option.

Recommended Reading

Azzopardi S, Wright TC. Novel strategies for managing infantile hemangiomas: a review. Ann Plast Surg. 2012;68(2):226–8.

Bertrand J, Sammour R, McCuaig C, Dubois J, Hatami A, Ondrejchak S, Boutin C, Bortoluzzi P, Laberge LC, Powell J. Propranolol in the treatment of problematic infantile hemangioma: review of 35 consecutive patients from a vascular anomalies clinic. J Cutan Med Surg. 2012;16(5):317–23.

Neri I, Balestri R, Patrizi A. Hemangiomas: new insight and medical treatment. Dermatol Ther. 2012;25(4):322–34.

Wollina U, Unger L, Haroske G, Heinig B. Classification of vascular disorders in the skin and selected data on new evaluation and treatment. Dermatol Ther. 2012;25(4):287–96.

Chapter 7
Branchial Cysts, Sinuses, and Fistulae

Introduction

- Branchial cysts are remnants of embryonic development and result from a failure of obliteration of the branchial clefts.
- They are a common cause of a congenital mass of the neck and an estimated 2–3 % of cases are bilateral.
- Branchial cysts are congenital cysts, which arise on the lateral aspect of the neck and commonly due to failure of obliteration of the second branchial cleft in embryonic development.
- Untreated branchial cleft cysts are prone to recurrent infection and abscess formation with resultant scar and sinus formation.
- There are rare case reports of malignancies that have been identified in branchial cleft lesions, including branchiogenic carcinoma and papillary thyroid carcinoma.

Embryology

- The branchial apparatus develops during the 2nd to 6th weeks of fetal life.
- At this stage, the neck develops like a hollow tube with circumferential ridges, which are termed branchial arches.
- The branchial arches subsequently develop into the musculoskeletal and vascular components of the head and neck.
- The regions between the arches are called branchial clefts (on the outside of the fetus) and branchial pouches (on the inside of the fetus).
- The branchial pouches subsequently develop into the middle ear, tonsils, thymus, and parathyroid glands.
- The first branchial cleft develops into the external auditory canal.
- The second, third, and fourth branchial clefts merge to form the sinus of His, which normally involutes.
- When a branchial cleft does not properly involute, a branchial cleft cyst develops.
- Occasionally, both the branchial pouch and branchial cleft fail to involute and a complete fistula forms between the pharynx and skin.
- Pathology:
  - Most branchial cleft cysts are lined with stratified squamous epithelium with keratinous debris within the cyst.
  - In a small number, the cyst is lined with respiratory (ciliated columnar) epithelium.

Fig. 7.1 A clinical photograph showing a branchial fistula. Note the location of the external opening at the anterior border of the lower third of the sternocleidomastoid muscle. The internal opening is usually upwards in the tonsillar fossa

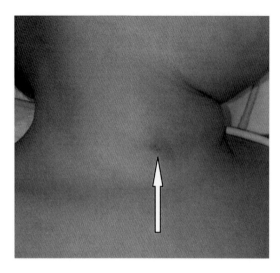

- Lymphoid tissue is often present in the wall of the cyst outside the epithelial lining which may form germinal centers.
- The cyst may contain granular and keratinaceous cellular debris.
- Cholesterol crystals may be found in the fluid extracted from a branchial cyst.
- Branchial fistula:
  - A branchial fistula forms when there is complete communication between the inside of the throat and outside of the skin.
  - Fistulas from the second and third pouches that have their external opening just in front of anterior border of the lower third of the sternocleidomastoid muscle while the internal opening may go up through the neck until it opens in the region of the tonsils (Fig. 7.1).
  - These fistulas may be bilateral in 10–15 % of the cases.

Types

- First branchial cleft cysts (10–20 %):
  - First branchial cleft cysts are divided into type I and type II.
  - Type-I cysts are located near the external auditory canal.
  - Most commonly, they are seen inferior and posterior to the tragus (base of the ear) but they may also be in the parotid gland or at the angle of the mandible.
  - Type-II cysts are associated with the submandibular gland or found in the anterior triangle of the neck.
- Second branchial cleft cysts (75–85 %):
  - This is the most common type.
  - They are found along the anterior border of the upper third of sternocleidomastoid muscle, passes through the carotid bifurcation, and opens into the tonsillar pillar.
  - These cysts may present anywhere along the course of a second branchial fistula, which proceeds from the skin of the lateral neck, between the internal and external carotid arteries, and into the palatine tonsil.

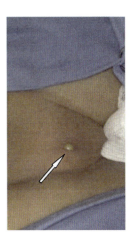

Fig. 7.2 A clinical photograph of a child with branchial fistula. Note its location and the discharge from the external opening

- Third branchial cleft cysts:
  - Third branchial cleft cysts are rare.
  - A third branchial fistula extends from the skin along the anterior border of the lower third of sternocleidomastoid muscle and courses posterior to the carotid arteries, under the glossopharyngeal nerve and over the vagus nerve and pierces the thyrohyoid membrane to enter the larynx, terminating on the lateral aspect of the pyriform sinus.
  - Third branchial cleft cysts occur anywhere along that course (e.g., inside the larynx), but they are characteristically located deep to the sternocleidomastoid muscle.

- Fourth branchial cleft cyst:
  - Fourth branchial cleft cysts are extremely rare.
  - A fourth branchial fistula arises from the lateral neck and parallels the course of the recurrent laryngeal nerve (around the aorta on the left and around the subclavian artery on the right), terminating in the apex of the pyriform sinus.
  - Fourth branchial cleft cysts occur in several locations, including the thyroid gland and mediastinum.
  - They may present as abscesses in the lower part of the neck, on the left side usually more than the right, and may be associated with infection of the thyroid gland.
  - Surgical removal may require excision of the upper pole of the thyroid gland along with the connection that goes into the pyriform sinus.

Clinical Features

- Most branchial cleft cysts are asymptomatic.
- Branchial cleft cysts are congenital in nature, but they may not present clinically until later in life, usually by early adulthood.
- A branchial cyst commonly presents as a solitary, painless mass in the neck of a child or a young adult.
- Discharge may be the presenting symptom if the lesion is associated with a sinus or fistula tract (Fig. 7.2).
- They may become infected and present as a tender, enlarged, or inflamed swelling or develop an abscess. This is especially during periods of upper respiratory tract infection, due to the lymphoid tissue located beneath the epithelium.

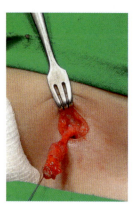

Fig. 7.3 An intraoperative photograph showing a branchial fistula being excised surgically. Note the big size of the fistula

- Depending on the size and the anatomical extension of the mass, local symptoms, such as dysphagia, dysphonia, dyspnea, and stridor, may occur.
- The possibility of carcinoma arising in a branchial remnant is controversial; some authors suggest that branchiogenic carcinoma is possible, but metastatic squamous cell carcinoma to regional lymph nodes that masquerade as a branchial cleft cyst is far more common.
- A patient who presents with an abscess of the thyroid gland probably has an underlying branchial cleft sinus or fistula communicating with the pyriform sinus.

Investigations

- Ultrasonography is the investigation of choice. It can confirm the cystic nature of the mass. It does not, however, adequately evaluate the extent and depth of the swelling.
- Both computed tomography (CT) scanning and magnetic resonance imaging (MRI) are useful in the evaluation of branchial cleft cysts.
- A sinogram may be obtained if a sinus tract exists to delineate the course and to examine the size of the cyst.

Treatment

- Surgical excision is the definitive treatment for branchial cleft cysts (Figs. 7.3, 7.4, 7.5).
- Complete excision may necessitate multiple horizontal incisions, known as a stair step or stepladder incision, to fully dissect out the occasionally tortuous path of the branchial cleft cysts.
- Definitive branchial cleft cyst excision should not be made during an episode of acute infection or if an abscess is present. Surgical incision and drainage of the abscesses are indicated if present, usually along with antimicrobial therapy.
- Endoscopic retroauricular approach may provide good surgical clearing with minimal scarring for second branchial cleft cysts.
- Alternatives to the open surgical excision have been proposed including sclerotherapy with OK-432 (picibanil) which has been reported to be an effective alternative to surgical excision of branchial cleft cysts.

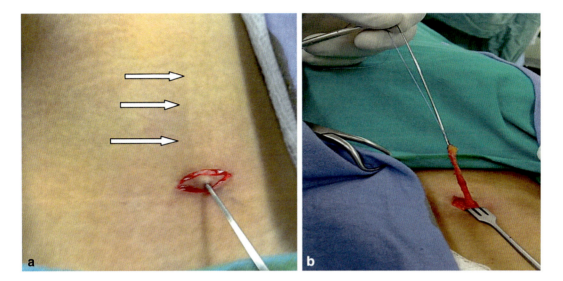

Fig. 7.4 A clinical intraoperative photograph showing a branchial fistula being excised via a single incision. Note the site of the external opening (**a**) and the course of the tract upwards (**b**)

Fig. 7.5 An intraoperative photograph showing a large branchial fistula being excised. Note the site of the insertion of the internal opening usually at the tonsillar fossa

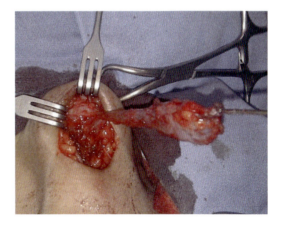

- Complications of surgical excision of branchial cleft cysts result from damage to nearby vascular or neural structures, which include carotid vessels and the facial, hypoglossal, vagus, and lingual nerves.
- Recurrence is uncommon, with a risk estimated at 3%.

Recommended Reading

Doi O, Hutson JM, Myers NA, McKelvie PA. Branchial remnants: a review of 58 cases. *J Pediatr Surg.* 1988;23(9):789–92.

Kim MG, Kim SG, Lee JH, Eun YG, Yeo SG. The therapeutic effect of OK-432 (picibanil) sclerotherapy for benign neck cysts. *Laryngoscope.* 2008;118(12):2177–81.

Rosa PA, Hirsch DL, Dierks EJ. Congenital neck masses. *Oral Maxillofac. Surg Clin North Am.* 2008;20:339–52.

Chapter 8
Sternomastoid Tumor of Infancy and Torticollis

Introduction

- Sternomastoid tumor of infancy is the most common neck mass in the neonatal period.
- The term sternomastoid tumor is a misnomer as this is not a true tumor but a muscle fibrosis.
- Commonly, it is seen in infants aged 2–3 weeks.
- The child usually presents with a visible or a palpable swelling on the lateral aspect of the neck.
- The mass is generally 1–3 cm in diameter.
- The tumor is more common in primipara and infants born with prolonged or difficult labor.
- The reported incidence of breech deliveries is about 20–30 % much higher than the normal incidence.
- In infants, the tumor is hard and the patient's head is tilted and flexed to the side of the fibrosis.
- It usually affects the middle or lower part of the sternomastoid muscle.
- In older children, the tumor is less discrete than it is in younger children and the sternocleidomastoid muscle appears thickened and foreshortened along its entire length. This thickening restricts rotation and lateral flexion of the neck.
- Torticollis is a result of unilateral tightness and shortening of one sternocleidomastoid muscle.
- Torticollis occurs in 0.4 % of all live births.
- The natural course is self-resolution of the torticollis in 80–90 % cases up to the age of 1 year.
- In about 10 %, the tumor and sternomastoid shortening persist beyond 12 months of age.

Etiology

- The etiology is not fully understood and several theories have been postulated. These include:
    - An idiopathic intrauterine embryopathy.
    - A manifestation of an intrauterine positional disorder with the development of sternocleidomastoid compartment syndrome.
    - Familial transmission of congenital muscular torticollis.
    - Approximately 20–30 % of patients presenting with sternocleidomastoid torticollis have a history of breech presentation at birth, with 60 % involved in a complicated birth.
    - An end-arterial branch of the superior thyroid artery supplies the middle part of the sternocleidomastoid muscle. Obliteration of this end artery may be responsible for the development of muscle fibrosis.

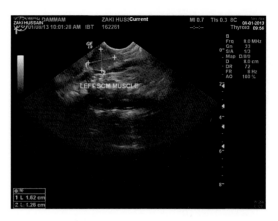

Fig. 8.1 Neck ultrasound showing left sternomastoid tumor

- A primary trauma that temporarily and acutely obstructs the veins may lead to intravascular clotting in the obstructed venous tree. This leads to the development of a sternocleidomastoid mass, which eventually disappears and is replaced by fibrous tissue.
- Abnormalities in the basal ganglia may be involved in the pathophysiology of spasmodic torticollis.

• It is important to differentiate muscular from nonmuscular torticollis.

Diagnosis

- The diagnosis is easily made clinically.
- Ultrasonography is used to confirm the diagnosis (Fig. 8.1).
- MRI may be useful in patients with nonmuscular causes of torticollis.
- Histopathologic findings include:
  - Fibrous replacement of skeletal muscle fibers that undergo atrophy.
  - The degree of fibrosis and its extent or distribution may vary.
  - Even in neonates, the fibrous tissue is mature.
  - This finding indicates that the disease began before birth.

Management

- Medical management of torticollis involves conservative treatment.
- Sternocleidomastoid fibrosis spontaneously resolves in the vast majority of infants (success rate of 80–95 %).
- The management for torticollis is primarily nonoperative, generally consisting of physiotherapy.
- Surgical management of congenital muscular torticollis is generally avoided until the child is aged at least 1 year.
- Only about 4–5 % of patients are surgically treated, generally after the age of 1 year.
- Indications for surgical management include:
  - Persistent sternocleidomastoid contracture limiting head movement
  - Persistent sternocleidomastoid contracture accompanied by progressive facial hemihypoplasia

- Craniofacial asymmetry and plagiocephaly
  - Conservative physiotherapy is unsuccessful
  - Torticollis in children older than 12 months

- Botulinum toxin type A has been used but the benefits with improved range of motion has been observed in very few patients.
- Surgical procedure:

  - It is performed under general anesthesia.
  - A 3–4-cm transverse skin incision is made about 1 cm over the sternal and clavicular origins of the affected sternomastoid muscle.

- An endoscopic or minimal access approach has also been used (endoscopic tenotomy).
- Recurrent torticollis after surgery is rare (5%).
- Secondary effects of untreated torticollis include:
- Plagiocephaly: an asymmetric skull deformity caused by flattening of one occiput that leads to the secondary flattening of the contralateral forehead
- Facial hemihypoplasia: inhibition in the growth of the mandible and maxilla due to muscle inactivity
- Compensatory ipsilateral elevation of the shoulder
- Cervical and thoracic scoliosis
- Wasting of additional muscles in the neck

Recommended Reading

Celayir AC. Congenital muscular torticollis: early and intensive treatment is critical. A prospective study. Pediatr Int. 2000;42(5):504–7.

Cheng JC, Tang SP, Chen TM, Wong MW, Wong EM. The clinical presentation and outcome of treatment of congenital muscular torticollis in infants—a study of 1,086 cases. J Pediatr Surg. 2000;35(7):1091–6.

Do TT. Congenital muscular torticollis: current concepts and review of treatment. Curr Opin Pediatr. 2006;18(1):26–9.

Tatli B, Aydinli N, Caliskan M, et al. Congenital muscular torticollis: evaluation and classification. Pediatr Neurol. 2006;34(1):41–4.

Chapter 9
Infantile Fibromatosis and Myofibromatosis

Introduction

- Infantile myofibromatosis is a rare benign mesenchymal tumor of infancy and early childhood.
- It refers to a family of soft-tissue lesions characterized by proliferation of benign fibrous tissue, which is composed of uniform, elongated, fusiform, or spindle-shaped cells surrounded and separated by abundant collagen (Fig. 9.1).
- Infantile myofibromatosis was first described by Stout in 1954 who called it congenital fibromatosis and subsequently several names were used to describe it.
- The term infantile myofibromatosis however was coined by Chung and Enzinger in 1981.
- Sixty percent of infantile myofibromatosis were diagnosed at or shortly after birth and 88 % occurred before 2 years of age.
- Infantile myofibromatosis is a relatively rare mesenchymal tumor characterized by the appearance of nodules at different sites of the body. Commonly, it is seen in infants and neonates but there are reports of myofibromatosis occurring in older children and adults.
- Commonly, it presents either as a solitary or as multiple nodules arising from the soft tissues of the head, neck, trunk, or extremities but it can affect the bones or to a lesser degree the lungs and gastrointestinal tract.
- There are however reports of infantile myofibromatosis affecting unusual sites such as the brain, myocardium, pancreas, spinal cord, omentum, and larynx.
- Accurate diagnosis and differentiating this from other more aggressive tumors is important.
- The exact pathogenesis of infantile myofibromatosis is not known. Intrauterine estrogen exposure was suggested as a possible etiology and based on familial occurrences; a genetic cause was also proposed.
- According to Enzinger and Weiss, infantile fibromatosis is classified into superficial and deep fibromatosis. Superficial tumors are usually purplish red as a result of intense vascularity. The intra-abdominal organ involvement is also known which carries worse prognosis.
- Fibromatosis is a group of related conditions having the following common features: proliferation of well-differentiated fibroblasts, infiltrative pattern of growth, presence of variable amount of collagen between the proliferating cells, lack of cytological features of malignancy and scanty or absent mitotic activity, and aggressive clinical behavior characterized by repeated local recurrences but lack of capacity to metastasize distantly.

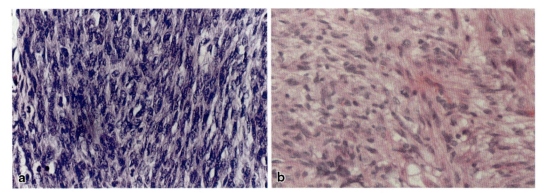

Fig. 9.1 Histological picture of infantile myofibromatosis showing uniform, elongated, fusiform, and elongated spindle-shaped cells surrounded by abundant collagen

Histopathology

- Diagnosis is usually made histologically.
- In infantile fibromatosis, the characteristic feature is the presence of small, round intracytoplasmic inclusions. They are periodic acid–Schiff (PAS) negative and they apparently consist of actin filaments. Morphologically, these lesions occur as unicentric gray white, firm, poorly demarcated masses varying from 1 to 15 cm in the greatest dimension.
- It is composed of uniform, elongated, fusiform, or spindle-shaped cells surrounded and separated by abundant collagen (Fig. 9.1).
- The lack of malignant cells on histology differentiates infantile fibromatosis from infantile fibrosarcoma.

Clinical Features

- Although histologically benign, this lesion tends to gradually infiltrate in skin subcutaneous tissue, muscles, nerves, blood vessels, and even bone. They are rubbery and tough.
- Clinically, the presentation is of a slow-growing, firm, poorly circumscribed mass.
- Clinically, there are three distinct forms of infantile myofibromatosis.

1. A localized form:
    - Presents as a solitary nodule (Figs. 9.2 and 9.3).
    - This is the commonest type seen in more than half of the cases.
    - It is usually seen in males.
    - The common sites for the nodules are the skin and subcutaneous tissues of the head and neck, extremities and trunk, as well as bones but there are reported cases of nodules occurring at unusual sites including the liver, pancreas, omentum, and gallbladder.
    - The common sites of bone involvement include the femur, tibia, ribs, pelvis, vertebrae, and skull.
    - Radiologically, the bony involvement is seen as well-circumscribed lytic lesions with a sclerotic margin. This can resemble a primary malignant tumor with multiple metastases.

Clinical Features

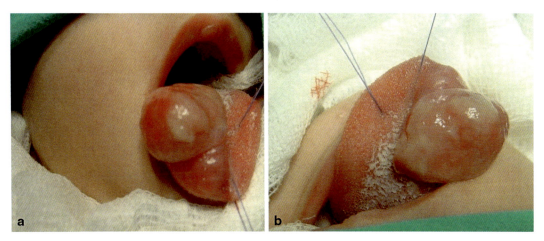

Fig. 9.2 a and **b** A clinical photograph of infantile fibromatosis of the tongue

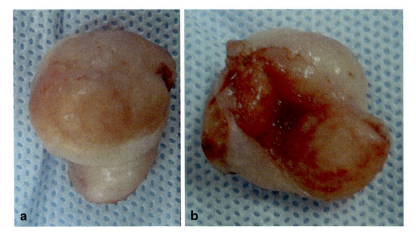

Fig. 9.3 a and **b** A clinical photograph of a resected infantile fibromatosis of the tongue

- The usual clinical course of the solitary form is initial rapid growth followed by spontaneous regression within the first 2 years.
- There is a 7–10% recurrence rate after excision of the solitary lesion.

2. A multicentric form without visceral involvement:
   - This is usually seen in females.
   - They present with multiple nodules in the skin and subcutaneous tissues and bones.

3. A generalized form:
   - In which there are multiple nodules as well as visceral involvement.
   - The visceral involvement is commonly seen in the lungs and gastrointestinal tract.
   - The presentation of gastrointestinal myofibromatosis is variable and depends on the extent of the disease. Diffuse myofibromatosis of the gastrointestinal tract causes a severe watery diarrhea while the solitary type may cause intestinal obstruction or perforation.

Fig. 9.4 Intraoperative photograph showing complete excision of infantile fibromatosis of the tongue for the patient in Figs. 9.2 and 9.3

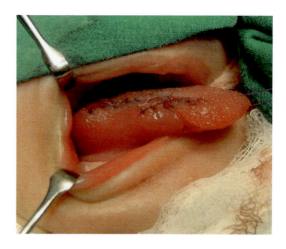

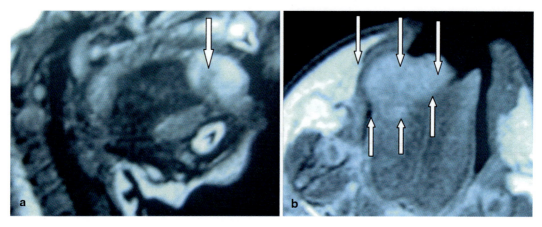

Fig. 9.5 a and **b** CT scan of a child with infantile fibromatosis of the tongue showing a localized mass of the tongue (infantile fibromatosis)

Treatment:

- Wide local excision is the treatment of choice. The primary goal of treatment for fibromatosis is complete surgical resection to achieve negative margins (Fig. 9.4).
- Imaging is required for surgical planning. Radiographic examination reveals a soft-tissue mass, usually noncalcified.
- Computed tomography (CT) appearances are nonspecific; magnetic resonance imaging (MRI) is the best modality for diagnosis and follow-up, specifically in deep fibromatosis (Fig. 9.5).
- The progression is unpredictable. Wide local excision can provide cure if excision is complete with an adequate resection margin but this may be difficult due to infiltrative nature.
- Local recurrence occurs usually within 18 months of original surgery.
- The management of children with unresectable or recurrent fibromatosis requires a multidisciplinary approach.

- Nonaggressive therapy with tamoxifen and diclofenac may be the first treatment choice in these patients, but in patients with progressive disease, cytotoxic chemotherapy is indicated. Weekly administration of vinblastine and methotrexate seems to be safe and effective in these children.
- For tumors that are not resectable or recurrent, conventional chemotherapy and alpha interferon with or without radiotherapy have been used.

Prognosis

- The prognosis of infantile myofibromatosis is variable depending on the extent of the disease.
- When the disease is localized or multicentric without visceral involvement, the prognosis is excellent and the disease is considered self-limiting as it can undergo spontaneous regression. This is usually within 1–2 years. The diagnosis needs however to be confirmed histologically and sometimes surgical excision becomes necessary because the lesion either is causing obstruction or becomes locally destructive.
- When there is visceral involvement, the prognosis however is poor and most of these patients die because of gastrointestinal complications in the form of severe watery diarrhea and perforations or cardiorespiratory arrest.

Recommended Reading

Chung EB, Ezinger FM. Infantile myofibromatosis. Cancer. 1981;48:1807–18.
Narchi H. Infantile myofibromatosis. Int Pediatr. 2001;16:238–9.

Chapter 10
Thyroglossal Cyst

Introduction

- Thyroglossal duct cysts are remnants of the embryonic thyroglossal duct.
- They are midline or just off the midline and move up and down upon swallowing and protrusion of the tongue.
- They may occur anywhere from the base of the tongue to the thyroid gland.
- The majority, however, are found at the level of the thyrohyoid membrane, under the deep cervical fascia.

Embryology

- The thyroid gland develops as a small group of cells at the base of the tongue (foramen cecum).
- These cells migrate downwards along the midline of the neck until they arrive at the final position of the thyroid gland where they grow into a butterfly-shaped gland (the thyroid gland).
- The thyroglossal tract usually becomes obliterated but any part of the tract can persist leading to the development of a cyst (thyroglossal cyst) as a result of the accumulation of thick mucus-like material.
- The thyroglossal duct, the path those thyroid cells travel through, goes just above, just below, or right through the hyoid bone. This is important to know when removing these cysts.
- Thyroglossal fistulae on the other hand are acquired following rupture or incision of infected thyroglossal cyst.
- Thyroglossal cysts are lined by variable tissues including columnar, cuboidal, and/or nonkeratinized pseudostratified squamous epithelium.
- Ectopic thyroid tissue is present in a proportion of thyroglossal cysts with estimates ranging widely, from 1.5 to 62%. Another ectopic tissue found in the thryroglossal cyst is the salivary gland tissue.

Sites

- Approximately 65% of thyroglossal cysts are located below the hyoid bone (between the hyoid bone and thyroid gland).
- Fifteen percent occur at the level of the hyoid bone.
- Twenty percent occur above the hyoid bone.
- Lingual thyroglossal cysts are rare, accounting for 1–2% of all thyroglossal cysts.

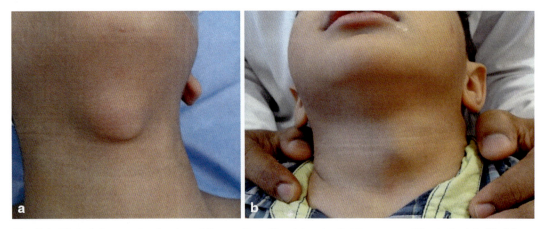

Fig. 10.1 Clinical photographs showing midline neck swelling (**a**) and a slightly more swelling to the left side (**b**)

Clinical Features

- Thyroglossal cysts are usually present as a midline neck swelling or a little to the left of the midline (Fig. 10.1).
- Usually painless, smooth, and cystic.
- A thyroglossal cyst will move upwards with protrusion of the tongue (Fig. 10.2).
- Thyroglossal cysts typically present in children and young patients, with an average age at the presentation of 6 years. About 50 % of patients are present before 20 years of age but a significant percentage (15 %) present after 50 years of age.
- They may become infected and present with pain, redness, and tenderness (Fig. 10.3).
- A thyroglossal cyst can develop anywhere along a thyroglossal duct, though cysts within the tongue or in the floor of the mouth are rare.
- The most common location for a thyroglossal cyst is midline or slightly off midline, between the isthmus of the thyroid and the hyoid bone, or just above the hyoid bone.
- In children, thyroglossal cysts are diagnosed clinically.
- Ultrasound is the most appropriate imaging to confirm the clinical diagnosis and identify the presence of the thyroid gland.
- There is controversy regarding the need for preoperative thyroid scintigraphy in patients with a thyroglossal duct cyst. Proponents argue that scintigraphy is sensitive for the detection of ectopic thyroid tissue in the neck and that the excision of a thyroglossal cyst in a patient with no additional functioning thyroid tissue might result in permanent hypothyroidism. Others feel that preoperative scintigraphy is not necessary.
- A properly performed Sistrunk procedure will remove all ectopic thyroid tissues regardless of whether it was identified on preoperative imaging and that scintigraphy results in an unnecessary radiation dose to the neck, especially in pediatric patients.

Treatment

- Sistrunk procedure, named for Dr. Walter Ellis Sistrunk who described it in 1920, is the procedure to remove thyroglossal cysts.
- The basis of this operation is to remove (all in one specimen) the thyroglossal cyst, the middle third of the hyoid bone, and follow the thyroglossal tract up to the base of tongue where it is ligated. This is to avoid recurrence.

Treatment 65

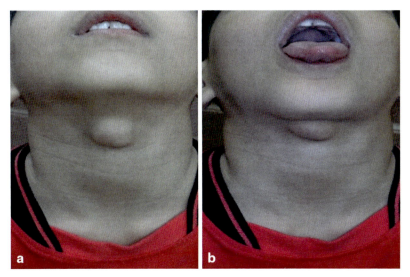

Fig. 10.2 Clinical photographs showing midline neck swelling (**a**) that moves with protrusion of the tongue (**b**)

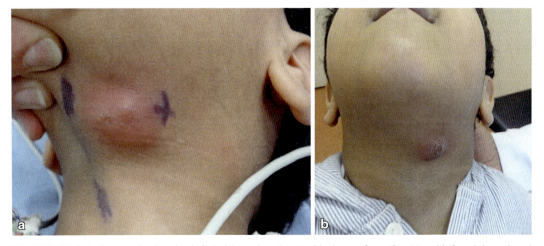

Fig. 10.3 Clinical photographs showing infected thyroglossal cyst with abscess formation (**a**) and infected thyroglossal cyst which formed a fistula (**b**)

- Although generally benign and mostly asymptomatic, thyroglossal cysts need to be removed. This is:
    - For cosmetic reasons if there is unsightly protrusion from the neck
    - To eliminate the chance of infection and abscess formation
    - To eliminate the risk of development of a carcinoma (very rare)
- The two most common complications of thyroglossal cysts are:
    - Infection
    - Malignancy (occurs in 1–4 % of cases)

- Every type of thyroid carcinoma has been identified within a thyroglossal cyst. These include:
  - Papillary, mixed follicular-papillary, squamous, follicular, anaplastic, and Hurthle cell carcinoma.
- In 80% of cases, thyroglossal cyst carcinoma is of papillary type.
- Invasion into surrounding soft tissue is seen in only 17% of thyroglossal cyst carcinomas.
- Metastasis is seen in 1.3%, which is much lower than the rate from carcinoma arising in the thyroid gland.
- Regional lymph nodes metastases occur in 8 % of cases.
- Coincidental thyroid gland carcinoma occurs in 14–25 % of cases.

Recommended Reading

Samara C, Bechrakis I, Kavadias S, Papadopoulos A, Maniatis V, Strigaris K. Thyroglossal duct cyst carcinoma: case report and review of the literature, with emphasis on CT findings. *Neuroradiology*. 2001;43:647–9.

Solomon J, Rangecroft L. Thyroglossal-duct lesions in childhood. *J Pediatr Surg*. 1984;19:555–61.

Chapter 11
Undescended Testes (Cryptorchidism)

Introduction

- Cryptorchidism (derived from the Greek κρυπτός, kryptos, meaning hidden and ὄρχις, orchis, meaning testicle) is the absence of one or both testes from the scrotum.
- Undescended testes are relatively common conditions affecting about 3% of full-term infants and 30% of premature infant boys are born with at least one undescended testis. However, about 80% of cryptorchid testes descend by the first year of life (the majority within 3 months), making the true incidence of cryptorchidism around 1% overall.
- Cryptorchidism can affect one or both testes and approximately 10% of cases are bilateral. For unilateral cases, the left testicle is more commonly affected (Fig. 11.1).
- In 90% of cases, an undescended testis can be palpable in the inguinal canal; in a minority, the testis or testes (impalpable) are in the abdomen or nonexistent.
- Undescended testes are associated with:
  - Reduced fertility.
  - Increased risk of testicular germ cell tumors.
  - Psychological problems at the time of puberty.
  - Undescended testes are more susceptible to testicular torsion and infarction.
  - Undescended testes are associated with inguinal hernias.
  - To reduce these risks, undescended testes are usually brought into the scrotum in infancy.
- Ascent of testes:
  - Although cryptorchidism nearly always refers to congenital absence or maldescent, a testis observed in the scrotum in early infancy can occasionally "reascend" into the inguinal canal.
- Retractile testis:
  - A testis which can readily move or be moved between the scrotum and the inguinal canal is referred to as retractile testis. Retractile testes are more common than truly undescended testes and do not need to be operated on.

Embryology

- Embryologically, the testes develop from primordial germ cells to form testicular cords along the genital ridge in the abdomen of the embryo. This is under the influence of the SRY gene on the short arm of the Y chromosome which influences the developing gonad (indifferent gonad) to become a testis rather than an ovary by the 2nd month of gestation.

Fig. 11.1 Clinical photograph showing left undescended testes

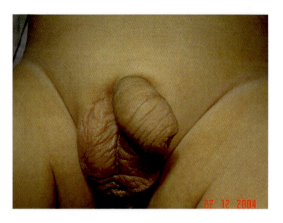

- The cells in the testes differentiate into Leydig cells (testosterone-producing cells) and Sertoli cells (müllerian-inhibiting hormone-producing cells). This occurs during the 3rd to 5th months of intrauterine life. The germ cells become fetal spermatogonia.
- Male external genitalia develop during the 3rd and 4th months of gestation.
- The testes remain high in the abdomen until the 7th month of gestation, when they move from the abdomen through the inguinal canals and into the scrotum.
- It has been proposed that the movement of the testes from the abdomen into the scrotum occurs in two phases.
- The first phase: movement of the testes across the abdomen to the entrance of the inguinal canal. This is influenced by anti-müllerian hormone (AMH).
- The second phase: movement of the testes through the inguinal canal into the scrotum. This is influenced by androgens (most importantly testosterone).
- In rodents, it has been shown that androgens induce the genitofemoral nerve to release calcitonin gene-related peptide (CGRP), which produces rhythmic contractions of the gubernaculum. This is a ligament which connects the testis to the scrotum and helps in its descend into the scrotum but a similar mechanism has not been demonstrated in humans.
- Maldevelopment of the gubernaculum or deficiency or insensitivity to either AMH or androgen therefore can prevent the testes from descending into the scrotum.
- In many infants with inguinal testes, further descent of the testes into the scrotum occurs in the first 6 months of life. This is attributed to the postnatal surge of gonadotropins and testosterone that normally occurs between the 1st and 4th months of life.
- Spermatogenesis continues after birth till about 5 years of age. Some of the fetal spermatogonia become type A spermatogonia and more gradually, other fetal spermatogonia become type B spermatogonia and primary spermatocytes. Spermatogenesis arrests at this stage until puberty.
- Most normal-appearing undescended testes are also normal by microscopic examination but reduced spermatogonia can be found. The tissues in undescended testes however start to degenerate and become abnormal microscopically between 2 and 4 years of age. There is some evidence that early orchidopexy reduces this degeneration.

A testis that is absent from the normal position in the scrotum can be:

1. Undescended (impalpable) and found anywhere along the "path of descent" from high posteriorly in the retroperitoneal space, just below the kidney, to the inguinal ring
2. Undescended (palpable) and found in the inguinal canal
3. Ectopic found away from the normal path of descent, usually outside the inguinal canal, and sometimes even under the skin of the thigh, the perineum, the opposite scrotum, or the femoral canal
4. Undeveloped (hypoplastic) or severely abnormal (dysgenetic; Fig. 11.2)
5. Vanished (anorchia)

Diagnosis

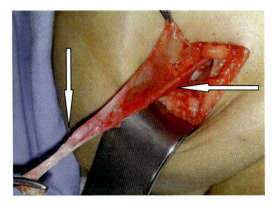

Fig. 11.2 Intraoperative photograph showing atrophic testes. Note the vas deferens and the small atrophic testes, indicated by arrows

Etiology

- In most full-term infant boys with cryptorchidism, a cause cannot be found.
- A combination of genetics, maternal, and other environmental factors may disrupt the normal development of the testes.
- Several factors may however increase the risk of cryptorchidism:
    - Prematurity.
    - Low birth weight.
    - Diabetes and obesity in the mother.
    - Regular alcohol consumption during pregnancy.
    - Cigarette smoking.
    - Family history of undescended testes.
    - Parents' exposure to some pesticides.
    - Cryptorcidism occurs at a much higher rate in those with Down's syndrome, Prader–Willi syndrome, and Noonan syndrome.
    - Spigelian hernia.

Diagnosis

- The diagnosis of undescended testis is a clinical one and normally for a palpable undescended testes no further investigations are require.
- In the minority of cases with bilaterally nonpalpable testes, further testing to locate the testes, assess their function, and exclude additional problems is often useful.
- Pelvic ultrasound or magnetic resonance imaging can often, but not invariably, locate the testes while confirming the absence of a uterus. The presence of a uterus by pelvic ultrasound suggests either persistent müllerian duct syndrome (AMH deficiency or insensitivity) or a severely virilized genetic female with congenital adrenal hyperplasia (Fig. 11.3).
- A karyotype can confirm or exclude forms of dysgenetic primary hypogonadism, such as Klinefelter syndrome or mixed gonadal dysgenesis.
- Hormone levels (especially gonadotropins and AMH) can help confirm that there are hormonally functional testes worth attempting to rescue.
- Stimulation with human chorionic gonadotropin (HCG) to elicit a rise of the testosterone level.

Fig. 11.3 Intraoperative photograph of an undescended testes being brought down

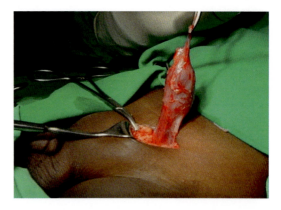

Fig. 11.4 Intraoperative photograph showing bilateral abdominal testes in a child with testicular feminization syndrome

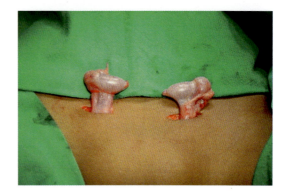

Treatment

- The primary management of cryptorchidism is surgery (orchidopexy).
- In cases where the testes are palpable, orchidopexy is often performed as an outpatient and has a very low complication rate.
- Orchidopexy is usually performed in infancy around 6–10 months of age. This age recommendation is based on (1) the rarity of spontaneous descent of testes after age 6 months and (2) the possible improvements in fertility that early intervention may confer (Fig. 11.4).
- Earlier orchidopexy is indicated in those with a clinically apparent associated inguinal hernia.
- When the undescended testis is in the inguinal canal, hormonal therapy is sometimes attempted and occasionally successful.
- The most commonly used hormone therapy is HCD. A series of HCG injections (5–10 injections over 2.5–5 weeks) is given and the status of the testis/testes is reassessed at the end.
- Although many trials have been published, the reported success rates of hormonal therapy vary widely. Success rates for the descent of testes into the scrotum following hormonal therapy are 25–55 % in uncontrolled studies but only 6–21 % in randomized blinded studies. This discrepancy is because of differences in patient age, treatment schedules, and possible inclusion of retractile testes.
- Hormonal therapy was reported to increase the size and vascularity of the testes which makes surgery easier.
- Agonistic analogs of gonadotropin-releasing hormone (GnRH) such as nafarelin or buserelin stimulate the release of the pituitary gonadotropins, luteinizing hormone (LH) and follicle-stimulating hormone (FSH), temporarily increasing gonadal steroidogenesis. Success rates in uncontrolled studies using GnRH range from 13 to 78 %, while better-controlled studies resulted in success rates

of 6–38%. Recent studies showed descent into the scrotum in 6% of the HCG-treated group and in 19% of the GnRH treated group. Higher descent rates were reported when the two therapies were combined.
- The cost of either type of hormone treatment is less than that of surgery and the chance of complications at appropriate doses is minimal.
- Adverse effects of HCG treatment include increased scrotal rugae, pigmentation, pubic hair, and penile growth, which regress after treatment cessation. A total dose of more than 15, 000 IU may induce epiphyseal plate fusion and retard future somatic growth.
- Nevertheless, despite the potential advantages of a trial of hormonal therapy, many surgeons do not consider the success rates high enough to be worth the trouble since surgery itself is usually simple and uncomplicated.
- Hormonal therapy however is worth in those with bilateral undescended testes especially if not palpable.
- In patients with intra-abdominal undescended testis, laparoscopy is useful to confirm the presence and position of the testis and decide upon surgery (single or staged laparoscopic Fowler-Stephens orchidopexy).
- The single-stage Fowler-Stephens procedure must be planned ahead to avoid devascularization of the secondary blood supply from the vas deferens and the cremaster muscles. It can be performed using the open or laparoscopic technique. The success rate is 67%.
- The two-stage Fowler-Stephens procedure theoretically allows improved collateral blood supply but a second stage is required. It may also be performed with an open or laparoscopic technique. The success rate is 77%.
- Based on the surgical approach, the success rates were as follows: 89% for inguinal orchidopexy, 84% for microvascular orchidopexy, 81% for transabdominal orchiopexy, 77% for staged Fowler-Stephens orchidopexy, and 67% for standard Fowler-Stephens orchidopexy. Microvascular orchidopexy allows adequate scrotal position with the preservation of the spermatic artery blood flow. However, it requires special expertise.
- The principal major complication of all types of orchidopexy is loss of the blood supply to the testis, resulting in loss of the testis due to ischemic atrophy or fibrosis.

Prognosis

Fertility

- Many men who were born with undescended testes have reduced fertility, even after orchidopexy in infancy.
- The reported reduction in fertility with unilateral cryptorchidism is about 10%. This is higher than the 6% report in the general population. The fertility reduction after orchidopexy for bilateral cryptorchidism is more marked, about 38%, or six times that of the general population.
- The degree to which this is prevented or improved by early orchidopexy is still uncertain.
- One contributing factor or reduced spermatogenesis in cryptorchid testes is temperature. The temperature of testes in the scrotum is at least a couple of degrees cooler than in the abdomen. Raising the temperature of the testes could damage fertility.
- Subtle or transient hormone deficiencies or other factors that impair testicular descent also impair the development of the spermatogenic tissue.
- An additional factor contributing to infertility is the high rate of anomalies of the epididymis in boys with cryptorchidism (over 90% in some studies). Even after orchidopexy, these may also affect sperm maturation and motility at an older age.

Testicular Cancer

- One of the strongest arguments for early orchidopexy is prevention of testicular cancer.
- About 1 in 500 men born with one or both undescended testes develop testicular cancer, roughly a 4–40-fold increased risk.
- The peak incidence of testicular cancer occurs in the 3rd and 4th decades of life.
- The risk is higher for intra-abdominal testes and somewhat lower for inguinal testes, but even the normally descended testis of a man whose other testis was undescended has about a 20% higher cancer risk than those of other men.
- The most common type of testicular cancer occurring in undescended testes is seminoma.
- Orchidopexy results in easier detection of testis cancer but does not lower the risk of actually developing cancer. There are however recent reports suggesting that orchidopexy performed before puberty resulted in a significantly reduced risk of testicular cancer than if done after puberty.
- The risk of malignancy in the undescended testis is 4–10-times higher than that in the general population and is approximately 1 in 80 with a unilateral undescended testis and 1 in 40 to 1 in 50 for bilateral undescended testes. The peak age for this tumor is 15–45 years.

Recommended Reading

Baker LA, Docimo SG, Surer I, Peters C, Cisek L, Diamond DL, et al. A multi-institutional analysis of laparoscopic orchidopexy. BJU Int. 2001;87:484–9.

Cortes D, Thorup JM, Visfeldt J. Cryptorchidism: aspects of fertility and neoplasms. A study including data of 1,335 consecutive boys who underwent testicular biopsy simultaneously with surgery for cryptorchidism. *Horm Res.* 2001;55(1):21–7.

Lee PA. Fertility in cryptorchidism. Does treatment make a difference? *Endocrinol Metab Clin North Am.* 1993;22:479–90.

Lindgren BW, Franco I, Blick S, Levitt SB, Brock WA, Palmer LS, Friedman SC, Reda EF. Laparoscopic Fowler-Stephens orchidopexy for the high abdominal testis. J Urol. 1999;162:990–4.

Tsujihata M, Miyake O, Yoshimura K, Kikimoto K, Matsumiya K, Takahara S, Okuyama A. Laparoscopic diagnosis and treatment of nonpalpable testis. Int J Urol. 2001;8:692–6.

Chapter 12
Varicocele

Introduction

- A varicocele is a mass of abnormally enlarged and dilated veins (the pampiniform plexus) in the testicle that essentially feels like a bag of worms.
- A varicocele is unusual in boys under 10 years of age and becomes more frequent at the beginning of puberty.
- It is found in 15–20 % of adolescent boys but can occur earlier.
- Varicocele almost always occurs on the left side (78–93 % of cases).
- Right-sided varicoceles are least common; they are usually noted only when bilateral varicoceles are present and seldom occur as an isolated finding.
- A unilateral right-sided varicocele should prompt an investigation for a retroperitoneal mass that causes obstruction of the right internal spermatic vein or thrombosis or occlusion of the inferior vena.
- Situs inversus is another cause of a right-sided varicocele.
- Varicoceles are one of the leading causes of male infertility and are detected in 35 % of adult males with primary infertility.
- In about 20 % of adolescents with varicocele, fertility problems will arise. Improvement in sperm parameters has been demonstrated after varicocelectomy. It has been reported that 71 % of patients who had varicocele ligation had improvements in their postoperative semen parameters.

Clinical Features

- Most varicoceles are asymptomatic; however, testicular pain or a mass may be a presenting symptom.
- It may be noticed by the patient or parents, or discovered by the pediatrician.
- The diagnosis depends upon the clinical finding of a collection of dilated and tortuous veins in the upright posture; the veins are more pronounced when the patient performs the Valsalva maneuver (Fig. 12.1).
- The size of both testicles should be evaluated during palpation to detect a smaller testis.

Classification

Varicocele is classified into three grades:

- Grade I: Varicocele palpable at Valsalva maneuver only.
- Grade II: Varicocele palpable without the Valsalva manoeuvre.

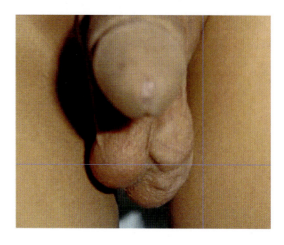

Fig. 12.1 A clinical photograph of a child with left varicocele that feels like a bag of worms

- Grade III: Visible varicocele.
- Grade 0: Subclinical varicocele cannot be detected clinically and venous reflux detected on ultrasound only.

The degree of testicular atrophy directly correlates with varicocele grade.

Etiology

- The etiology of varicocele is unknown and most likely multifactorial. These include:
  - Congenital absence of the valves in the left testicular vein.
  - Abnormal variations in venous drainage of the testes.
  - The right testicular vein drains directly into the inferior vena cava and the left testicular vein drains at a right angle into the left renal vein. This pattern predisposes to slower drainage in the left testicular vein. This may explain the high incidence of varicocele on the left side compared to the right.
- The "nutcracker" phenomenon: The left renal vein is occasionally compressed between the superior mesenteric artery and the aorta. This creates higher pressure in the left testicular vein, which drains into the renal vein.
- Increased length of the left testicular vein: The left vein is 8–10 cm longer than the right testicular vein.

Diagnosis

- The diagnosis of varicocele is made clinically (feeling a bag of worms).
- Venous reflux into the pampiniform plexus is diagnosed using Doppler color flow both in the supine and upright positions.
- The ultrasound examination includes assessment of the testicular volume to document testicular atrophy.
- In adolescents, a testis that is smaller by more than 2 mL compared to the other testis is considered to be hypoplastic.

- Venography is the study of choice to detect a subclinical varicocele in the evaluation of infertile adult patients but has a limited role in children and adolescents.

Treatment

- The treatment of varicocele is still controversial regarding when to operate and on whom to operate.
- Ipsilateral testicular growth retardation is the most frequent indication for varicocele repair in adolescents.
- Varicocele associated with decreased ipsilateral testicular size (a 20% volume deficit in the involved testis detected by an orchidometer or ultrasonography) is an indication for surgical repair.
- Histological studies have revealed seminiferous tubule sclerosis, small vessel degenerative changes, and abnormalities of Leydig, Sertoli, and germ cells. These changes have been documented in patients as young as 12 years.
- The recommended indication criteria for varicocelectomy in children and adolescents are:
  - Symptomatic varicocele.
  - Bilateral varicocele.
  - Varicocele associated with a small testis.
  - In older adolescent: decreased sperm quantity and quality (decreased sperm motility, lower total sperm counts, and increased number of abnormal sperm forms).
  - A large varicocele causing physical or psychological discomfort.
- Surgical treatment is aimed at ligation or occlusion of the internal spermatic veins.
- Several methods are used, differing primarily in the level at which the vessels are approached. These include:
  - Abdominal retroperitoneal (Palomo).
  - Inguinal (Ivanissevitch).
  - Subinguinal approach.
- Microsurgical techniques and laparoscopic-assisted transperitoneal or retroperitoneal approaches are also currently used.
- Angiographic occlusion. This is accomplished by percutaneous embolization of the internal spermatic veins. Although this method is less invasive, it appears to have a higher failure rate (10–25%).
- Complications of varicocelectomy regardless of the technique used, include:
  - Hydrocele formation.
  - Recurrent or persistence of the varicocele.
  - Testicular atrophy.
  - Hydrocele formation is the most common complication and most likely results from lymphatic obstruction.
  - The frequency of hydrocele varies with the surgical method used.
    - The microscopic-assisted procedures carry the lowest complication rates (<1%).
    - Inguinal, retroperitoneal, and laparoscopic ligations carry a postoperative hydrocele risk of less than 10%.
    - Embolization is very infrequently associated with hydrocele formation.
  - Less common complications include testicular atrophy, hematoma, injury to the vas deferens, chronic testicular pain, and recurrence or persistence of the varicocele.

- Recurrence rates following varicocele ligation vary with the technique used.
    - Microsurgical approaches recur in fewer than 5% of cases.
    - A 13–16% recurrence rate is observed with inguinal, retroperitoneal, and laparoscopic ligations.
    - Embolization has an 80–90% success rate and a recurrence rate of approximately 10–25%.

Recommended Reading

Niyogi A, Singh S, Zaman A, Khan A, Nicoara C, Haddad M, et al. Varicocele surgery: 10 years of experience in two pediatric surgical centers. J Laparoendosc Adv Surg Tech A. 2012;22(5):521–5.

Chapter 13
Acute Scrotum

Introduction

- Acute scrotum is one of the common conditions in the pediatric age group.
- Early diagnosis is of paramount importance to avoid the drastic sequelae of testicular loss.
- The most common diagnoses encountered in a child with acute scrotal swelling and pain are testicular torsion, torsion of a testicular appendage, epididymitis and epididymoorchitis, and idiopathic scrotal edema. Other conditions to be considered in the differential diagnosis are hernia, tumors, Henoch–Schönlein purpura, trauma, varicocele, and hydrocele.
- Common causes of acute scrotum:
  - Torsion of testis
  - Epididymitis and epididymoorchitis
  - Trauma
  - Torsion of testicular appendage
  - Idiopathic scrotal edema

Testicular Torsion

- Torsion of testis occurs when an abnormally mobile testis twists on the spermatic cord, obstructing its blood supply.
- Testicular torsion is a true surgical emergency and must be considered in any patient who complains of acute scrotal pain and swelling and the likelihood of testicular salvage decreases as the duration of torsion increases. Delay in diagnosis and management can lead to loss of testes.
- Conditions that may mimic testicular torsion, such as torsion of a testicular appendage, epididymitis, trauma, hernia, hydrocele, varicocele, and Schönlein–Henoch purpura, generally do not require immediate surgical intervention.
- Testicular torsion can occur at any age including the prenatal and perinatal periods but commonly seen in adolescents.
- Torsion is most frequent among adolescents with about 65 % of cases presenting between 12 and 18 years of age.
- Testicular torsion presentation includes:
  - An acute onset of severe scrotal pain
  - Scrotal swelling and erythema
  - Nausea and vomiting
  - Local scrotal redness and pain

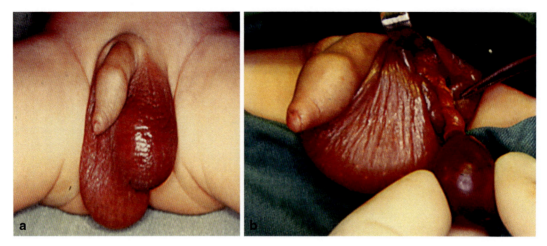

Fig. 13.1 a A clinical photograph of a newborn with left testiculat torsion. Note the swelling and discoloration of the scrotum. **b,** An intraoperative photograph of a newborn with left testicular torsion. Note the extravaginal type of torsion

- Predisposing conditions to testicular torsion include:
  - The most common underlying cause for testicular torsion is a congenital malformation known as a "bell-clapper deformity."
    ◦ The tunica vaginalis normally attaches to the posterolateral surface of the testes and allows very little mobility of the testes within the scrotum.
    ◦ In the "bell-clapper deformity," there is an inappropriately high attachment of the tunica vaginalis which is inadequately affixed allowing it to move and rotate freely on the spermatic cord within the tunica vaginalis.
    ◦ It is present in 12 % of males and accounts for 90 % of all cases of intravaginal torsion.
  - Cryptorchid testes are at significantly higher risk of torsion than scrotal testes.
  - A horizontal lie of the testes.
  - Polyorchidism.
  - Epididymal anomalies.
  - Torsions are sometimes called "winter syndrome" because they are more frequent in cold conditions.
- Types of testicular torsion:
  - There are two types of testicular torsion.
  - Extravaginal torsion:
    ◦ A torsion which occurs outside of the tunica vaginalis (Fig. 13.1a).
    ◦ This type occurs exclusively in newborns.
    ◦ Extravaginal torsion constitutes approximately 5 % of all torsions and of these cases of testicular torsion, 70 % occur prenatally and 30 % occur postnatally.
    ◦ Neonates with extravaginal torsion present with scrotal swelling, discoloration, and a firm, painless mass in the scrotum (Fig. 13.1b).
    ◦ It is commonly unilateral but can present bilaterally (Fig. 13.2a).
    ◦ Such testes are usually necrotic from birth and must be removed surgically (Fig. 13.2b).
    ◦ It is also believed that torsion occurring during fetal development can lead to the vanishing testis, and is one of the causes of an infant being born with monorchism.
    ◦ The fact that 30 % of these cases occur postnatally calls for early surgical exploration.

Introduction

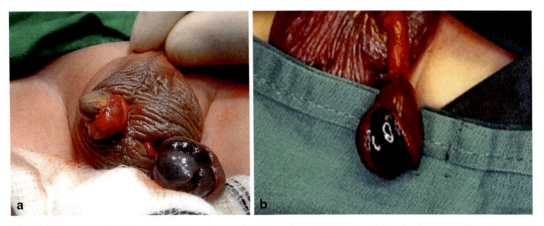

Fig. 13.2 Intraoperative photograph of a newborn with bilateral testicular torsion (**a**) and an intraoperative photograph of a newborn with testicular torsion (**b**). Note the already necrotic testis

- Intravaginal torsion:
    - Torsion occurring within the tunica vaginalis.
    - The peak incidence of intravaginal torsion occurs at age 13–14 years.
    - The left testis is more frequently involved.
    - Bilateral cases account for 2% of all torsions.
- Clinical features:
    - Testicular torsion usually presents with an acute onset of diffuse testicular pain and tenderness. There is a rapid onset of testicular pain.
    - The age of the patient may be helpful as torsion of the appendix testis is more common in prepubertal boys (Table 13.1).
    - Nausea is common and usually afebrile but may have a low-grade fever.
    - The scrotum is generally neither swollen nor discolored, and the affected testis may have a horizontal lie.
    - Prehn's sign: The physical lifting of the testicles relieves the pain of epididymitis but not pain caused by testicular torsion. This was once believed to be helpful in determining whether the presenting testicular pain is caused by acute epididymitis or from testicular torsion but it is not reliable.
    - The cremasteric reflex is generally absent in cases of testicular torsion.
    - Many of the symptoms of testicular torsion are similar to epididymitis though epididymitis is usually characterized by discoloration and swelling of the testis, often with fever, and the cremasteric reflex is not affected.

Diagnosis:

- The diagnosis of testicular torsion is often made clinically.
- Emergency diagnosis and treatment are usually necessary within 4–6 hours from the onset of symptoms in order to prevent necrosis.
- The most widely used imaging modality for evaluation of testicular torsion is ultrasonography with Doppler scanning for blood flow (Fig. 13.3).
- In general, a Doppler ultrasound should be obtained only in low-suspicion cases to rule out torsion while in those cases with a convincing history and physical examination immediate surgical detorsion is the treatment of choice.
- A Doppler ultrasound scan is nearly 100% accurate at diagnosing torsion. There is absence of blood flow in the twisted testicle, which distinguishes the condition from epididymitis.

Table 13.1 Differential diagnosis and management of the acute scrotum

Type	Onset of symptoms	Age at diagnosis	Site of tenderness	Urinalysis	Cremasteric reflex	Treatment
Testicular torsion	Acute	Early puberty	Diffuse	Negative	Negative	Surgical exploration
Appendiceal torsion	Subacute	Prepubertal	Localized to upper pole	Negative	Positive	Bed rest and scrotal elevation
Epididymitis	Insidious	Adolescence	Epididymal	Positive or negative	Positive	Antibiotics

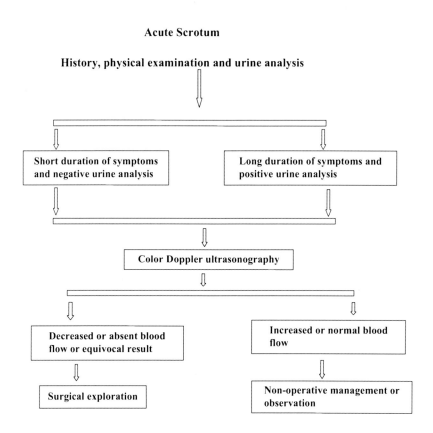

Fig. 13.3 An algorithm of the diagnosis and management of acute scrotum

- Radionuclide scanning (technetium-99 m pertechnetate) of the scrotum:
    - This is the most accurate imaging technique to diagnose testicular torsion.
    - It is however not widely available, and even in centers with functioning nuclear medicine facilities, they may not have these available at all hours.
    - Radioisotope scanning has been reported to be highly accurate for the diagnosis of testicular torsion.
    - The ischemic area is seen as a photopenic zone in testicular ischemia.
    - In cases of inflammation and infection, increased uptake is seen.

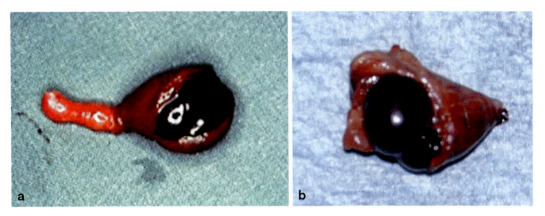

Fig. 13.4 a and b Necrotic testis after orchiectomy

Treatment

- The two most important determinants of early salvage rate of the testis are:
  - The time between onset of symptoms and detorsion
  - The degree of twisting of the cord thus, time is of the essence
- Time should not be wasted attempting to arrange for imaging studies, laboratory testing, or other diagnostic procedures as this results in lost testicular tissue.
- Salvage rate depends on the time between onset of symptoms and detorsion:
  - Between 90 and 100%, if detorsion is done within 6 h of onset of symptoms.
  - Between 20 and 40% after 12 h.
  - From 0 to 10% if >24 h.
- Testicular torsion classically develops as a medial rotation; however, in up to one-third of cases, a lateral rotation has been described.
- When manual detorsion is contemplated, the testis is typically rotated laterally ("opening the book"); however, if the testis is already laterally rotated, this maneuver worsens the condition. So, manual detorsion is not a commonly performed procedure.
- Manual detorsion is successful between 26.5 and 80% of patients.
- Surgical detorsion is the definitive treatment for testicular torsion. If the testis is necrotic, perform an orchiectomy.
- Always perform contralateral orchiopexy when testicular torsion is confirmed intraoperatively, in order to prevent future torsion of the other testicle.
- If viability of the testis is in question after detorsion, the testis should be left in the scrotum and followed up clinically and radiologically. If necrotic it will ultimately atrophy.
- Neonatal torsion is treated surgically with exploration and contralateral orchiopexy because bilateral (synchronous or asynchronous) neonatal testicular torsion, while rare, has been described. If the testis is necrotic, perform an orchiectomy (Fig. 13.4).
- Patients requiring an orchiectomy because of a nonviable testis may benefit from the placement of a testicular prosthesis. This is done through an inguinal incision and usually 6 months following torsion to allow for healing and inflammatory changes to resolve.

Intermittent Testicular Torsion

- Intermittent testicular torsion is a chronic condition characterized by all of the symptoms of full torsion but is followed by eventual spontaneous detortion and subsequent resolution of pain.
- Nausea or vomiting may also occur.
- These patients are at significant risk of developing a complete torsion and possible subsequent orchiectomy.
- The treatment for intermittent testicular torsion is elective bilateral orchiopexy.

Torsion of the Testicular Appendix

- In a child with an acute scrotum, testicular torsion is not the most common condition. Torsion of testicular appendices represents the more common cause of scrotal pain.
- The appendix testis: A müllerian duct remnant located at the superior pole of the testicle is the most common appendage to undergo torsion.
- The epididymal appendix: A Wolffian duct remnant located on the head of the epididymis.
- Torsion of either appendage produces pain similar to that experienced with testicular torsion, but the onset is more gradual.
- This type of torsion is the most common cause of acute scrotal pain in boys aged 7–14 years.
- Its appearance is similar to that of a full torsion but the onset of pain is more gradual. Typically, it has a more gradual onset than testicular torsion and patients may endure pain for several days before seeking medical attention.
- Palpation reveals a small firm nodule on the upper portion of the testis which displays a characteristic "blue dot sign." This is the appendix of the testis which has become discolored and is noticeably blue through the skin.
- The cremasteric reflex is preserved.
- Torsion of the appendix testis may present similarly to testicular torsion. The age of the patient may be helpful, as torsion of the appendix testis is more common in prepubertal boys.
- Color Doppler ultrasonography demonstrates normal or increased blood flow.
- Torsion of a testicular appendage may be misinterpreted as epididymitis. However if the urinalysis is normal, no antibiotic therapy is required.
- Management consists of:
    - Bed rest.
    - Analgesia.
    - Scrotal elevation to minimize inflammation and edema.
    - Nonsteroidal anti-inflammatory drugs (NSAIDs) generally are not helpful and thus are not routinely used.
- The condition usually resolves within 3–5 days.
- In the acute setting, differentiating testicular torsion from torsion of the appendix is sometimes impossible, and scrotal exploration should be performed whenever the diagnosis is uncertain.

Epididymitis and Epididmoorchitis

- Epididymitis is the most common inflammatory process involving the scrotum and more common in adults.

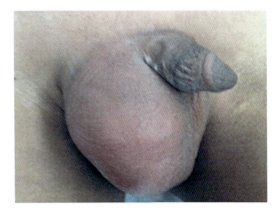

Fig. 13.5 A clinical photograph of a child with severe epididymitis complicated by abscess formation

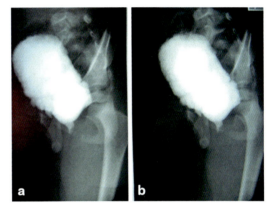

Fig. 13.6 a and **b** A micturating cystourethrogram showing neurogenic bladder with high intravesical pressure which may lead to reflux epididymitis

- Infections generally originate in the lower urinary tract from the bladder, urethra, or prostate and are typically caused by urinary tract pathogens or sexually transmitted organisms (chlamydia or gonorrhea).
- Epididymitis in adolescents and young adults is often related to sexual activity and does not present with a urinary tract infection.
- In prepubertal boys, however, epididymitis is almost always associated with a urinary tract anomaly.
- Epididymitis also occurs in children, but is due to infection with Streptococcus or Staphylococcus (Fig. 13.5).
- In urinary tract abnormalities also infection with E. coli is seen.
- In those with increased bladder pressure and contractions against a closed sphincter, there is reflux not only into the left ureter and prostate but also into the epididymis, which resulted in epididymitis (Fig. 13.6).
- Any episode of epididymitis and urinary tract infection should be investigated with a renal/bladder sonogram and a voiding cystourethrogram to rule out structural problems.
- Treatment includes empiric antibiotic therapy until the results of a urine culture are known.
- If the culture is negative, the symptoms are most likely due to nonbacterial epididymitis caused by urinary reflux.
- A sterile chemical epididymitis can result from reflux of sterile urine through the ejaculatory ducts, for instance, if the ureter inserts in the prostatic urethra or a utricular cyst, this may lead to increased pressure in the vas deferens (Fig. 13.7).
- Clinically, the epididymis is swollen and heterogeneous. There is usually a small hydrocele and scrotal wall thickening.

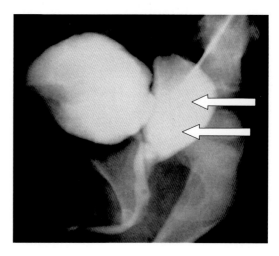

Fig. 13.7 Micturating cystourethrogram in a child who presented with epididymitis showing a large utricular cyst (*arrows*)

- Color Doppler show increased flow (Fig. 13.8).
- Bed rest and scrotal elevation are often helpful.
- NSAIDs and analgesics can be used to alleviate symptoms.
- The pain and swelling generally resolve within a week. Resolution of epididymal induration however may require several weeks.

Idiopathic Scrotal Edema

- Acute idiopathic scrotal edema is another possible cause of an acute scrotum.
- Idiopathic scrotal edema is seen in school-aged boys.
- The etiology of this condition remains unknown.
- It is characterized by the rapid onset of significant scrotal edema usually without tenderness.
- Erythema may be present.
- Clinically, the child is usually afebrile, and the testes and epididymes feel normal.
- All diagnostic tests including WBC and urine analysis are normal.
- Ultrasound shows only scrotal skin edema with normal testes and epididymes.
- Treatment consists of bed rest and scrotal elevation. Analgesics are rarely needed.

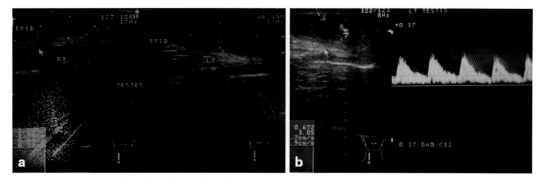

Fig. 13.8 a Ultrasound of a child with epididymitis. Note the enlarged left epididymis when compared to the right one. **b** A Doppler ultrasound of a child with epididymitis. Note the increased flow

Other Causes of Acute Scrotum

Scrotal Trauma

- Trauma to the testis can cause severe pain, bruising, and/or swelling.
- Severe testicular injury is uncommon and usually results from either a direct blow to the scrotum or a straddle injury and rarely a penetrating injury.
- A rare type of testicular trauma, called testicular rupture, occurs when the testicle receives a direct blow or is squeezed against the hard bones of the pelvis.
- A spectrum of injuries may occur. These include:
  - Intratesticular hematoma
  - Hematocele (blood collection between the leaves of the tunica vaginalis)
  - Laceration of the tunica albuginea (testicular rupture)
- Traumatic epididymitis is a noninfectious inflammatory condition that usually occurs within a few days after a blow to the testis.
- Color Doppler ultrasonography is the imaging technique of choice.
- The treatment depends on the ultrasound findings and usually conservative.
- Testicular rupture on the other hand requires immediate exploration, drainage, and repair.

Henoch–Schönlein Purpura

- Henoch–Schönlein purpura is a systemic vasculitis with manifestations usually involving the skin, gastrointestinal tract, kidneys, and joints.
- The "classic triad" of Henoch–Schönlein purpura (Fig. 13.9) include:
  - Purpura
  - Arthritis
  - Abdominal pain

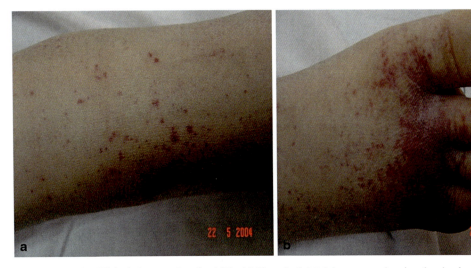

Fig. 13.9 a and **b** Clinical photographs of a child with Henoch–Schönlein purpura showing the classic rash

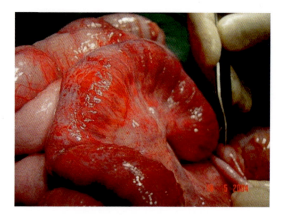

Fig. 13.10 Intraoperative photograph of a child with Henoch–Schönlein purpura. Note the intestinal hemorrhage

- Purpura occurs in all cases, joint pains, and arthritis in 80%, and abdominal pain in 62%.
- Some include gastrointestinal hemorrhage as a fourth criterion; this occurs in 33% of cases, sometimes, but not necessarily always, due to intussusception (Fig. 13.10).
- Acute scrotal swelling may accompany Henoch–Schönlein syndrome and may be the presenting manifestation mimicking testicular torsion. This may cause the patient to undergo unnecessary surgery, because the patient may have complained of severe scrotal pain and swelling.

Inguinal Hernia

- Inguinal hernia should be suspected in a child who has a history of intermittent groin swelling. If the diagnosis is unclear, ultrasound examination can be helpful. An incarcerated or strangulated hernia requires urgent surgical intervention, whereas a reducible hernia should be repaired electively (Fig. 13.11).

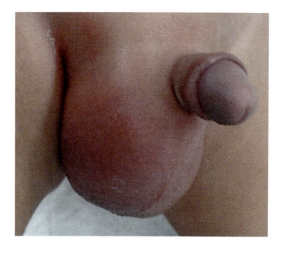

Fig. 13.11 A clinical photograph of a child with strangulated inguinal hernia that may be confused with acute scrotum

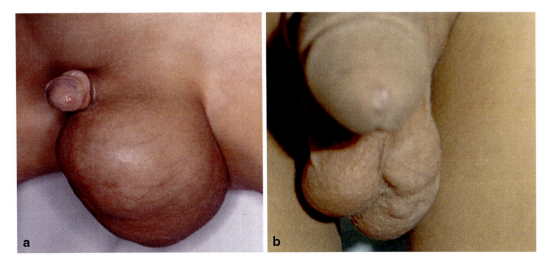

Fig. 13.12 a A clinical photograph of a child with a hydrocele. This is usually diagnosed clinically. **b** A clinical photograph of a child with left varicocele that may cause scrotal discomfort and pain

Hydrocele

- A hydrocele occurs because of a patent processus vaginalis. Most hydroceles resolve spontaneously. Therefore, an infant with a hydrocele and no evidence of a hernia is usually just observed for the first 1 or 2 years of life. If the hydrocele persists beyond this time, surgical repair is recommended (Fig. 13.12a).

Varicocele

- Occasionally, a varicocele causes mild to moderate scrotal discomfort. No changes in the scrotal skin occur, but the affected hemi-scrotum may have a full appearance. On physical examination, a varix is palpable as a "bag of worms" above a palpably normal testis and epididymis. Varicoceles can affect both testicular growth and fertility and should be treated surgically (Fig. 13.12b).

Recommended Reading

Lewis AG, Bukowski TP, Jarvis PD, et al. Evaluation of acute scrotum in the emergency department. J Pediatr Surg. 1995;30:277.

Schalamon J, Ainoedhofer H, Schleef J, et al. Management of acute scrotum in children—the impact of Doppler ultrasound. J Pediatr Surg. 2006;41:1377.

Sessions AE, Rabinowitz R, Hulbert WC, et al. Testicular torsion: direction, degree, duration and disinformation. J Urol. 2003;169:663.

Chapter 14
Esophageal Atresia and/or Tracheoesophageal Fistula

Introduction

- Esophageal atresia (EA) with or without tracheoesophageal fistula (TEF) is a fairly common congenital disorder.
- The exact incidence of EA with or without TEF is not known, but an incidence of 1 in 3000 to 1 in 4500 live births has been reported worldwide.

Embryology

- The esophagus and trachea are derived from the primitive foregut.
- During the fourth and fifth weeks of embryologic development, the trachea forms as a ventral diverticulum from the primitive pharynx. A tracheoesophageal septum develops at the site where the longitudinal tracheoesophageal folds fuse together.
- This septum then divides the foregut into a ventral portion, the laryngotracheal tube, and a dorsal portion (the esophagus).
- EA results if the tracheoesophageal septum is deviated posteriorly. This deviation causes incomplete separation of the esophagus from the laryngotracheal tube and results in a concurrent TEF.
- EA as an isolated congenital anomaly may occur, rarely.
- In these cases, the atresia is attributable to failure of the recanalization of the esophagus during the eighth week of development and is not associated with TEF.
- Embryologically, many anatomic variations of EA with or without TEF have been described.

Anatomy

- The most common variant of this anomaly consists of EA (a blind esophageal pouch) with a distal TEF (a fistula between the trachea and the distal esophagus). This is estimated to occur in 84–87 % of the cases.
- The second most common anomaly is pure EA without TEF seen in 6–8 % of the cases. This condition is usually associated with an underdeveloped distal esophageal remnant, making surgical repair more cumbersome.
- The third most common variation is the H-type fistula, which consists of a TEF without EA. This is seen in 4–5 % of the cases and is more difficult to diagnose clinically. If the fistula is long and oblique, the symptoms may be minimal, and the condition may not be identified for many years.

Fig. 14.1 The different anatomic variants of EA/TEF

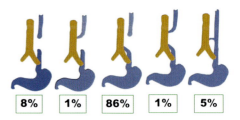

- The different anatomic variants of EA with or without TEF are shown in Fig. 14.1.
- Type c (EA with distal TEF) is the commonest type making up to 86 % of the cases. This is followed by pure EA which forms about 8 %. The H-type TEF makes about 4–5 % of the cases.

Clinical Features

EA is usually detected shortly after birth and should be suspected in an infant with drooling (excessive salivation) that is frequently accompanied by choking, coughing, and sneezing.

- The infant may become cyanotic and may stop breathing as the overflow of fluid from the blind pouch is aspirated into the trachea.
- These patients should not be fed but when feeding is attempted the infant coughs, chokes, and becomes cyanotic.
- Prompt recognition, appropriate clinical management to prevent aspiration, and urgent referral to an appropriate tertiary care center have resulted in a significant improvement in the rates of morbidity and mortality in these infants.
- The presentation of those with H-type TEF is variable and nonspecific and a high index of suspicion is important in this regard.
- Commonly, these patients present with recurrent chest infection, cyanosis, and choking during feeds.
- Any newborn, infant, or child who presents with repeated attacks of choking and coughing during feeding, abdominal distension, and recurrent attacks of chest infection should raise suspicion of congenital H-type TEF and must be investigated accordingly.
- In many of these patients, the diagnosis is difficult and occasionally delayed until late childhood or even up to adulthood.

Diagnosis

- Prenatally, ultrasonographic findings of polyhydramnios, proximal dilated upper pouch, and a small or absent gastric bubble is suggestive but not confirmatory sign of isolated EA or EA and TEF as many other conditions are associated with polyhydramnios. This however must be confirmed postnatally.
- The diagnosis can easily be confirmed by simply passing a nasogastric tube. Failure to pass the nasogastric tube and coiling of the tube in the upper pouch confirms the diagnosis of EA. A plain chest and abdominal x-ray will confirm this (Fig. 14.2).

Diagnosis

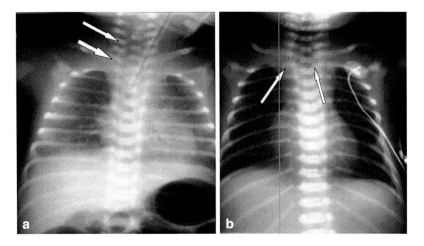

Fig. 14.2 Chest x-ray showing an N/G coiled in the upper esophageal pouch. Note the gas in the stomach and intestines denoting an associated tracheoesophageal fistula in the first and absence of gas denoting an isolated esophageal atresia in the second

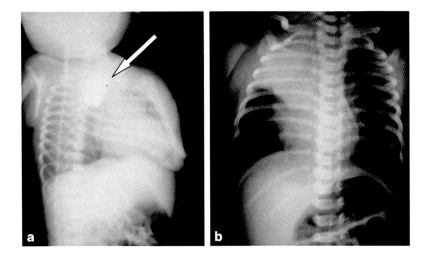

Fig. 14.3 a and **b** Chest x-rays showing esophageal atresia and aspiration pneumonia

- The presence of gas in the stomach and intestines with a coiled nasogastric tube in the proximal pouch confirms the diagnosis of EA with distal TEF. The level of nasogastric tube in relation to the vertebra can be used to determine the height of the upper pouch. This is important to plan the surgical repair (Fig. 14.2b).
- The use of contrast esophagogram to confirm the diagnosis should be abandoned as this will not only delay their transfers but also increase the risk of hypothermia and aspiration pneumonia (Figs. 14.3 and 14.4).
- An echocardiogram is important to establish associated cardiac anomalies and a normal left-sided aortic arch.
- Contrast-enhanced studies are necessary to identify or locate an H-type TEF (Fig. 14.5).
- This requires an experienced radiologist who should perform contrast-enhanced studies (pull out esophagogram) with fluoroscopic control.
- The study may have to be performed more than once to establish the diagnosis. Endoscopy and/or bronchoscopy may be performed to locate or rule out H-type TEF.

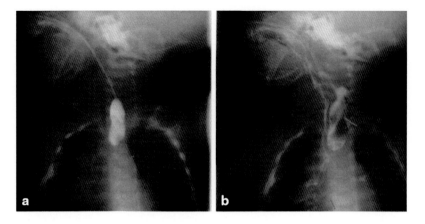

Fig. 14.4 Upper pouch esophagogram showing esophageal atresia (**a**). Note the spillage of contrast into the tracheobronchial tree (**b**)

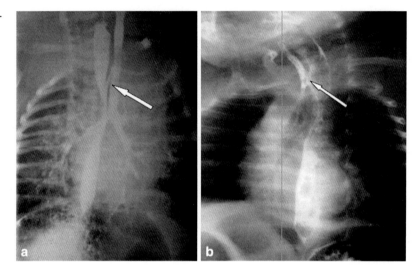

Fig. 14.5 a and **b** Esophagogram showing H-type tracheoesophageal fistula (*arrows*)

Associated Anomalies

- Associated anomalies are frequent with EA, occurring in more than 50% of patients (Table 14.1).
- Most infants have more than one malformation. Infants with isolated EA have a higher incidence of other malformations than EA with TEF while the associated anomalies are less often in those with pure H-type TEF.
- Congenital heart malformations such as ventricular septal defect, patent ductus arteriosus, or tetralogy of Fallot are the commonest seen in 30% of patients.
- In general, about 5% of infants with EA have a right-sided aortic arch and if this is detected preoperatively, a left thoracotomy is advocated to achieve repair.
- A preoperative echocardiogram is valuable in this regard.
- Gastrointestinal anomalies, including imperforate anus, duodenal atresia, and malrotation, occur in approximately 15% of infants with EA (Fig. 14.6).
- Musculoskeletal defects are common and include vertebral abnormalities and defects of the ribs and extremities.

Table 14.1 Associated anomalies in esophageal atresia

System	Potential anomalies	%
Cardiovascular	Ventricular septal defect, patent ductus arteriosus, Fallot tetralogy, right-sided aortic arch, atrial septal defect, coarctation of the aorta	30–35
Musculoskeletal	Multiple or single hemi vertebrae, scoliosis, rib deformities, radial dysplasia, absent radius, radial-ray deformities, syndactyly, polydactyly, lower-limb tibial deformities	10–15
Gastrointestinal	Imperforate anus, duodenal atresia, malrotation, intestinal malformations, Meckel's diverticulum, annular pancreas	14–20
Genitourinary	Renal agenesis or dysplasia, horseshoe kidney, polycystic kidney, ureteral and urethral malformations, hypospadias, undescended testicles	14–20
Chromosomal abnormalities	*Trisomies 13, 21, or 18*	4–5
Multiple	*VATER/VACTERL*	10

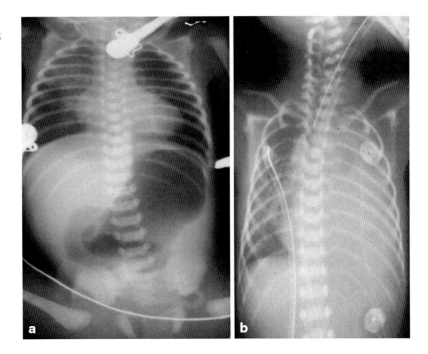

Fig. 14.6 Chest and abdominal x-ray showing EA/TEF associated with jejunal atresia in one and left congenital diaphragmatic hernia in the other

- Urinary tract malformations, such as hypospadias, horseshoe kidney, and renal agenesis, can also occur.
- Approximately 10% of patients with EA have an abnormality of the urinary tract or the musculoskeletal system.
- The acronym VATER (vertebral defects, anorectal malformations, tracheoesophageal fistula, renal anomalies, renal dysplasia) or VACTERL (vertebral defect, anorectal malformation, cardiac defect, tracheoesophageal fistula, renal anomaly, radial dysplasia, and limb defects) has been used to describe the condition of multiple anomalies in these infants. Up to 10% of infants with EA have the VATER syndrome (Fig. 14.7).
- Several chromosomal abnormalities are associated with EA/TEF. Among these, trisomy 18 and 21 are the commonest (Fig. 14.8).

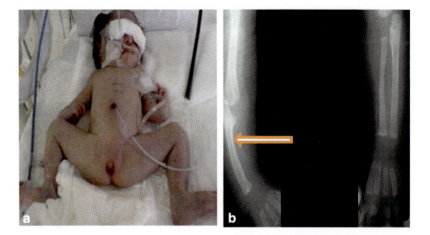

Fig. 14.7 Clinical photograph (**a**) and upper arms x-rays (**b**) showing radial agenesis in patient with VATER association

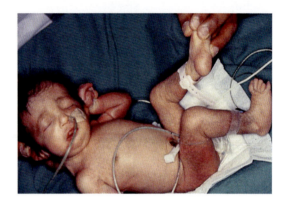

Fig. 14.8 Clinical photograph showing a patient with esophageal atresia and Edward's syndrome (Trisomy 18)

Treatment

- EA is not a surgical emergency and repair of the esophagus should be done as soon as the baby is stabilized.
- Those with a large TEF need to be treated more urgently as the fistula may compromise their ventilation or the stomach may markedly distend and perforate (Fig. 14.9).
- As a rule, a child's own esophagus is better than any substitution and every attempt should be made to preserve it.
- In the majority of cases of EA with TEF, joining the two ends of the esophagus is straightforward.
- This is usually done through a right thoracotomy and via an extrapleural approach.
- In general, patients with EA and a distal TEF have adequate esophageal length to allow primary reconstruction.
- Surgery involves division of the fistula after ligating its tracheal end, stretching the two ends of the esophagus and primary single layer end-to-end anastomosis.
- There may be mild to moderate tension at the site of anastomosis. The anastomosis is done over a nasogastric tube which is passed into the stomach and can be used to decompress the stomach or for early postoperative feeding.
- An extrapleural chest tube is left after surgery to allow for drainage of secretions if a leak occurs at the surgical site. This can be removed early if there is no drainage but most surgeons will remove it after doing a postoperative contrast study which is usually done on the sixth or seventh postoperative day.

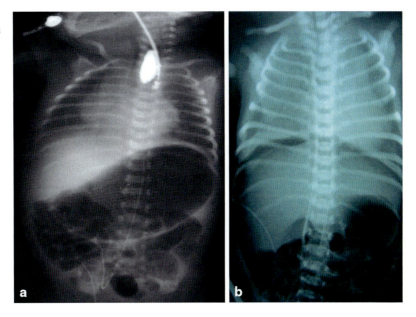

Fig. 14.9 Contrast study showing esophageal atresia in a patient with large distal tracheoesophageal fistula. Note the markedly dilated stomach on the *left* (**a**) and pneumoperitoneum as a result of gastric perforation on the *right* (**b**)

- In some infants, however, the esophageal ends are so far apart (long gap) they cannot be easily connected.
- Long gap EA is usually defined as a gap length exceeding 4 cm, a gap greater than two vertebral bodies, or an upper pouch level above the thoracic inlet.
- To solve this, a variety of techniques were adopted. These include delayed repair (waiting for the esophageal ends to grow closer) or esophageal lengthening procedures such as the Kimura, Livaditis, Scharli, or Foker techniques.
- The Foker technique involves two thoracotomies. First, anchoring sutures are placed securely at the two ends of the atretic esophagus and are brought out diagonally to the chest wall. Over a period of days to weeks, the two ends are brought closer together by a series of daily lengthening by traction on the exposed sutures. The closure of the gap is monitored radiologically with radio-opaque markers at the atretic ends. A second thoracotomy is then performed to achieve a tension-free anastomosis.
- Rarely, primary gastric pull up or subsequent esophageal replacement procedure (gastric, jejunal, colonic) is necessary following primary esophagostomy and gastrostomy in the neonatal period. These procedures are associated with a higher prevalence of long-term respiratory complications and substitution-related complications (Figs. 14.10 and 14.11).
- With the recent advances in minimal invasive surgery, pediatric surgeons are gaining experience in repairing EA using minimal invasive thoracoscopic approach. This approach should be undertaken only by those who have extensive experience in pediatric thoracoscopic surgery.

Prognosis and Outcome

- Over the past 50 years, refinements in neonatal surgical technique, preoperative support, anesthesia, and neonatal intensive care have improved the outcome. It is also recognized that prompt diagnosis with appropriate clinical management and expeditious referral to a tertiary care center has had a dramatic impact on the improved survival of these infants.
- Estimates today suggest that, in the absence of other severe anomalies, survival rates in these infants approach 100%.

Fig. 14.10 Upper contrast study in a patient post gastric replacement for esophageal atresia

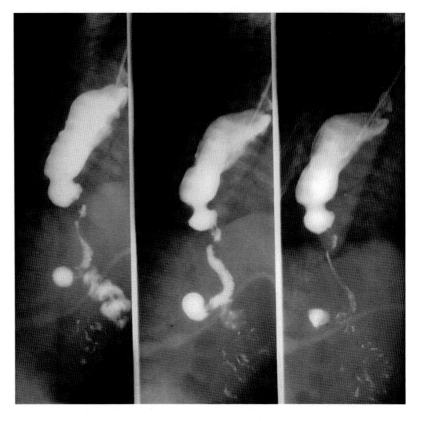

Fig. 14.11 Upper contrast study showing colonic replacement in a patient with esophageal atresia

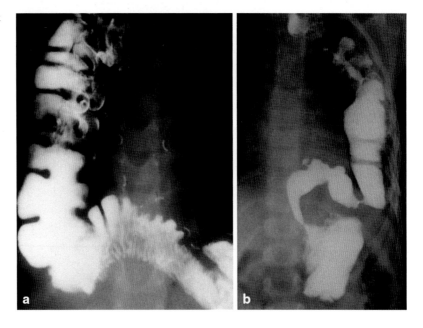

Prognosis and Outcome

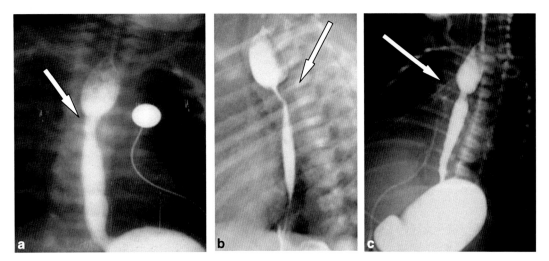

Fig. 14.12 Upper contrast study in a patient post EA/TEF repair. **a**, Note the slight narrowing at the site of anastomosis which is normal and upper contrast study in two patients (**b, c**) with esophageal stricture following repair of EA/TEF

Fig. 14.13 Upper contrast study showing anastomotic leak in a patient post repair of EA/TEF

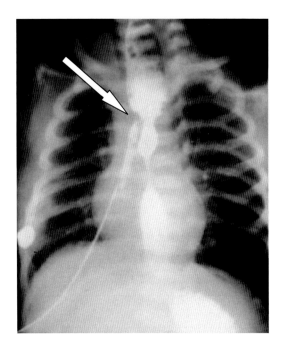

- Current overall survival rates are generally in the 85–90 % range.
- Mortality is usually secondary to associated severe anomalies.
- Postoperatively, these patients are liable to develop early and late complications.
- Early complications include:
  - Anastomotic leak seen in 10–20 %
  - Recurrent TEF in 3–10 %
  - Esophageal stricture seen in 15–40 % depending on the definition of stricture (Figs. 14.12 and 14.13

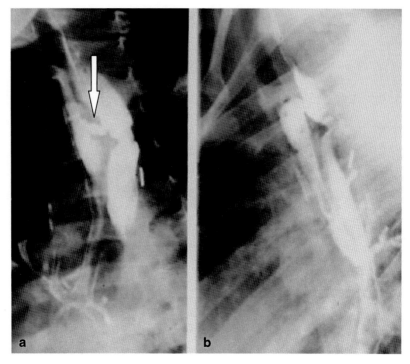

Fig. 14.14 a and b Upper contrast study showing recurrent tracheoesophageal fistula (*arrow* in **a**)

Esophageal stricture is a common complication of esophageal atresia repair seen in up to 50 % of patients.

- Several factors contribute to its development. These include:
  - Anastomosis techniques and suture materials
  - Repair under tension
  - Ischemia at the anastomosis
  - Leakage of anastomosis
  - Gastroesophageal reflux
- Repeated dilatations are necessary in nearly 40 % of patients who develop esophageal stricture.
- Patients who do not respond to the dilatation program or have long length of the stricture and in those complicated by gastroesophageal reflux, surgical intervention may be necessary. In case of gastroesophageal reflux, fundoplication may also be required.
- Anastomotic leak is an uncommon early complication following the repair of EA/TEF occurring in 10–20 % of patients. However, it has potentially significant long-term consequences.
- Major disruption is rare and is usually manifest by an early pneumothorax and salivary drainage from the chest drain.
- The majority of leaks are small and resolve spontaneously with or without pleural drainage. While 95 % resolve spontaneously or with pleural drainage, esophageal stricture follow in 50 % of cases. They can also be followed by a recurrence of the TEF (Fig. 14.14).
- Late complications include:
  - Gastroesophageal reflux occurring in up to 35–58 % of children
  - Esophageal motility dysfunction seen in more than 75 % of patients
  - Tracheomalacia which is clinically significant in 10–20 % of patients (Fig. 14.15)
- In 1962, Waterston proposed a prognostic classification system for patients with EA/TEF.
- Category A includes patients who weigh >5.5 lb (2.5 kg) at birth and who are otherwise well.

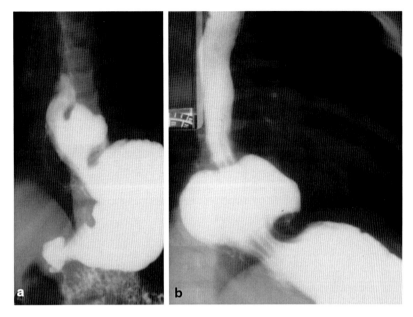

Fig. 14.15 Upper contrast study showing gastro-esophageal reflux (**a**) and hiatal hernia (**b**) in a patient following repair of EA/TEF

- Category B includes patients who weigh 4–5.5 lb (1.8–2.5 kg) and are well or who have higher birth weights, moderate pneumonia, and congenital anomalies.
- Category C includes patients who weigh < 4 lb (1.8 kg) or have higher birth weights, severe pneumonia, and severe congenital anomalies.
- This classification is no longer used.
- In 1994, Spitz et al. recognized that the presence or absence of cardiac anomalies is a proven major prognostic factor and suggested the following classification system:

    - Group I: Birth weight > 1.5 kg and no major cardiac disease.
    - Group II: Birth weight < 1.5 kg or major cardiac disease.
    - Group III: Birth weight < 1.5 kg and major cardiac disease.

- The overall survival in each of these classifications is as follows:
- Spitz classification:

    - Group I: Mortality rate of 3 %
    - Group II: Mortality rate of 41 %
    - Group III: Mortality rate of 78 %

- Waterston classification:

    - Category A: Mortality rate of 0 %
    - Category B: Mortality rate of 4 %
    - Category C: Mortality rate of 11 %

Recommended Reading

Foker JE, Krosch TCK, Catton K, Munro F, Khan KM. Long-gap esophageal atresia treated by growth induction: the biological potential and early follow-up results. Semin Pediatr Surg. 2009;18:23–9.
Spitz L. Esophageal atresia. Lessons I have learned in a 40-year experience. J Pediatr Surg. 2006;41(10):1635–40.
Spitz L, Ruangtrakoo R. Esophageal substitution. Semin Pediatr Surg. 1998;7:130–3.

Chapter 15
H-type Tracheoesophageal Fistula

Introduction

- Esophageal atresia (EA) with or without tracheoesophageal fistula (TEF) is a relatively common congenital malformation with an estimated incidence of about one per 3000–4000 live births.
- Several anatomical variants have been described. The most common type is EA with distal TEF, comprising 75% of cases.
- H-type TEF fistula on the other hand is rare comprising 2–4% of all cases of EA with or without TEF.
- The rarity of H-type TEF as well as the nonspecific clinical presentation which can mimic other respiratory illnesses are contributing factors for delayed diagnosis.
- It is well known that EA with distal TEF is associated with a high incidence of associated anomalies. H-type TEF on the other hand is rarely associated with other congenital anomalies. There is however an association between H-type TEF and anorectal malformations.

Etiology

- H-type TEF is a rare condition and the majority of cases reported in the literature are congenital.
- There are however case reports of acquired TEF fistula secondary to:
  - Ingestion of a caustic substance
  - Esophageal foreign body
  - Disc battery
  - A high intracuff pressure of an endotracheal tube

Presentation and Diagnosis

- In 1873, Lamb described the first case of congenital H-type TEF, a condition that continues to be missed and the diagnosis is often delayed.
- One reason for this is the presentation of H-type TEF which is variable and nonspecific.

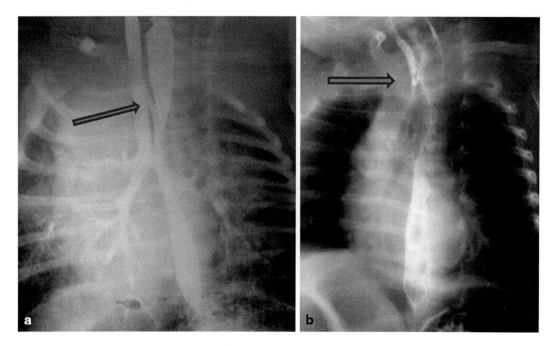

Fig. 15.1 Barium swallow showing an N-type rather than H-type TEF in (**a**) and an H-type TEF in (**b**)

- Commonly, these patients present with recurrent chest infection, cyanosis, and choking during feeds.
- To obviate delay in diagnosis, a high index of suspicion is important in this regard.
- Any newborn, infant, or child who presents with the following should raise suspicion of congenital H-type TEF and must be investigated accordingly:
  - Repeated attacks of choking and coughing during feeding
  - Abdominal distension
  - Recurrent attacks of chest infection
    Should raise suspicion of congenital H-type TEF and must be investigated accordingly.
- In many of these patients, the diagnosis is difficult and occasionally delayed until late childhood or even up to adulthood.
- Several investigative techniques have been used to diagnose H-type TEF including:
  - Upper gastrointestinal contrast studies
  - Bronchoscopy
  - Computed tomography (CT) scan
  - Measurement of intragastric oxygen tension
- The diagnosis may however necessitate several upper gastrointestinal studies.
- One reason for this is the way the fistula connects to the trachea which may be in the form of an N rather than an H (Fig. 15.1). This makes the flow of contrast from the esophagus into the trachea difficult as the tracheal connection is higher than the esophageal connection.

Treatment

- Definitive preoperative diagnosis of H-type TEF is important and, once this is made, localization of the level of the fistula becomes a priority for the proper choice of operative approach.
- This can be ascertained from the contrast study or via a preoperative bronchoscopy.
- To treat H-type TEF, a variety of techniques have been used including:
  - An open approach
  - Thoracoscopic approach
  - Endoscopic closure
- The treatment of H-type TEF is traditionally through an open approach via a cervical or thoracic incision.
- Although a low H-type TEF should be repaired by a transthoracic approach, the majority of cases, however, can be repaired via a transcervical approach which is less invasive than a thoracotomy and has a low morbidity and mortality.
- Add to this the fact that the transthoracic approach may not be an adequate approach for all the cases.
- The transcervical approach is however not without complications. One of the serious complications is damage to the recurrent laryngeal nerve. This must be borne in mind at the time of surgery and postoperatively, as these patients may develop postoperative strider.
- To facilitate ligation and division of TEF, intraoperative localization is important.
- Bronchoscopic cannulation of the fistula with a Fogarty or ureteric catheter has been recommended to aid ready identification at the time of surgery, but this is not always successful.
- Transillumination of the H-type TEF via a flexible miniature bronchoscopy for operative localization was also used.
- With the recent advances in minimal invasive surgery, thoracoscopic repair of H-type TEF has been reported to be feasible and safe for low fistulas.
- Endoscopic closure of fistulae has been reported with various techniques such as:
  - Tissue adhesives
  - Electrocautery
  - Sclerosants
  - Laser
  - The use of flexible ball electocautery and injection of histoacryle glue either on their own or in combination.

Recommended Reading

Brookes JT, Smith MC, Smith RJ, Bauman NM, Manaligod JM, Sandler AD. H-type congenital tracheoesophageal fistula: University of Iowa experience 1985 to 2005. Ann Otol Rhinol Laryngol. 2007;116(5):363–8.
Sundar B, Guiney EJ, O'Donnell B. Congenital H-type tracheoesophageal fistula. Arch Dis Child. 1975;50(11):862–3.
Yazbeck S, Dubuc M. Congenital tracheoesophageal fistula without esophageal atresia. Can J Surg. 1983;26(93):239–41.

Chapter 16
Congenital Esophageal Stenosis

Introduction

- Congenital esophageal stenosis (CES) is a rare clinical entity that is often associated with other congenital anomalies, namely esophageal atresia with or without tracheoesophageal fistula.
- It is an interesting clinical entity because of its diverse clinical manifestation and complex treatment.
- In those patients undergoing repair of TEF/EA soon after birth, and due to the strong association with CES, close attention should be paid to the postoperative course which can reveal this.

Incidence

- The incidence of CES is estimated at 1:25,000 to 50,000 live births.
- The incidence of other congenital anomalies associated with CES ranges from 17 to 33 %. These include:
    - Esophageal atresia with or without tracheoesophageal fistula
    - H-type tracheoesophageal fistula
    - Cardiac anomalies
    - Intestinal atresias
    - Malrotation
    - Anorectal malformations
    - Hypospadias
    - Chromosomal anomalies

Classification

CES is divided into three different types based on pathological findings:

1. Congenital fibromuscular hyperplasia:
    - CES due to fibromuscular hyperplasia commonly affect the middle third of the esophagus.

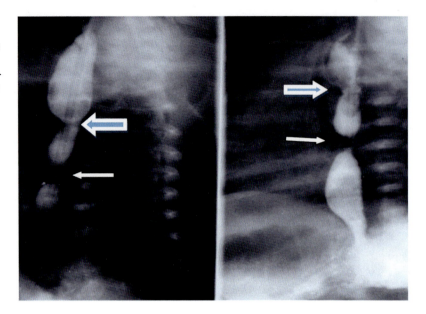

Fig. 16.1 Congenital esophageal stenosis (*left arrows*) in a postoperative patient with esophageal atresia and tracheoesophageal fistula (*right arrows*)

2. Congenital membranous web:
   - Congenital esophageal web or diaphragm is the rarest of the three forms of CES and may be analogous to membranes in other parts of gastrointestinal tract (GIT).
   - It is commonly located in the middle or lower third of esophagus.
3. Congenital tracheobronchial remnants:
   - CES due to tracheobronchial remnants commonly involves the lower third of the esophagus.

Clinical Features

- The symptoms of CES include dysphagia, excess salivation, regurgitation, aspiration episodes, and failure to thrive.
- The majority of patients with CES are detected at the time of introduction of solid food at the age of 4 months onwards.
- It is not uncommon for these patients to present with food impaction or foreign body impaction at the site of stenosis.

Diagnosis

- The main diagnostic investigations are esophagogram and esophagoscopy (Figs. 16.1 and 16.2).
- It is important to rule out other diagnosis like achalasia and stricture secondary to gastroesophageal reflux
- Esophageal pH monitoring is valuable in this regard.

Fig. 16.2 Congenital esophageal stenosis affecting the middle third of the esophagus (*arrows*)

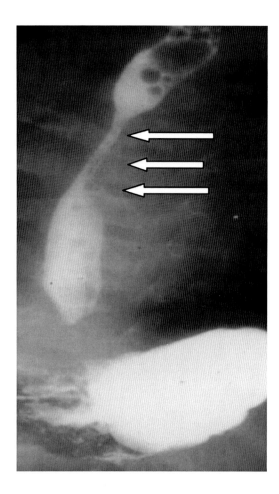

- Investigations such as pH monitoring, manometry, and endoscopic biopsy are performed to rule out other conditions mimicking CES such as acquired esophageal stenosis and achalasia. It is not uncommon for achalasia to be confused with CES.
- Radiologically, it is difficult to differentiate between the three types but membranous (web) obstruction is more localized affecting a much shorter segment, but in the presence of severe proximal dilatation this may be difficult to demonstrate.
- The diagnosis of the different types of CES is based on histological findings. This however is not the case for those with CES secondary to fibromuscular hyperplasia where the diagnosis is made by exclusion. The majority of patients with fibromuscular hyperplasia respond to dilatation, and very rarely surgical resection is necessary.

Treatment

- CES is managed with forceful dilatation using bougienage or hydrostatic balloon dilatation (Fig. 16.3).
- Resection with anastomosis is reserved for those with intractable (fibromuscular hyperplasia) cases and those harboring tracheobronchial rests.

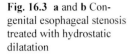

Fig. 16.3 a and b Congenital esophageal stenosis treated with hydrostatic dilatation

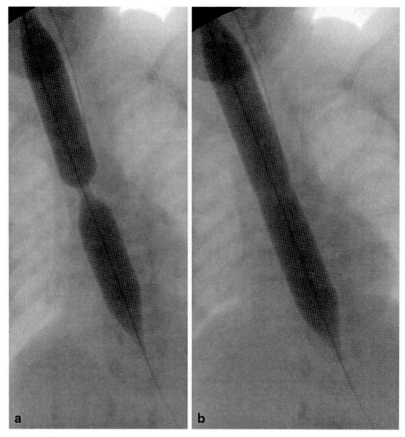

- Successful endoscopic excision using laser or electrocautery of congenital esophageal webs has been reported.
- Most intractable cases are due to the presence of tracheobronchial rest. These are treated with resection and end-to-end anastomosis.

Recommended Reading

Nihoul-Fekete C, De Backer A, Lortat-Jacob S, et al. Congenital esophageal stenosis. Pediatr Surg Int. 1987;2:89–92.
Yeung CK, Spitz L, Brereton RJ, et al. Congenital esophageal stenosis due to tracheo-bronchial remnants: a rare but important association with esophageal atresia. J Pediatr Surg. 1992;27:852.

Chapter 17
Achalasia

Introduction

- Achalasia is a relatively rare disease of the esophagus.
- The term achalasia means "failure to relax" and achalasia is characterized by inability of the lower esophageal sphincter to relax and ineffective peristalsis, resulting in functional obstruction of the esophagus.
- As a result, patients with achalasia have difficulty in swallowing both solid and liquid food.

Incidence

- The exact incidence of achalasia is unknown.
- An incidence of 0.5–1.0 per 100,000 population per year has been reported.

Etiology

- Achalasia is an esophageal motility disorder.
- The exact etiology of achalasia is unknown.

Clinical Features

- The most common symptom of achalasia is difficulty in swallowing (dysphagia).
- The dysphagia is for both liquid and solid foods and often the patients describe feeling that food "gets stuck" in the chest after it is swallowed.
- In achalasia, dysphagia occurs with both solid and liquid food, whereas in esophageal stricture, the dysphagia typically occurs only with solid food and not liquids, until very late in the progression of the obstruction.
- Food regurgitation (or vomiting) of usually undigested food.
- Heartburn and difficulty belching are common.
- Symptoms usually get steadily worse.
- Nighttime cough.
- Weight loss.
- Recurrent aspiration pneumonia.

Fig. 17.1 Barium swallow and meal showing the classic narrowing of the lower esophagus (bird's beak sign)

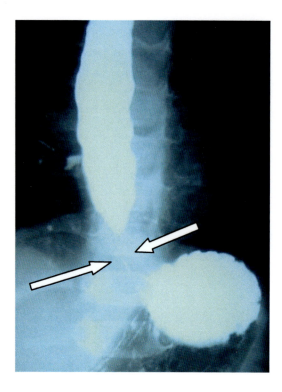

Diagnosis

- Chest X-ray: The dilated esophagus may be seen on chest X-ray as an air-filled tube or sometimes as an air fluid level.
- The diagnosis of achalasia is suggested by contrast esophagram and confirmed by esophageal manometry.
- Esophageal manometry usually shows repetitive contraction waves, a high-pressure lower esophageal sphincter (LES) with incomplete LES relaxation upon swallowing.
- The esophagus is dilated, widened with a characteristic tapered narrowing of the lower end, sometimes likened to a "bird's beak" (Figs. 17.1 and 17.2).
- Endoscopy is helpful in the diagnosis of achalasia although it can be normal in early stages of achalasia. Often, there is inflammation of the esophagus, which is caused by the irritating effect of food and fluids that collect in the esophagus.

Treatment

Achalasia is still not a curable disease and the goals of therapy are:

- To relieve symptoms
- To improve esophageal emptying
- To prevent the development of megaesophagus

The following treatment options are available:

1. Pharmacologic treatment:

Treatment

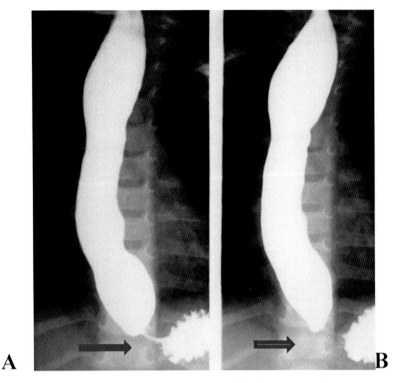

Fig. 17.2 Barium swallow showing bird's beak sign. Note also the dilated tortuous esophagus

- A group of oral medications that help to relax the lower esophageal sphincter has been used to treat achalasia.
- This includes drugs like nitrates (isosorbide dinitrate, Isordil) and calcium channel blockers (nifedipine, Procardia; verapamil, Calan; sildenafil, Viagra).
- Although some patients with achalasia, particularly early in the disease, have improvement of symptoms with medications, most do not.
- By themselves, oral medications are likely to provide only short-term relief of symptoms and many patients experience side effects (nausea, headache, low blood pressure). These are rarely used in children.
- Because of this, the use of pharmacologic treatment is rather limited to the beginning of the disease and for patients who did not respond to interventional or surgical treatment.

2. Pneumatic balloon dilatation of the lower esophageal sphincter:

   - The advantage of this is that no operation is needed as this can be done during endoscopy (Fig. 17.3).
   - However, there is a 5% risk of esophageal perforation leading to mediastinitis.
   - Moreover, one dilatation is usually not enough and there is the need for further dilatations, which can be a disadvantage for later surgical treatment.
   - The success of forceful dilation has been reported to be between 60 and 90% (mean overall success rate is 78%).

3. Injection of botulinum toxin in the sphincter muscle:

   - Botulinum toxin, a substance that leads to relaxation of the sphincter muscle.

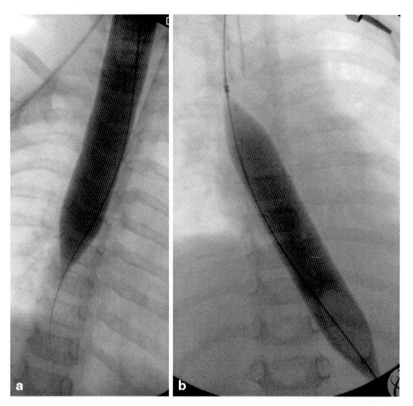

Fig. 17.3 a and b Pneumatic balloon dilatation of achalasia

- The responder rate (65–100%) is initially good. However, long-term results are rather disappointing.
- Injection is quick, nonsurgical, and requires no hospitalization.
- Treatment with botulinum toxin is safe, but the effects on the sphincter often last only for months, and additional injections with botulinum toxin may be necessary.
- Injection is a good option for patients who are very elderly or are at high risk for surgery.
- Injection of botulinum toxin is not used in the pediatric age group.

4. Operative treatment (Heller's myotomy):

- Esophagomyotomy was first described in 1903 by Heller and since then has been used as the standard procedure to treat achalasia.
- The surgery can be done using:
  - An open technique (traditionally, surgery was accomplished via a transthoracic or transabdominal approach)
  - A more preferable approach is the laparoscopic approach (Fig. 17.4)
- The myotomy is begun approximately 3 cm below the gastroesophageal junction (GEJ) and extended superiorly into the dilated esophagus for about 6–8 cm above the GEJ.
- In general, the laparoscopic approach is used with uncomplicated achalasia.
- Esophagomyotomy is more successful than forceful balloon dilation, probably because the pressure in the lower sphincter is reduced to a greater extent and more reliably.
- Eighty to ninety percent of patients have good results.
- With prolonged follow-up, however, some patients develop recurrent dysphagia. Thus, esophagomyotomy does not guarantee a permanent cure.

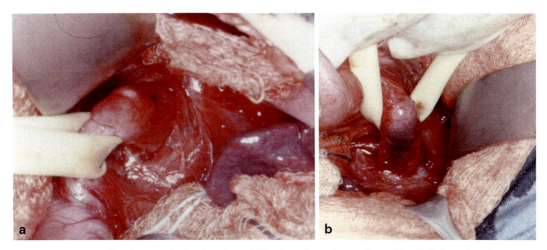

Fig. 17.4 Intraoperative photograph showing the mobilized esophagus in a patient with achalasia and Heller's myotomy (**a**). Note the bulging mucosa after dividing the muscles (**b**)

- The most important side effect with esophagomyotomy is gastroesophageal reflux.
- In order to prevent this, anti-reflux surgery (fundoplication) is performed with the Heller's myotomy.
- Laparoscopic myotomy, usually combined with a partial fundoplication, has an overall success rate of 87%.

Recommended Reading

Lee CW, Kays DW, Chen MK, Islam S. Outcomes of treatment of childhood achalasia. J Pediatr Surg. 2010;45(6):1173–7.

Tannuri AC, Tannuri U, Velhote MC, Romão RL. Laparoscopic extended cardiomyotomy in children: an effective procedure for the treatment of esophageal achalasia. J Pediatr Surg. 2010;45(7):1463–6.

Chapter 18
Infantile Hypertrophic Pyloric Stenosis

Introduction

- Infantile pyloric stenosis is a relatively common condition that causes severe projectile non-bilious vomiting in the first few weeks of life.
- It results from hypertrophy of the muscles surrounding the pylorus leading to its narrowing and gastric outlet obstruction.

Epidemiology and Etiology

- Infantile pyloric stenosis occurs in the first 3–6 weeks of life.
- Infantile pyloric stenosis has also been reported in the first few days of life and in utero.
- Males are more commonly affected than females, with firstborn males affected about four times as often.
- It is commonly associated with people of Jewish ancestry.
- Pyloric stenosis is more common in Caucasians than Hispanics, Blacks, or Asians.
- The incidence of infantile hypertrophic pyloric stenosis is variable. It is:
    - 2.4 per 1000 live births in Caucasians.
    - 1.8 per 1000 live births in Hispanics.
    - 0.7 per 1000 live births in Blacks.
    - 0.6 per 1000 live births in Asians.
    - Less common among children of mixed race parents.
    - Caucasian babies with blood type B or O are more likely than other types to be affected.
- The exact cause is not known.
- It appears to be inherited in a multifactorial manner.
- Infantile hypertrophic pyloric stenosis has been reported in twins and several members of the same family suggesting genetic predisposition or familial component.
- There is a fivefold increase in the risk of developing infantile hypertrophic pyloric stenosis in first-degree relatives if one member of the family is affected.
- Nitric oxide is an essential chemical transmitter responsible for relaxation of the pyloric sphincter muscles. Studies have shown deficiency in nitric oxide synthase in the myenteric plexus in patients with infantile hypertrophic pyloric stenosis.

Fig. 18.1 Pathophysiology of infantile hypertrophic pyloric stenosis

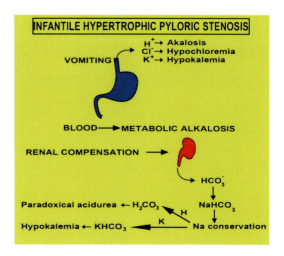

Pathophysiology

- There is hypertrophy and hyperplasia of the two (circular and longitudinal) muscular layers of the pylorus.
- This leads to narrowing of the pyloric canal and gastric outlet obstruction.
- The pyloric canal becomes lengthened, and the whole pylorus becomes thickened. The mucosa is usually edematous and thickened.
- Infantile pyloric stenosis is characterized by persistent, non-bilious projectile vomiting due to gastric outlet obstruction.
- This results in loss of gastric acid with subsequent hypochloremia (chloride loss) and metabolic alkalosis (acid loss).
- Prolonged vomiting leads to loss of large quantities of gastric secretions rich in hydrogen and chloride. As a result of dehydration, the kidneys attempt to conserve Na^+ to maintain volume by exchanging Na^+ for K^+ and hydrogen secreted as $KHCO_3$ and H_2CO_3 (paradoxical aciduria). There is a metabolic alkalosis, but instead of having an alkalotic urine, it is acidic (Fig. 18.1).

Signs and Symptoms

- There is progressively projectile and non-bile-stained vomiting. The child remains hungry and takes food immediately after vomiting.
- Poor weight gain and malnutrition (Fig. 18.2).
- Ninety-five percent have a palpable pyloric mass (olive sign) which is felt in the right upper abdomen, especially after vomiting and during a test feed.
- May be dehydrated.
- Visible peristalsis in the epigastrium travelling from left to right (Fig. 18.3).
- Indirect hyperbilirubinemia may be seen in 1–2 % of affected infants.

Treatment

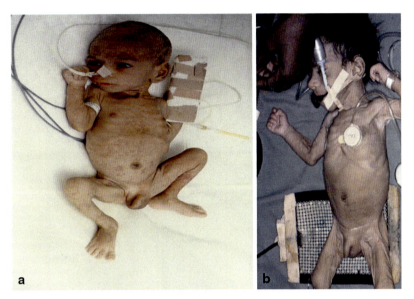

Fig. 18.2 a and **b** Clinical photograph of patients with infantile hypertrophic pyloric stenosis with poor weight gain, malnutrition, dehydration, and epigastric fullness

Diagnosis

- Diagnosis is via a careful history and physical examination, often supplemented by radiographic studies.
- Abdominal radiographs are not necessary and may show a fluid-filled or air-distended stomach, suggesting the presence of gastric outlet obstruction. A markedly dilated stomach with exaggerated incisura (caterpillar sign) may be seen (Figs. 18.3 and 18.4).
- Current imaging techniques, particularly ultrasonography, are noninvasive and accurate for identification of infantile hypertrophic pyloric stenosis. Ultrasonography is the method of choice for the diagnosis of hypertrophic pyloric stenosis, because it has a sensitivity and specificity of almost 100 %.
- Ultrasonography confirms hypertrophic pyloric stenosis when the pyloric muscle thickness is >4 mm and the pyloric channel length is >15 mm.
- An upper gastrointestinal (GI) series is also not necessary and should be done only in doubtful cases when other imaging tests are inconclusive or when the infant presents with atypical clinical features. It is diagnostic when showing the narrowed pyloric canal filled with a thin stream of contrast material, a "string sign" or the "railroad track sign" (Fig. 18.5).
- Blood tests will reveal hypokalemic, hypochloremic metabolic alkalosis.

Treatment

- The mortality and morbidity of infantile pyloric stenosis comes from the dehydration and electrolyte disturbance. Therefore, the infant must be initially stabilized by correcting the dehydration and hypochloremic alkalosis with IV fluids. This can usually be accomplished in about 24–48 h using ½ normal saline with K^+ supplements.
- Infantile pyloric stenosis is typically managed with surgery.

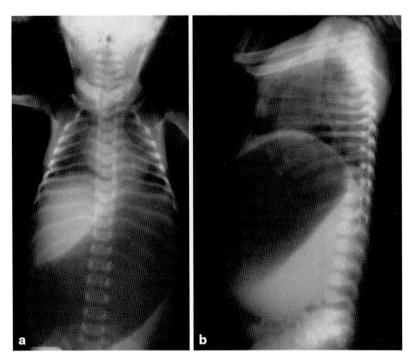

Fig. 18.3 a and **b** Abdominal X-ray showing markedly dilated stomach

- Intravenous and oral atropine has been used to treat pyloric stenosis; however, it requires prolonged hospitalization, skilled nursing, and careful follow-up during treatment. It might be an alternative to surgery in children who have contraindications for anesthesia or surgery.
- The Ramstedt pyloromyotomy remains the standard procedure for pyloric stenosis.
- Pyloromyotomy can be done by open procedure or laparoscopically depending on the surgeon's experience and preference. Care should be taken to avoid duodenal perforation during the procedure and, if this happens, the perforation should be closed and covered with an omental patch (Fig. 18.6).
- Traditionally, the pyloromyotomy is performed through a right upper quadrant transverse incision.
- Recent studies have compared the operative time, cost, and hospital stay associated with the traditional right upper quadrant transverse incision, a circumumbilical incision (believed to have better cosmesis), and a laparoscopic procedure. The laparoscopic pyloromyotomy has been found to be safe and effective, with shorter operative times and hospital stay.
- Feeding can be initiated 4–8 h after recovery from anesthesia. Infants who are fed earlier than 4 h do vomit more frequently and more severely, leading to significant discomfort for the patient and anxiety for the parents.
- As many as 80 % of patients continue to regurgitate after surgery; however, patients who continue to vomit 5 days after surgery may warrant further radiologic investigation.
- Patients should be observed for surgical complications:
  - Incomplete pyloromyotomy
  - Mucosal duodenal perforation
  - Bleeding
- The prognosis of infantile pyloric stenosis is very good, with complete recovery.

Treatment

Fig. 18.4 Erect abdominal X-ray showing dilated stomach with air fluid level in a patient with infantile hypertrophic pyloric stenosis. Note the scanty gas in the distal bowel

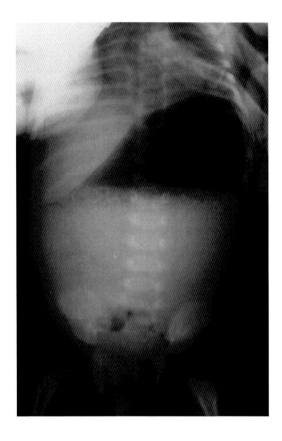

Fig. 18.5 Barium meal in a patient with infantile hypertrophic pyloric stenosis showing dilated stomach and pyloric stenosis. Note the string sign

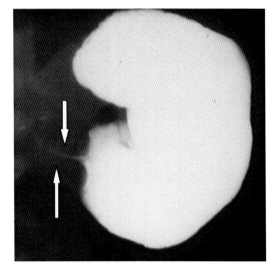

Fig. 18.6 Intraoperative photograph showing the pyloric tumor and the pyloromyotomy being performed

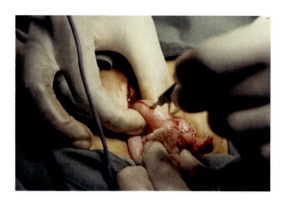

Recommended Reading

Kawahara H, Imura K, Nishikawa M, Yagi M, Kubota A. Intravenous atropine treatment in infantile hypertrophic pyloric stenosis. Arch Dis Child. 2002;87(1):71–4.

Ohshiro K, Puri P. Pathogenesis of infantile hypertrophic pyloric stenosis: recent progress. Pediatr Surg Int. 1998;13:243–52.

Rollins MD, Shields MD, Quinn RJ, Wooldridge MA. Pyloric stenosis: congenital or acquired? Arch Dis Child. 1989;64(1):138–9.

Spitz L. Vomiting after pyloromyotomy for infantile hypertrophic pyloric stenosis. Arch Dis Child. 1979;54(11):886–9.

Chapter 19
Congenital Gastric Outlet Obstruction (Pyloric and Antral Atresia and Web)

Introduction

- Congenital pyloric atresia (CPA) which was first described by Calder in 1749 is a very rare condition.
- Its incidence is approximately 1 in 100,000 newborns and constitutes about 1 % of all intestinal atresias.
- Its exact etiology is not known, but embryologically, it is thought to result from developmental arrest between the fifth and twelfth weeks of intrauterine life.
- CPA commonly occurs as an isolated lesion. This type generally has an excellent prognosis.
- It has however been reported in association with other anomalies which are common seen in 30–45 % of the cases including:
  - Epidermolysis bullosa (EB)
  - Aplasia cutis congenital (ACC)
  - Multiple hereditary intestinal atresias

Anatomy

The anomaly is present in either the pyloric or the antral region.

- Antral membranes (web or diaphragm):
  - Are thin, soft, and pliable, composed of mucosa/submucosa
  - Located eccentrically 1–3 cm proximal to the pyloroduodenal junction
  - Can present as a wind sock (Fig. 19.1)
- Rarely, there is an antral atresia with a gap (Fig. 19.2).
- Pyloric atresia is divided into three types:
  - Type 1: Pyloric atresia with a membrane (Fig. 19.3a)
  - Type 2: Pyloric atresia with a solid cord between the two ends (Fig. 19.3b)
  - Type 3: Pyloric atresia with a gap between the stomach and duodenum (Fig. 19.4)
- Type 1 is the commonest.

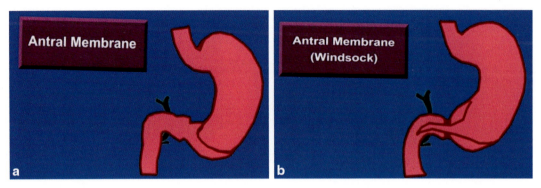

Fig. 19.1 Diagrammatic representation of antral membrane (**a**) and antral membrane forming a windsock (**b**)

Fig. 19.2 Diagrammatic representation of antral gap atresia

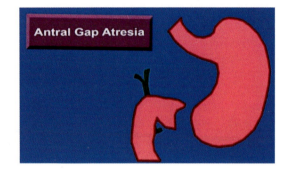

Associated Anomalies

- Epidermolysisbullosa (Fig. 19.5; the association of CPA with EB should not preclude surgical treatment).
- ACC.
- Hereditary multiple intestinal atresia (HMIA).
- CPA in association with HMIA is universally fatal as so far none of the reported cases survived.
- Recently, a combined immunodeficiency syndrome was reported in patients with HMIA.

Presentation

- Recurrent nonbilious vomiting in a newborn.
- Respiratory problems are common, and dyspnea, tachypnea, cyanosis, and excessive salivation may be the presenting findings that can be mistaken for esophageal atresia (Fig. 19.6).
- The presence of an abnormally dilated gastric bubble on prenatal sonogram should alert the physician toward the diagnosis of congenital gastric outlet obstruction.

Investigation

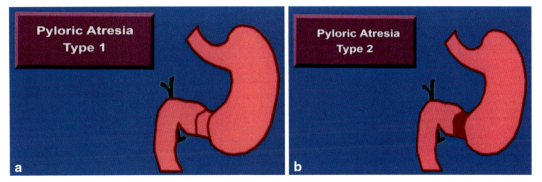

Fig. 19.3 a and **b** Diagrammatic representation of types 1 and 2 pyloric atresia

Fig. 19.4 Diagrammatic representation of type 3 pyloric atresia

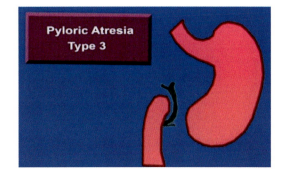

Clinical Examination

- The dilated stomach may be visible clinically. The lower abdomen remains scaphoid (Fig. 19.7).
- Look for associated anomalies. An associated esophageal atresia can be confirmed by failure to pass a nasogastric tube in to the stomach.

Investigation

- X-ray abdomen: Single large gastric air bubble with no distal gas (Fig. 19.8a). This can be confirmed further by a barium meal (Fig. 19.8b).
- If the air is noted distal to the stomach, a contrast study is required to look for incomplete membrane.
- The possibility of associated intestinal atresias must always be kept in mind and to exclude or locate associated colonic atresia, a preoperative barium enema is advocated.

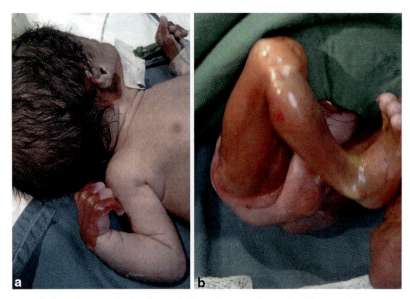

Fig. 19.5 a and **b** Clinical photograph showing aplasia cutis congenita and epidermolysisbullosa in a patient with congenital pyloric atresia

Fig. 19.6 Diagrammatic representation of a patient with congenital pyloric atresia, duplication cyst, and multiple intestinal atresia

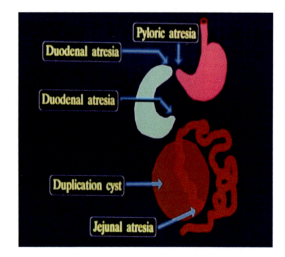

Management

The treatment of CPA is surgical as follows:

- Pyloric diaphragms and pyloric atresia without a gap are treated by excision and Heineke–Mikulicz pyloroplasty.
- For pyloric atresia with a gap, the treatment is pyloro-duodenostomy.
- Dessanti et al. described pyloric sphincter reconstruction for those with CPA without a gap.

Management 125

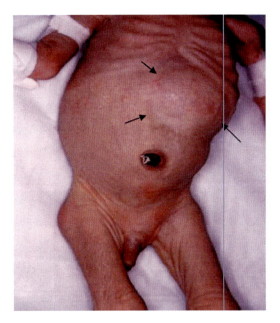

Fig. 19.7 Clinical photograph showing a visible dilated stomach in a patient with congenital pyloric atresia

- Gastrojejunostomy and gastrostomy should be avoided as they are associated with a high morbidity.
- An alternative where facilities are available is endoscopic balloon dilatation or resection of the web.
- Intraoperatively it is important to make sure that only one pyloric diaphragm is present as these can be multiple.
- It is also important to check for the patency of the remaining intestines using saline injection and exclude associated intestinal atresias which are often multiple.

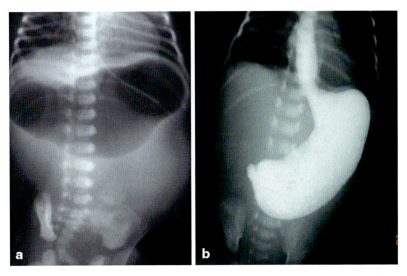

Fig. 19.8 Plain abdominal x-ray showing a large single air bubble with no gas distally in a patient with congenital pyloric atresia. This is confirmed with contrast study

Prognosis

- The prognosis of CPA is variable.
- Isolated CPA has an excellent prognosis.
- The overall mortality however is very high exceeding 50%.
- This is attributed to the high incidence of severe and often fatal associated anomalies.

Recommended Reading

Al-Salem A, Nawaz A, Matta H, Jacobsz A. Congenital pyloric atresia: the spectrum. Int Surg. 2002;87:147–51.

Dessanti A, Iannucelli M, Dore A, Meloni GB, Niolu P. Pyloric atresia: an attempt at anatomic pyloric sphincter reconstruction. J Pediatr Surg. 2000;35:1372–4.

Ilce Z, Erdogan E, Kara C, Celayir S, Sarimurat N, Senyüz OF, Yeker D. Pyloric atresia: 15-year review from a single institution. J Pediatr Surg. 2003;38:1581–4.

Sencan A, Mir E, Karace I, Günşar C, Sencan A, Topçu K. Pyloric atresia associated with multiple intestinal atresias and pylorocholedochal fistula. J Pediatr Surg. 2002;37:1223–4.

Chapter 20
Gastric Volvolus

Introduction

- Gastric volvolus is a rare clinical entity defined as an abnormal rotation of the stomach around one of its axis of >180°.
- The majority is seen in adults and 10–20% of cases occur in children usually before age 1 year.
- The classic triad associated with acute gastric volvolus was described by Borchardt in 1904 and includes:
  - Severe epigastric pain
  - Retching without vomiting
  - Inability to pass a nasogastric tube

Classification

- There are several classifications of gastric volvolus.
- The most frequently used classification of gastric volvolus was proposed by Singleton.
- This is based on the axis around which the stomach rotates and is classified as follows (Fig. 20.1):
- Organoaxial:
  - The stomach rotates around an axis that connects the gastroesophageal junction and the pylorus.
  - The antrum rotates in opposite direction to the fundus of the stomach.
  - This is the most common type of gastric volvolus (Fig. 20.2).
- Mesentericoaxial:
  - The stomach rotates around an axis that connects the lesser and greater curvatures. The antrum rotates anteriorly and superiorly so that the posterior surface of the stomach lies anteriorly (Fig. 20.3).
- Mixed (Combined):
  - This is a rare form in which the stomach twists mesentericoaxially and organoaxially.
  - Combined gastric volvulus is usually observed in patients with chronic volvulus.
  - The mixed variety is extremely rare and difficult to differentiate both radiologically and intraoperatively.

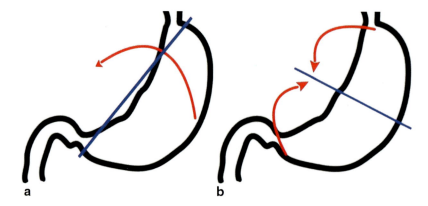

Fig. 20.1 Organoaxial (**a**) and mesentericoaxial (**b**) gastric volvolus. Note the axis of rotation marked by the *blue line*

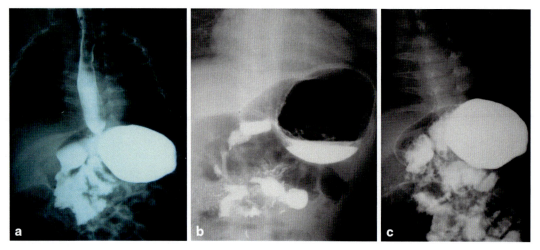

Fig. 20.2 Barium meal showing organo-axial gastric volvolus. Note the associated gastroesophageal reflux in (**a**) and the air fluid level in (**b**). Note the absence of gastroesophageal reflux in (**c**)

According to etiology, gastric volvolus is divided into two types:

- Type 1 (Idiopathic):
  - This type comprises two thirds of cases and is presumably due to abnormal laxity of the gastrosplenic, gastroduodenal, gastrophrenic, and gastrohepatic ligaments. These ligaments anchor the stomach and their laxity leads to volvolus of the stomach.
- Type 2 (Secondary or acquired):
  - This type is found in one third of patients and is usually associated with congenital or acquired abnormalities that result in abnormal mobility of the stomach. These include:
    ◦ Diaphragmatic defects
    ◦ Congenital asplenia
    ◦ Pyloric stenosis
    ◦ Colonic distension
    ◦ Abnormal attachments, adhesions, or bands

Fig. 20.3 Barium meal showing mesentericoaxial gastric volvolus

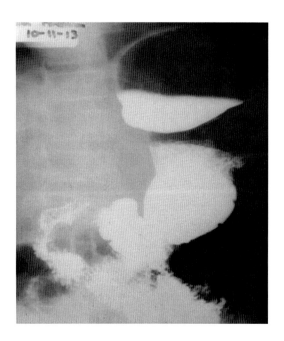

- Congenital paraesophageal hernia
- Neuromuscular disorders
- Congenital defects of the gastric ligaments

Gastric volvolus can be classified depending on the presentation into:

1. Acute gastric volvolus:
   - Acute gastric volvolus is extremely rare and life-threatening if not recognized and treated promptly.
   - The presenting symptoms depend on the degree of twisting and the rapidity of onset.
     - Acute gastric volvolus commonly manifests as sudden onset of severe epigastric or left upper quadrant pain.
     - Occasionally, some patients present with hematemesis secondary to mucosal ischemia. This can rapidly progress to hypovolemic shock from loss of blood and fluids.
     - The Borchardt triad (pain, retching, and inability to pass a nasogastric tube) is diagnostic of acute gastric volvolus but these are commonly seen in adults.

2. Chronic gastric volvolus:
   - Patients typically present with nonspecific symptoms including repeated attacks of vomiting, intermittent epigastric pain, and abdominal fullness following meals. Recurrent attacks of vomiting are the most common presenting symptom.
   - Patients may present with repeated attacks of chest infections.
   - Because of the nonspecific nature of the symptoms, the diagnosis is often delayed.
   - Upper gastrointestinal (GI) series can be diagnostic.
   - To obviate delay in diagnosis, chronic gastric volvolus must be kept in mind and should be included in the differential diagnosis of infants and children with:
     - Recurrent attacks of vomiting
     - Abdominal distension
     - Failure to thrive
     - Recurrent chest infection secondary to aspiration

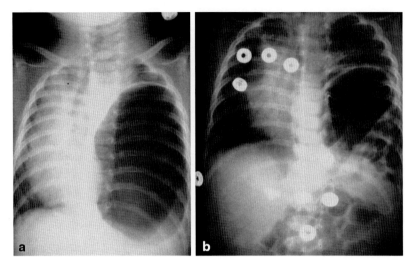

Fig. 20.4 Chest X-ray showing intrathoracic gastric volvolus in a patient with diaphragmatic hernia (**a**). Note the markedly dilated stomach as a result of the volvolus and decompression following insertion of a NG tube (**b**)

Gastric volvolus can also be classified depending on the site of the volvolus into:

1. Intra-abdominal gastric volvolus:
   - This is the commonest type.
2. Intrathoracic gastric volvolus:
   - This is extremely rare.
   - It is seen in infants and children with diaphragmatic hernia and intrathoracic stomach.
   - It may be associated with cardiopulmonary compromise from severe gastric distension.
   - Passing a nasogastric tube can be life-saving but care should be taken when placing the nasogastric tube, as aggressive placement may cause perforation; this is especially true in the pediatric age group (Figs. 20.4 and 20.5).

Treatment

- The treatment of gastric volvolus is variable depending on the type of the volvolus.
- Acute gastric volvolus requires an emergency surgery.
- Chronic gastric volvolus on the other hand should be treated conservatively unless the symptoms are severe.
- This consists of:
  - Keeping the patient in the prone position with slight head up rather than the usual supine position with head up.
  - Metachlopromide is given to enhance esophageal and gastric emptying.
  - H_2 blockers to prevent esophageal ulceration due to associated gastroesophageal reflux.
- The surgical treatment of chronic gastric volvolus is still controversial.
- Anterior gastropexy: There are those who advocate anterior gastropexy only. This alone, however, may aggravate the already existing gastroesophageal reflux.

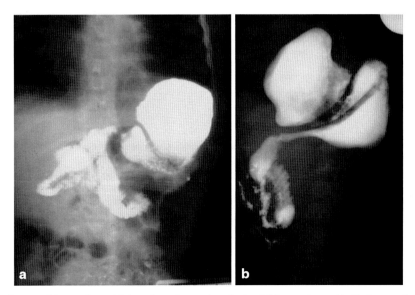

Fig. 20.5 Barium meal in a patient with intrathoracic gastric volvolus (**a**) in a patient with diaphragmatic hernia (**b**)

- Fundal gastropexy: Others perform only fundal gastropexy, while some advocate adding an antireflux procedure to overcome the associated gastroesophageal reflux.
- Combined anterior and fundal gastropexy: This is usually done without adding an antireflux procedure.
- The addition of fundal gastropexy not only fixes the stomach and eliminates volvolus but also helps in eliminating the associated gastroesophageal reflux by reforming the angle of His without performing a formal antireflux procedure.
- There have been increasing reports of the use of minimally invasive techniques for the treatment of gastric volvolus. These have the potential to decrease the morbidity associated with the open gastropexy

Recommended Reading

Al-Salem AH. Acute and chronic gastric volvulus in infants and children: who should be treated surgically? Pediatr Surg Int. 2007;23(11):1095–9.

Al-Salem AH. Congenital paraesophageal hernia with intrathoracic gastric volvolus in two sisters. ISRN Surg. 2011;1:856568. [Epub 2011 Apr 19].

Chapter 21
Congenital Duodenal Obstruction

Introduction

- Congenital duodenal atresia is a congenital bowel obstruction, usually affecting the second part of duodenum.
- The overall incidence is about one in 6000 births.
- Approximately one-third of patients with duodenal obstruction have trisomy 21 (Down's syndrome).
- The widely accepted theory regarding the embryogenesis of duodenal atresia is failure of recanalization of the solid part of the gastrointestinal (GI) tract.

Anatomy

- There are three types of congenital duodenal obstruction as outlined by Gray and Skandalakis (see chapter on intestinal atresia).
- Annular pancreas may cause extrinsic duodenal obstruction but more often underlying web, stenosis, or atresia is the cause of obstruction.
- Duodenal obstruction can also result from extrinsic causes such as Ladd's bands, duplication cyst, portal vein passing anterior to duodenum, etc.
- Congenital duodenal obstruction is also classified into:
    - Complete: caused by duodenal atresia or complete duodenal diaphragm
    - Incomplete (Partial): caused by duodenal stenosis, duodenal diaphragm with a central hole, or extrinsic causes.

Presentation

- Congenital duodenal obstruction is increasingly recognized antenatally by the classic double bubble appearance on ultrasound and associated maternal polyhydramnios (30–65 % of cases).
- Early onset of bilious vomiting and feeding intolerance (Fig. 21.1).
- Rarely, the vomiting is non-bilious if the obstruction is proximal to ampulla of Vater.
- Features of trisomy 21 (Down's syndrome).
- Milder degree of partial duodenal obstruction as in those with duodenal diaphragm with a hole or duodenal stenosis may be recognized late in infancy or childhood (Fig. 21.2).

Fig. 21.1 a and **b**, Bile-stained vomiting in a newborn with congenital duodenal obstruction

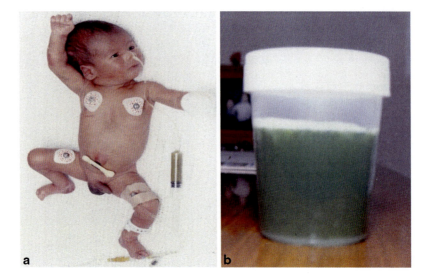

Examination

- Upper abdominal distension or scaphoid abdomen if the stomach is empty or the child is on nasogastric drainage.
- Bilious aspirate in the nasogastric tube.
- Look for evidence of Down's syndrome, dehydration, and associated cardiac malformation.

Associated Anomalies

- Trisomy 21 (Down's syndrome) → 28.2%
- Congenital heart disease → 22.6%
- Annular pancreas → 23.1%
- Intestinal malrotation → 19.7%
- Esophageal atresia/tracheoesophageal fistula → 8.5%

Diagnosis

- A plain abdominal X-ray showing double bubble is sufficient to confirm the diagnosis of complete duodenal obstruction (Fig. 21.3). Further contrast studies are not necessary.
- If the plain abdominal X-ray shows distal bowel gas, the diagnosis is less certain and needs a contrast study especially to rule out the presence of malrotation (refer to algorithm in chapter on intestinal obstruction; Fig. 21.4).
- The presence of a duodenal diaphragm with a central aperture is confirmed by the incomplete duodenal obstruction in absence of malrotation (Fig. 21.5).
- Small amount of distal gas in the presence of complete duodenal obstruction is explained by passage of air through ampulla of Vater, which bifurcates to open on either side of a duodenal web.

Fig. 21.2 Contrast study showing partial duodenal obstruction (duodenal diaphragm with a central hole). Note the thin contrast seen distally

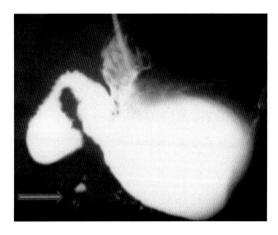

Preoperative Preparation

- Surgical correction of congenital duodenal obstruction is not an emergency and should be performed in a semi-elective manner in a stable child.
- Steps outlined in the general approach should be followed.
- A nasogastric tube placement rules out associated esophageal atresia seen in an occasional patient.
- It is important to place a peripherally inserted central catheter (PICC) at the outset as it is needed for parenteral nutrition in the postoperative period.
- Associated cardiac anomaly should be investigated.

Operative Management

- Open surgery or laparoscopic correction of congenital duodenal obstruction can be performed.
- Open surgery.
    - Once the normal rotation of the bowel is ascertained, the duodenum is mobilized and the cause and site of obstruction is appraised.
        1. A diamond-shaped duodeno-duodenostomy (as described by Kimura) or a simple duodeno-duodenostomy is performed in cases of type 2 atresia and with annular pancreas.
        2. A continuous serosal lining points towards a duodenal web (type 1 atresia) and a duodenotomy with excision of the web taking care to avoid injury to ampulla of Vater (position of the ampulla is identified by pressing the gallbladder and observing the flow of bile) is the treatment of choice. The duodenum is closed transversely. Duodeno-duodenostomy also can be performed in this situation but care should be taken to perform the anastomosis between the correct segments across the web.
        3. A side-to-side duodeno-jejunostomy may be a preferred technique in cases of a type 3 atresia with a wide gap or if the atresia is in the third or fourth parts of duodenum (Fig. 21.6).
            - A soft transanastomotic tube along with a nasogastric tube may be left across the anastomosis to initiate early feeding but is not necessary.
            - The presence of a second distal atresia (unusual) is ruled out by gently injecting saline distally.
            - Tapering duodenoplasty may be required in cases with gross dilatation of proximal duodenum and can be accomplished with plication, excision and suturing or GIA stapler (Fig. 21.7).

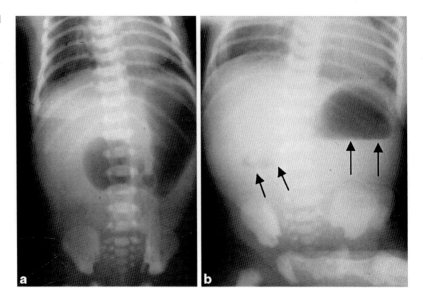

Fig. 21.3 Plain abdominal X-ray showing dilated stomach (**a**) and double bubble sign (**b**; *arrows*) indicative of congenital duodenal obstruction

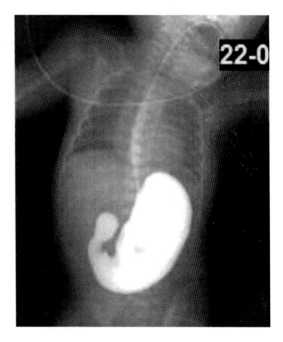

Fig. 21.4 Contrast study showing complete duodenal obstruction. Note the absence of air or contrast distally

- Laparoscopic repair of congenital duodenal obstruction in experienced hands is safe and gives the same results. It is performed by a three-port approach and a combination of 3 and 5 mm instruments. The principles of surgery remain the same. Distal atresia is ruled out by inspecting the bowel.

Postoperative Care

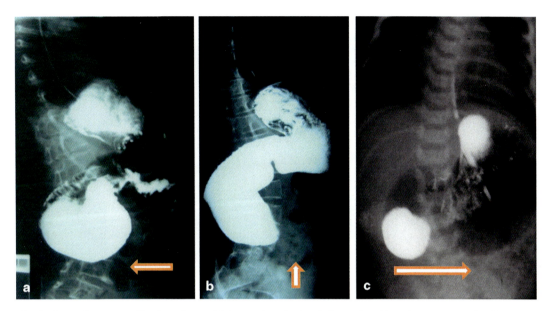

Fig. 21.5 a–c Contrast studies in patients with incomplete duodenal obstruction. Note the scanty gas distally and the passage of small amount of contrast distally (*arrows*)

Fig. 21.6 Contrast study showing congenital duodenal obstruction in the third part of duodenum

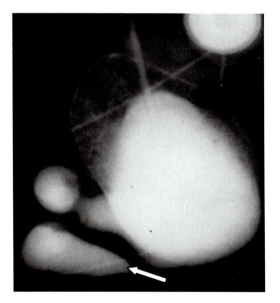

Postoperative Care

- All infants are maintained on bowel rest and parenteral nutrition.
- Nasogastric aspirates are monitored and fluid losses are replaced.
- If a transanstomotic tube is in place, continuous jejunal feeds are started on second postoperative day.

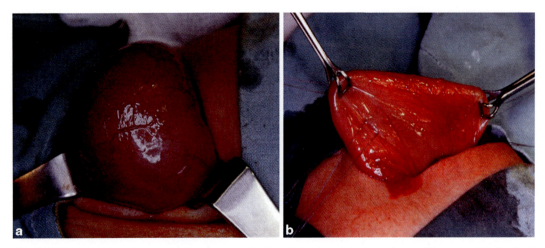

Fig. 21.7 Intraoperative photograph showing grossly dilated duodenum in a newborn with congenital duodenal obstruction (**a**) which will need a tapering duodenoplasty (**b**)

- Once nasogastric aspirates are no longer bilious, gradual feeding can be started through nasogastric tube and advancement as tolerated. Full feeding is usually achieved by 1.5–2 weeks.

Complications

- Anastomotic leak.
- Wound infection.
- Delayed gastric emptying with consequent delayed feeding are usual short-term complications.
- Long-term complications include:
    - Adhesive bowel obstruction
    - Anastomotic narrowing with proximal duodenal dilatation requiring open surgery with tapering or endoscopic balloon dilatation.

Recommended Reading

Gray SW, Skandalakis JE. Embryology for surgeons: the embryological basis for treatment of congenital defects. Philadelphia: WB Saunders; 1986.

Kimura K. Diamond shaped anastomosis for duodenal atresia: an experience with 44 patients over 15 years. J Pediatr Surg. 1990;25:977–8.

Chapter 22
Neonatal Intestinal Obstruction

Introduction

- Neonatal intestinal obstruction is one of the common pediatric emergencies.
- The diagnosis and general treatment of common causes of small and large bowel obstruction in a neonate are discussed here. Individual conditions will be discussed separately.
- In most cases of neonatal intestinal obstruction, the diagnosis is obvious after the plain abdominal x-ray and further contrast studies may not be necessary but in certain cases it is performed to arrive at a diagnosis or to exclude certain conditions. This is shown in Fig. 22.1.

Differential Diagnosis

- Atresia and stenosis involving duodenum, small bowel, and colon
- Intestinal malrotation
- Meconium ileus (associated and not associated with cystic fibrosis)
- Hirschsprung's disease (HD)
- Small left colon
- Meconium plug syndrome
- Volvulus, internal herniation
- Late-presenting cases of anorectal malformations (ARM)
- Necrotizing enterocolitis (NEC)

Rare causes include:

- Large retroperitoneal masses
- Intussusception
- Missed (late presenting) obstructed inguinal hernia

Remember to exclude nonsurgical causes of abdominal distension.

Presentation

- "A neonate with bilious vomiting or aspirate has intestinal obstruction until proved otherwise."
- The presenting symptoms could be any combination of the following:

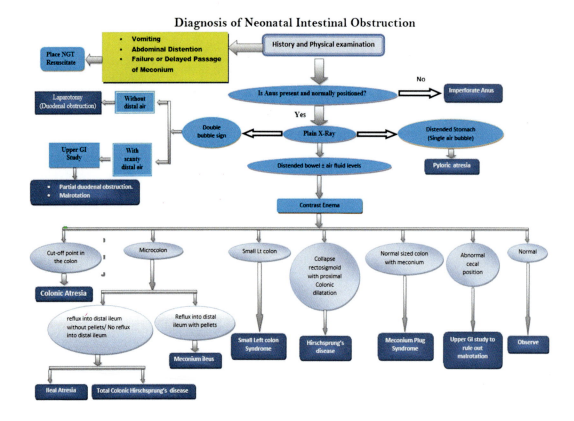

Fig. 22.1 Diagnosis of neonatal intestinal obstruction

- Bilious vomiting
- Abdominal distension (Fig. 22.2)
- Delayed passage of meconium
- Passage of grayish white pellets only
- Sepsis

History should include:

- Length of pregnancy
- Antenatal (presence of polyhydramnios may indicate intestinal obstruction) and family history (relevant in cases of HD and cystic fibrosis)
- Maternal diabetes (relevant in cases of small left colon syndrome)
- Passage of meconium (assisted or unassisted) and its timing (delayed passage of meconium beyond 24 h is a presenting symptom of HD or small left colon syndrome and needs to be investigated)
- Passage of a plug of meconium
- If the baby has passed anything rectally? If yes, color and consistency of the content (in intestinal atresia the baby may pass greenish white pellets)
- Results of antenatal ultrasound (dilated bowel loops indicating bowel obstruction)

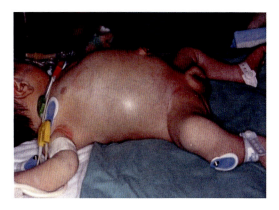

Fig. 22.2 A newborn with marked abdominal distension suggesting distal intestinal obstruction, necrotizing enterocolitis, or sepsis. The more marked the abdominal distension, the more distal is the obstruction

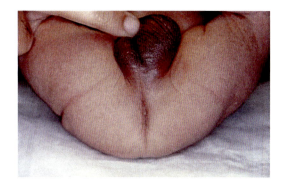

Fig. 22.3 A clinical photograph showing absent anus diagnostic of anorectal malformation

Examination

In the examination, look for and note:

- The presence of a normal anus (Fig. 22.3).
- A normal anus may be seen in cases of congenital rectal atresia (Fig. 22.4).
- Extent of abdominal distension, if any.
  - No distension with duodenal obstruction.
  - Early and upper abdominal distension with proximal intestinal obstruction.
  - With more distal obstruction distension is generalized and slow to appear.
- Visible and palpable bowel loops.
- Erythema and tenderness of abdominal wall (denotes NEC with perforation or gangrene of bowel or volvulus. It may also be seen in cases of a meconium cyst).
- Extent of dehydration (judged by reduced urine output, dryness of tongue, sunken fontanels).
- Associated anomaly (e.g., Down's syndrome can be a pointer to duodenal atresia or HD).

Investigations

- Complete blood count (CBC).
- Serum electrolytes, creatinine, and blood urea nitrogen (BUN).

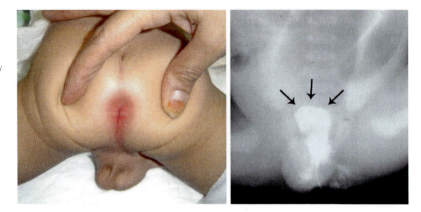

Fig. 22.4 A clinical photograph showing a normal looking anus in a newborn with congenital rectal atresia confirmed by barium enema

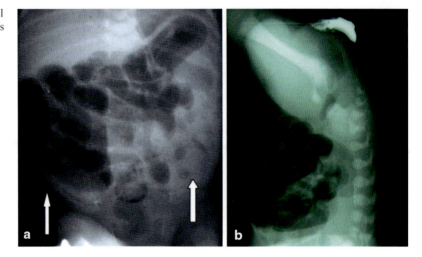

Fig. 22.5 Plain abdominal x-ray showing oedamatous bowel loops and pneumatosis intestinalis in a patient with necrotizing enterocolitis (**a**) and an invertogram in a patient with low anorectal agenesis (**b**)

- Serum bilirubin.
- Prothrombin time (PT) and partial thromboplastin time (PTT).
- Blood group and cross match (packed red blood cell, PRBC, and fresh frozen plasma, FFP, are kept available for the surgery).
- Blood for genetic studies in appropriate cases.

Imaging Studies

- Plain x-ray abdomen: usually a supine film but a lateral decubitus film in NEC and an invertogram or a prone cross-table lateral film for anorectal malformations (Fig. 22.5).

Note:

- Bowel gas pattern (In a normal abdomen the gas pattern looks like small equal-sized hexagons distributed uniformly across the abdomen. Any loop dilated more than the size of the thumb is abnormal.)

Imaging Studies

Fig. 22.6 Plain abdominal x-ray showing dilated stomach with little air distally suggesting partial duodenal obstruction secondary to malrotation, duodenal diaphragm with a hole, or duodenal stenosis

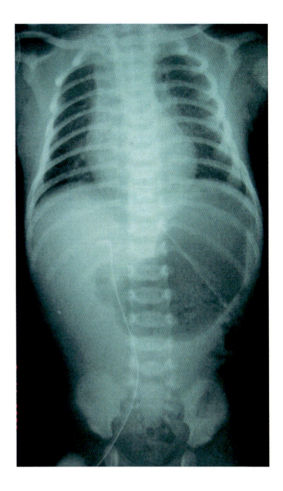

Fig. 22.7 Plain abdominal x-ray showing dilated stomach and proximal duodenum suggesting congenital duodenal obstruction (**a**). Note the absence of air distally indicating complete obstruction and upper contrast study showing complete duodenal obstruction (**b**)

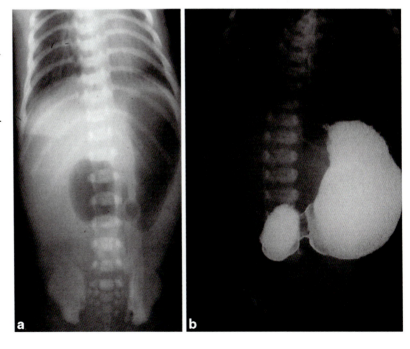

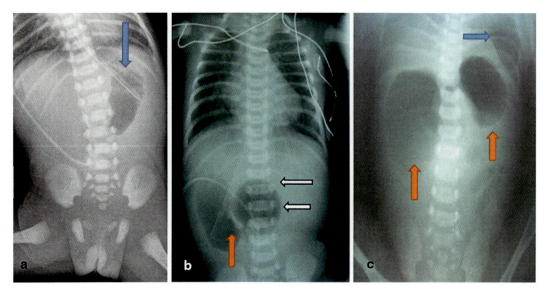

Fig. 22.8 Plain abdominal x-rays showing a single air bubble (**a**), double bubbles (**b**), and triple bubbles (**c**)

Fig. 22.9 Plain abdominal x-ray showing marked dilatation of bowel loops with air–fluid level indicative of distal intestinal obstruction. In the second one, plain abdominal x-ray showing dilated bowel loops with no gas distally suggesting small bowel obstruction. Note the small number of bowel loops suggesting upper small bowel obstruction

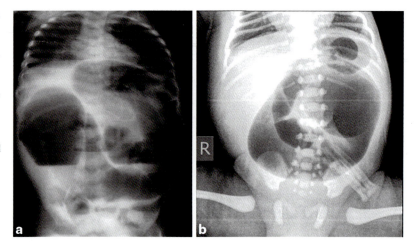

- Amount of abdominal air (Very little distal air could indicate malrotation or duodenal obstruction secondary to a diaphragm with a central hole or duodenal stenosis when associated with double bubble; Figs. 22.6 and 22.7)
- A single gastric bubble denotes gastric outlet obstruction, double bubbles are indicative of duodenal obstruction, and triple bubbles suggests upper jejunal obstruction (Fig. 22.8).
- Number of fluid levels (Double bubbles with absence of or very little air in the distal bowel identifies duodenal obstruction; the more the number of fluid levels the more distal the obstruction; Fig. 22.9)
- Dilated bowel loops without fluid levels and a hyaline or soap bubble appearance of right lower abdomen may be indicative of meconium ileus.
- Bowel wall thickening (indicated by increased separation of loops of bowel).

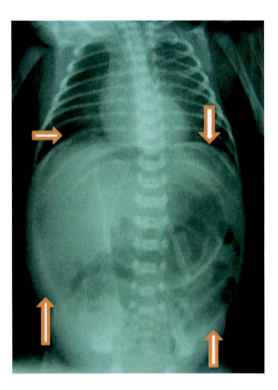

Fig. 22.10 Abdominal x-ray with perforated necrotizing enterocolitis showing free air (*football sign*)

- Free air due to perforation from any cause is suspected on supine film when the bowel wall is sharply delineated (pencil lining). A large pocket of air overlying liver and the ligamentum teres is known as a "football sign"(Fig. 22.10).
- Calcification may be noted suggestive of antenatal perforation. A curvilinear calcification may indicate the presence of meconium cyst.
- Ultrasound and other studies are not needed for routine cases. Ultrasound may be helpful to look for other associated anomalies and helps to diagnose free or loculated intra-abdominal fluid collection denoting perforation or a meconium cyst.

Contrast Studies

- The first enema a neonate receives should be a contrast enema.
- The contrast enema acts not just a diagnostic tool but works as a therapeutic measure in cases of meconium plug, small left colon syndrome, and meconium ileus (Fig. 22.11).
- Contrast upper gastrointestinal (GI) studies are needed in cases where malrotation is suspected and sometimes to characterize the duodenal obstruction. A good thought is given prior to ordering an upper GI study and if two studies are ordered the upper GI study should always be done after the contrast enema (Figs. 22.12 and 22.13).
- One cannot overemphasize that the surgeon should remain present during the study.

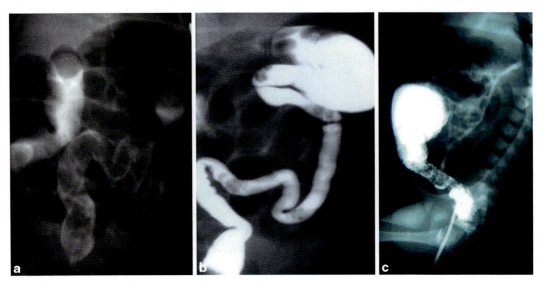

Fig. 22.11 Lower contrast study showing meconium plug syndrome (**a**), small left colon syndrome (**b**), and Hirschsprung's disease (**c**)

Fig. 22.12 a Lower contrast study showing small unused colon suggesting small bowel obstruction or total colonic Hirschsprung's disease. **b** Note the dilated proximal bowel loops

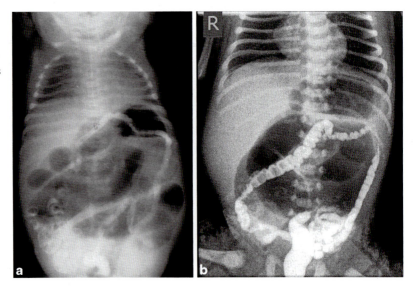

Important Things to Remember While Doing the Contrast Study

- These are almost always performed with a water soluble contrast (dilute Gastrografin where available, metrizamide, or Urografin).
- Make sure the baby is well hydrated; the radiology suit temperature is warm enough for the baby.
- Avoid using Foley catheter with the bulb inflated.
- Perform the study using image intensifier.
- Make sure not to inject more contrast than necessary (osmotic action of the contrast can draw a lot of fluid in the bowel causing volume imbalance in a small baby).

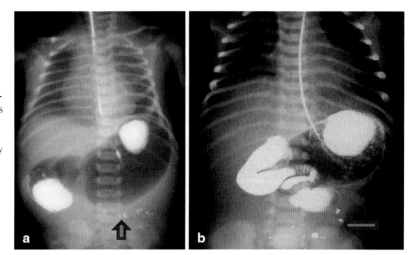

Fig. 22.13 Upper contrast study showing congenital duodenal obstruction. Note the passage of small amount of contrast material distally indicative of incomplete obstruction secondary to duodenal stenosis or duodenal diaphragm with a hole (**a**). In the second upper contrast study showing proximal jejunal obstruction with small amount of contrast passing distally suggesting incomplete jejunal obstruction or more commonly malrotation with volvulus (**b**)

Treatment

- This is individualized according to the diagnosis and will be discussed with each condition separately but certain principals remain common.
- The baby is cared for in the neonatal care unit with regulation of temperature and adequate monitoring.
- Ensure there is a good intravenous access (a PICC can be inserted preoperatively or should be inserted under anesthesia before the surgery).
- The child should be on appropriate intravenous fluid containing dextrose 10% and electrolyte mix appropriate for age.
- A well-positioned nasogastric tube should be in place.
- Avoid use of suppository or enema.
- Anticipate the need for postoperative ventilation and discuss it with the anesthetist and neonatologist.
- The baby should receive broad spectrum antibiotic cover including anaerobes.
- The baby should be transported in an incubator to and from the operating room (OR). The OR temperature should be kept high and measures should be taken to keep the baby warm during surgery. (Cover the baby's head and exposed limbs with cotton or space blankets, use warm air blowing devices like "Bairhugger," or warm blankets.)
- Warm saline is used during the procedure and all the fluids given to the baby are warmed appropriately.
- A urinary catheter is not necessary for every case but may be inserted for longer procedures or to monitor the output closely in critical babies.

Chapter 23
Congenital Intestinal Stenosis and Atresia

Jejunoileal Stenosis and Atresia

Introduction

- The word atresia comes from the Greek a, which means no or without, and tresis, which means orifice.
- Intestinal atresia or stenosis can occur anywhere along the gastrointestinal tract, and the site of the obstruction determines the clinical presentation.
- Most newborns with intestinal obstruction present with bilious vomiting which in the neonatal period should be considered secondary to a mechanical intestinal obstruction until proven otherwise.
- Jejunoileal atresias and stenoses are major causes of neonatal intestinal obstruction.
- The incidence of jejunal and ileal atresia ranges from 1 in 1500 to 12,000 live births.
- Atresia accounts for 95 % of jejunoileal obstructions and stenosis accounts for the remaining 5 % of cases.
- The ileum is slightly more affected than jejunum (55–45 %).
- Unlike duodenal atresia, jejunoileal atresias are not commonly associated with Down syndrome.
- Patients with intestinal atresia are characterized by young gestational age and low birth weight.
- There is no correlation between jejunoileal atresia and parental age.
- There is an increased prevalence of intestinal atresias in infants born to teenage mothers.
- Jejunoileal atresias affect females as equally as males.
- Associated anomalies are found in only 10 % of neonates with jejunoileal atresias. These are more common in those with jejunal atresia.
- The survival of patients with neonatal intestinal obstruction has markedly improved over the past 20 years. This is attributed to several factors including improved perioperative care of newborns, pediatric anesthesia, and surgical techniques.

Etiology

- Multiple theories regarding the etiology of jejunoileal atresias have been proposed including:
    - In utero intussusception
    - Intestinal perforation
    - Segmental volvulus
    - Thromboembolism

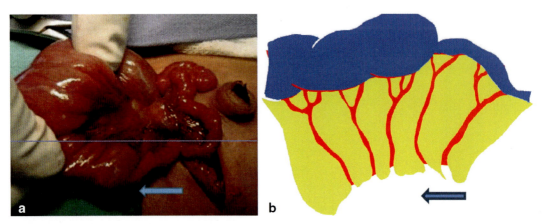

Fig. 23.1 Operative (**a**) and diagrammatic (**b**) representation of type I intestinal atresia. There is continuity of bowel, no defect in the mesentery and an intraluminal diaphragm

- Atresias can also develop in patients with gastroschisis and in those with meconium ileus.
- In 1955, Louw and Barnard demonstrated the role of late intrauterine mesenteric vascular accidents as the likely cause of jejunoileal atresias, rather than the previously accepted theory of inadequate recanalization of the intestinal tract.
- The most accepted theory is that of an intrauterine vascular accident which leads to a decreased intestinal perfusion and ischemia of the respective segment of intestine. This leads to narrowing of the bowel or in most severe cases, complete obliteration of the intestinal lumen leading to atresia.
- Genetic factors: Familial cases of various types of intestinal atresia have been described. This association is presumably an autosomal dominant type.

Classification

- There are two broad types of jejunoileal defects:

    1. Stenoses
    2. Atresias

- A stenosis:

    – A localized narrowing of the bowel without loss of bowel continuity and an intact mesentery.
    – The proximal dilated intestine is in continuity with the distal nondilated bowel, and a narrow segment with a small lumen is present between them.
    – The small-bowel length is normal and no defect in the mesentery present.

- Atresias are further subdivided into four types.
- The different types represent a spectrum of severity, from a simple web to full atresia with loss of bowel length.
- Type I atresia (Fig. 23.1):

    – In type I atresias, there is an intraluminal diaphragm (membrane).
    – As in duodenal webs, a windsock effect may be seen secondary to an increase in intraluminal pressure in the proximal dilated bowel causing a prolapse of the web into the distal part of the bowel.
    – There is no defect in the mesentery.

Classification

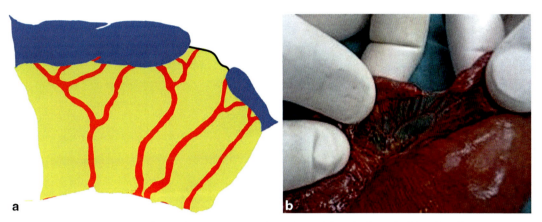

Fig. 23.2 Diagrammatic (**a**) and operative (**b**) representation of type II intestinal atresia. There is a fibrous cord connecting the two intestinal segments with an intact mesentery. This is in a patient with multiple intestinal atresias. Note the dilated segment of bowel proximal to another atresia

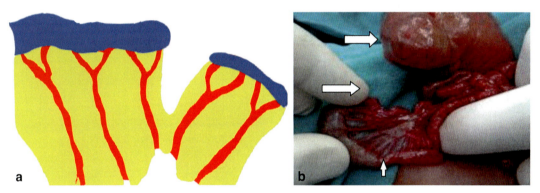

Fig. 23.3 Diagrammatic (**a**) and operative (**b**) representation of type IIIa atresia. Note the defect in the mesentery and the two atretic ends separated with no fibrous cord between them. Note also the distal type I atresia (*thin arrow*)

- The bowel length is normal.
- Type II (Fig. 23.2):
  - In type II atresia, the affected segments of intestines are separated from each other and the dilated proximal portion has a bulbous blind end connected by a fibrous cord to the blind end of the distal collapsed bowel.
  - The mesentery is intact.
  - The bowel length is usually normal.
- Type IIIa (Fig. 23.3):
  - In type IIIa atresia, the affected segments of intestines are separated from each other without a connecting fibrous cord and the dilated proximal portion has a bulbous blind end which is separated from the blind end of the distal collapsed bowel.
  - A V-shaped mesenteric defect is present.
  - The intervening bowel has undergone intrauterine resorption, and, as a result, the bowel is variably shortened.

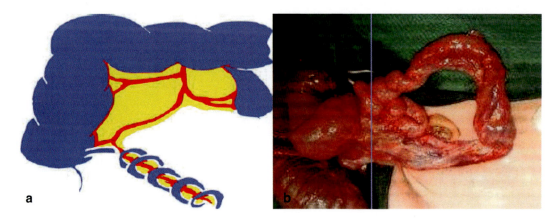

Fig. 23.4 Diagrammatic (**a**) and operative (**b**) representation of type IIIb atresia (apple peel deformity). There is a single feeding vessel around which the intestines are twisted

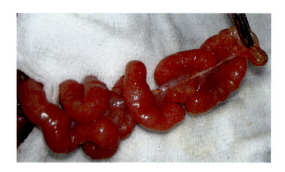

Fig. 23.5 Intraoperative photograph showing apple peel deformity. Note the single feeding artery

- Type IIIb (Figs. 23.4 and 23.5):
    - Type IIIb atresia is also known as a Christmas tree or apple peel deformity because of the appearance of the bowel as it wraps around a single feeding vessel.
    - There is a large defect in the mesentery.
    - The bowel length is significantly shortened.
    - The distal small bowel receives its blood supply from a single ileocolic or right colic artery.
    - Many patients with this type of intestinal atresia have low birth weight (70 %) and are premature (70 %).
    - They may also have malrotation (54 %), multiple intestinal atresias, and an increased number of other associated anomalies that increase the prevalence of complications (63 %) and mortality rate (54–71 %).

- Type IV (Figs. 23.6 and 23.7):
    - Type IV involves multiple small-bowel atresias of any combination of types I–III.
    - This defect has the appearance of a string of sausages because of the multiple lesions.
    - This type of intestinal atresia may occur in several members of the same family which suggest a possible autosomal recessive transmission.
    - Multiple intestinal atresias have been reported in association with cystic dilatation of the bile ducts.

Classification

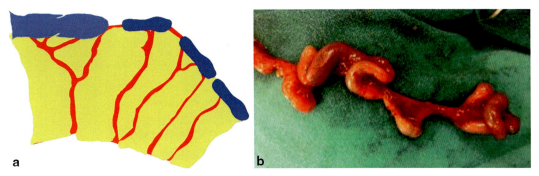

Fig. 23.6 Diagrammatic (**a**) and operative (**b**) representation of type IV atresia

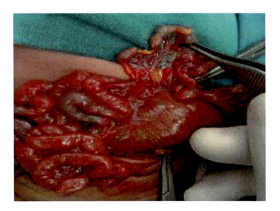

Fig. 23.7 Intraoperative photograph showing type IV atresia

- Multiple intestinal atresias have also been reported in rare association with pyloric atresia and pylorocholedochal fistula.
- The intestinal length is invariably and considerably shortened.

Pathophysiology

- In small intestinal atresias, the ileum (55%) is slightly affected more than the jejunum (45%).
- In more than 90% of patients, the atresia is single; however, multiple atresias are reported in 6–20% of cases.
- Jejunoileal atresia can be associated with:
  - Intrauterine volvulus (27%)
  - Gastroschisis (16%)
  - Meconium ileus (12%)
- Sixty-two percent of atresia and stenosis cases were noted in the jejunum, 30% in the ileum, and 8% in both the jejunum and the ileum.
- The frequency of atresia is as follows:
  - Stenosis (7%)
  - Type I atresia (16%)
  - Type II atresia (21%)

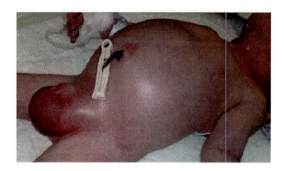

Fig. 23.8 Clinical photograph showing severe abdominal distension in a patient with low intestinal obstruction

- Type IIIa atresia (24%)
- Type IIIb atresia (10%)
- Type IV atresia (22%)

- The mean birth weight and gestational age are significantly lower in patients with jejunal atresia than in those with ileal atresia.
- Most jejunal atresias were multiple, whereas most ileal atresias were single.
- Antenatal perforation is seen more frequently in ileal atresia but less in jejunal atresia.
- The postoperative course is often prolonged, and the mortality rate is more in patients with jejunal atresia.

Clinical Features

- History of polyhydramnios during prenatal ultrasonographic evaluation is common (30%). This is more in those with upper jejunal atresia.
- Prematurity (35%). This is more in those with jejunal atresia.
- Low birth weight (25–50%). This is more in those with jejunal atresia.
- Bilious vomiting. The more proximal the obstruction the more is the vomiting.
- Abdominal distension. This is more common in those with distal obstruction (Fig. 23.8).
- Jaundice (30%). This is secondary to indirect hyperbilirubinemia and it is more in those with ileal atresia.
- Failure to pass meconium in the first day of life. The passage of meconium does not however rule out intestinal atresia.
- Clinically, intestinal loops as well as peristalsis may be visible.
- An excessively dilated proximal bowel segment may undergo torsion, necrosis, and/or perforation. In these cases, the patient appears septic and dehydrated, and the abdominal wall may be erythematous.
- Clinically, neonates with a proximal atresia develop bilious vomiting within hours, whereas patients with more distal obstruction may take longer to start vomiting.
- A normal or scaphoid like abdomen in a neonate with bilious vomiting is indicative of a proximal obstruction.
- Abdominal distension is more marked in those with distal obstruction.

Fig. 23.9 Plain abdominal x-ray showing dilated bowel loops and absent gas distally indicative of intestinal obstruction

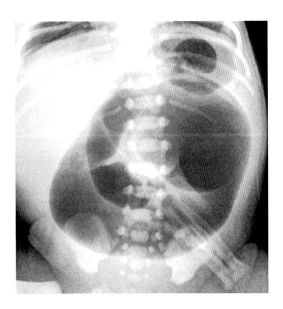

Diagnosis

- Antenatal ultrasound:
    - The diagnosis of intestinal atresias should be suspected antenatally during a routine ultrasound when it shows a dilated intestinal segment.
    - This is specially so in the presence of polyhydramnios.
    - These abnormalities are indicative of intestinal obstruction.
    - Persistently dilated bowel loops on serial ultrasounds have shown a 66.7% positive correlation with intestinal atresia diagnosed after birth. This more so in those with proximal atresia.
- Plain abdominal x-ray (Fig. 23.9):
    - Plain abdominal radiograph of a newborn patient with small-bowel atresia demonstrates diffuse bowel distension, with gasless pelvis and air–fluid levels.
    - The more distal the obstruction, the more is the gaseous distension.
    - With more proximal atresias, few air–fluid levels are seen with no apparent gas in the lower part of the abdomen.
    - The more distal the obstruction, the more air–fluid levels are seen and distal intestine remains gasless.
    - In jejunal atresia, plain abdominal radiograph reveals a dilated gastric bubble and a massively dilated duodenum and proximal jejunum with a gasless abdomen distal to the level of the obstruction.
    - Peritoneal calcifications, seen in 12% of patients, suggest meconium peritonitis, asign of in utero intestinal perforation.
- Stenosis in a neonate is difficult to diagnose and it may not manifest for some time. These patients have a history of intermittent vomiting and failure to thrive. An upper gastrointestinal study with small-bowel follow-through is indicated in these patients.
- Barium enema (Fig. 23.10):
    - A contrast enema can be useful to:
        - Distinguish large-bowel obstruction from small-bowel obstruction.

Fig. 23.10 Barium enema showing small unused colon

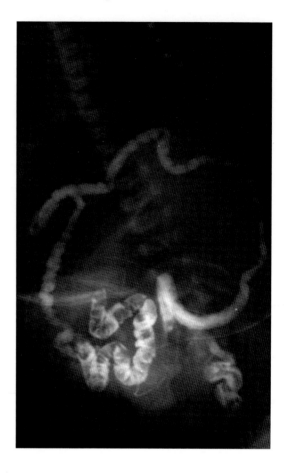

- Identify the site of colonic or distal ileal obstruction.
- Determine the presence of a microcolon.
- Identify the position of the cecum. This is useful in cases of abnormal rotation and fixation of the intestine.
- Barium enema is used to define a microcolon (unused colon) indicative of a small-bowel obstruction.
- Most neonates with jejunoileal atresia have an unused microcolon, except when the vascular accident leading to atresia occurs late in gestation, as in the case of idiopathic in utero intussusception.
- Patients with meconium ileus also present with a microcolon.
- Barium enema is also useful to establish the diagnosis of other causes of lower obstruction, such as Hirschsprung's disease or a meconium plug.
- The contrast enema may also reflux into the small bowel and help define the level of a distal obstruction or meconium ileus.

- Upper gastrointestinal contrast study:
  - Is seldom required.
  - This study is typically performed to rule out partial obstruction or malrotation, which is present in 10 % of patients with jejunoileal atresia.
  - When performed, the study shows gastric dilatation and an enlarged small bowel up to the level of the atresia, where a blind pouch can be seen.

Classification

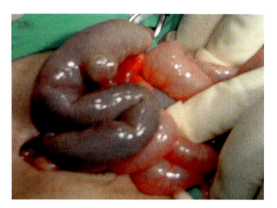

Fig. 23.11 Intraoperative photograph showing Meckel's diverticulum in a patient with congenital intestinal atresia

- In cases of intestinal stenosis, the prestenotic segment appears dilated, a transition point is evident, and contrast material can be seen in the distal bowel.
- In jejunal atresia, upper-gastrointestinal contrast study demonstrates a dilated stomach and duodenum, with an enlarged upper jejunum and a lack of passage of contrast agent to the distal small bowel.
• Video capsule endoscopy: Although in use for more than 10 years in specific gastrointestinal conditions in adults, this has been recently used in the diagnosis of small intestinal atresias in neonates.

Treatment

• The treatment of neonates with intestinal atresia and its success depends on several factors. These include:
    - Early diagnosis
    - Proper preoperative stabilization
    - The right choice of surgical procedure
    - Good postoperative care
• Preoperative care:
    - Once the diagnosis of neonatal intestinal obstruction is made, the patient should be fully resuscitated.
    - Gastric decompression via an orogastric or a nasogastric tube.
    - The use of umbilical lines should be avoided because of the increased risk of infection and because they interfere with the incision for laparotomy.
    - 1 mg of vitamin K is given intramuscularly.
    - Broad-spectrum antibiotics are given intravenously.
    - Fluid resuscitation.
    - Control of temperature to avoid hypothermia.
• Operative approach:
    - A transverse supraumbilical incision is used as it affords adequate exposure of the abdominal contents.
    - Laparoscopic approaches for the management of intestinal atresias have been reported lately but these require advanced laparoscopic skills.

Fig. 23.12 Intraoperative photograph showing type I jejunal atresia. Note the dilated proximal jejunum

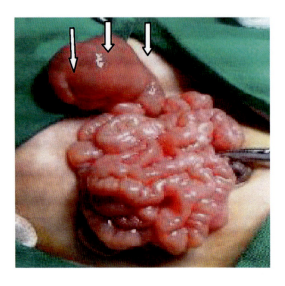

Fig. 23.13 Intraoperative photograph showing type I atresia

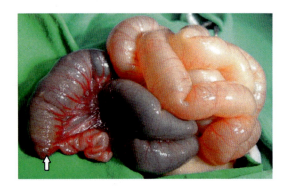

- The full length of the bowel is manually explored for malrotation, other atresias, or stenoses (Fig. 23.11).
- Care is taken to keep the bowel moist and protected with warm gauze at all times.
- Intraoperatively, every effort should be made to prevent or correct hypothermia, hypovolemia, hypoglycemia, and hypoxemia.
- The length of intestine that appears functional is measured as this affects the choice of operative procedure and overall prognosis.
- Distal atresias, which occur in 6–21 % of patients, must be excluded. This checked by the saline test (irrigate normal saline solution into the distal pouch and milk it caudally to ensure patency of the distal collapsed bowel).
- When the intestinal length is normal, the dilated proximal pouch can be resected, by removing 10–15 cm of dilated bowel proximal to the atresia, to avoid postoperative physiologic obstruction due to lack or abnormal peristalsis (Figs. 23.12 and 23.13).
- If the bowel length is limited, a tapering enteroplasty should be considered rather than resection (Fig. 23.14).
- A single layer, end-to-oblique or end-to-end anastomosis is performed. The mesenteric gap is then approximated with fine absorbable sutures, taking care not to kink the anastomosis or damage the mesenteric vessels (Fig. 23.15).

Classification

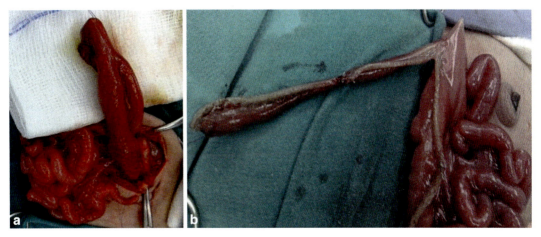

Fig. 23.14 Intraoperative photograph showing a markedly dilated jejunum (**a**) and reduction jejunoplasty using GIA (**b**)

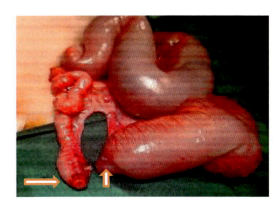

Fig. 23.15 Intraoperative photograph showing intestinal atresia. Note the marked discrepancy in size between the two bowel segments

- Patency of the anastomosis can be tested by milking intestinal air or intestinal contents through it.
- In type IV atresia with minimal remnant bowel, stenting of multiple bowel segments has been performed with success.
- Gastrostomy tubes are not to be used, and postoperative nasogastric suction is sufficient for gastric decompression.
- Some authors recommend using a gastrostomy tube in a very high jejunal atresia for stomach decompression and to pass a transanastomotic tube for early postoperative enteral drip feeding.
- When bowel length is reduced (for type III or IV atresias) and there is a danger of having a short-bowel syndrome, an antimesenteric tapering jejunoplasty may be performed. This can be performed manually or using a gastrointestinal anastomosis (GIA) stapler and oversewing the staple line with Lembert nonabsorpable sutures (Figs. 23.16 and 23.17).
- A central venous catheter is placed if the need for long-term total parenteral nutrition (TPN) is anticipated.
- In case of multiple atresias, one must decide whether all atresias can be managed at the same time or a staged repair is necessary. In the latter case, a temporary proximal ileostomy is made.
- A single-stage repair of multiple atresias with restoration of intestinal continuity and preservation of maximal bowel length is the preferred operative management.

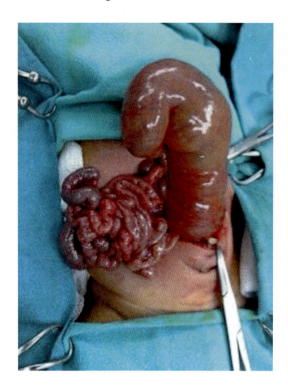

Fig. 23.16 Intraoperative photograph showing a markedly dilated jejunum in a patient with jejunal atresia

- Postoperative management:
  - The patient is admitted to the neonatal intensive care unit.
  - Nothing by mouth (NPO).
  - The baby should be kept warm.
  - Oxygen saturation should be monitored.
  - Vital signs should be assessed frequently.
  - Intubation for respiratory support should be considered for those with severe abdominal distension or sepsis.
  - An orogastric tube should be placed for gastric decompression. This should continue until the return of bowel function.
  - Gastric output must be replaced volume for volume.
  - Blood transfusion is administered if indicated.
  - A bladder catheter is used to ensure a urinary output of 1–2 mL/kg/h.
  - TPN should be started shortly after surgery and continued until enteral feeds are tolerated.
- Intestinal failure is now defined as the presence of malabsorption after clinically significant small-bowel resection.
- The minimal length of intestines necessary to maintain nutritional status is not exactly fixed. Newborns require at least 10–20 cm of postduodenal small bowel to avoid short-bowel syndrome if the ileocecal valve and colon are preserved but when the ileocecal valve is resected, this requirement increases to 40–50 cm. The loss of the ileum is the most difficult part to compensate.
- Surgical bowel-lengthening procedures and small-bowel transplantation are beneficial in patients of short-bowel syndrome.

Classification

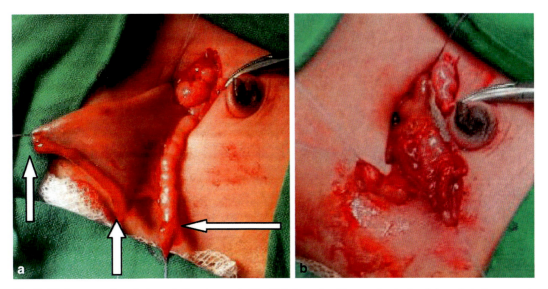

Fig. 23.17 Intraoperative photograph showing markedly dilated proximal loop and reduction jejunoplasty (**a**; *arrows*). Note the marked difference in size prior to reduction jejunoplasty using GIA (**b**)

Outcome and Prognosis

- Currently, the overall survival rates of newborns with intestinal atresias have reached 90%, with a surgical mortality rate of less than 1%.
- The most common cause of death in infants with jejunoileal atresia is infection related to pneumonia, peritonitis, or sepsis.
- The most important surgical complications are anastomotic leaks and functional intestinal obstruction at the level of the anastomosis; these occur in as many as 15% of patients.
- Short-bowel syndrome may occur in patients born with multiple atresias or in those with the apple-peel deformity type. This result in longer hospital stay, more feeding problems, and higher morbidity and mortality rates.
- Today, the survival rate for patients with short-bowel syndrome is 80 da%.
- The overall prognosis depends upon the amount of residual functional bowel.
- The presence or absence of the ileocecal valve does not appear to affect the mortality rate. However, it does notably affect the length of time that TPN is required and, therefore, affects the complications related to its use.
- The use of the longitudinal intestinal lengthening and tailoring (LILT) procedure, proposed by Bianchi and modified by Aigrain, can allow the child to be weaned from parenteral nutrition.
- Malabsorption and steatorrhea are most severe in patients with terminal ileal resection, particularly those in whom the ileocecal valve is excised. Vitamin B supplements are useful in these patients.
- Prematurity, birth weight < 2 kg, and associated anomalies are independent risk factors for prolonged hospital stay and higher mortality rate.

Atresia and Stenosis of the Colon

Introduction

- Colonic atresia is the least common type of intestinal atresias and comprises 1.8–15% of all intestinal atresias and stenoses.
- Colonic atresia was first described in 1673.
- It is very rare and various incidences have been reported, ranging from 1 in 1500 live births to 1 in 66,000 live births. The most accepted incidence of colonic atresia is 1 in 20,000.
- Colonic atresias may occur at any site in the colon; however, atresias proximal to the splenic flexure and distal to the vascular watershed area are the most common.
- Colonic atresias are frequently associated with other anomalies, including jejunoileal atresia, Hirschsprung's disease, and genitourinary malformations.
- Patients usually present with abdominal distention and failure to pass meconium.
- Stenosis of the colon is much more common than atresia.
- In congenital stenosis, a narrow segment of colon is observed, but bowel continuity is maintained.
- Multiple colonic atresias are uncommon; however, colonic atresia may be overlooked when small intestinal atresia is present.
- Rare cases of familial colonic atresia have been described. Hereditary multiple intestinal atresia affects both the large and small intestine, whereas nonhereditary multiple intestinal atresia usually spares the colon.
- The incidence of colonic stenosis is not known because most cases are acquired. Necrotizing enterocolitis is the most common cause of postnatal colonic stenosis (10–25%).

Etiology

- In 1955, Louw and Barnard hypothesized that small-bowel atresias are caused by prenatal vascular interruption.
- The same mechanism is believed to cause colonic atresia.
- Similar to jejunoileal atresia, colonic atresia is believed to be caused by an in utero vascular accident resulting in ischemic injury.
- Thrombosis, volvulus, and herniation with strangulation are all mechanisms that may cause in utero vascular injury and bowel necrosis with subsequent reabsorption.
- The colon receives its blood supply from the superior mesenteric artery and inferior mesenteric artery. The splenic flexure is the most vulnerable site to ischemia. Nevertheless, atresia and stenosis occur throughout the colon.
- Prenatal maternal use of vasoconstrictive medications, such as cocaine, amphetamines, nicotine, or decongestants, has been suggested to be a risk factor for intestinal atresia formation.
- Congenital stenosis occurs when the bowel injury is incomplete.
- Acquired colonic stenosis is more common than atresia or congenital stenosis.
- Acquired colonic stenosis occur:
  - In necrotizing enterocolitis
  - At the anastomotic site following colonic resection
  - In Crohn's disease
  - Post-cardiac catheterization ischemia
  - In left-sided colonic tuberculosis

Associated Anomalies

- Colonic atresia has been associated with abdominal wall defects and abnormalities of the genitourinary tract.
- Nonfixation of the colon.
- Anal atresia and *imperforated anus.*
- Hirschsprung's disease.
- O*mphalocele.*
- Absence of a hand.
- Additional conditions reported in patients with colonic stenosis include:
  - Cryptophthalmia syndrome (cleft lip and palate, microphthalmia, dysplastic kidneys, proximal jejunal atresia)
  - Arthrogryposis
  - Proximal intestinal atresia
  - Malrotation
  - Riley–Day syndrome (familial dysautonomia)
  - Coloboma
  - Cataracts
  - Facial hemihypertrophy
  - Facial asymmetry with palsy
  - Microphthalmia with partial iridial coloboma, exophthalmia, and bilateral optic nerve hypoplasia

Clinical Features

- Patients with colonic atresia or congenital stenosis may sometimes have findings on prenatal ultrasonography, such as dilated bowel loops or the presence of polyhydramnios.
- Initial physical examination findings are normal in the absence of associated conditions.
- The anus usually appears normal.
- Progressive abdominal distention develops.
- Rectal examination reveals white or pale mucus rather than pigmented meconium.
- Failure to completely pass meconium suggests atresia, whereas delayed passage of meconium (>24 h) suggests Hirschsprung's disease.
- Patients with colonic atresia may pass meconium normally because the incident that caused the atresia may have occurred after the colon had become filled with meconium.
- Colonic stenosis behaves like colonic atresia when the lesion is very tight. In less severe cases, the child may have chronic problems like bloating with feeds, cramping, or poor weight gain. The abdomen may become distended with feeding, and stool production is scant, if present.
- Colonic perforation may occur. This is caused by overdistension of closed colonic loop, between a competent ileocecal valve proximally and the blind-ending colon distally.

Classification

- Colon atresia is typically classified using the 1989 descriptions of intestinal atresia by Bland-Sutton and the 1964 descriptions by Louw.
- Type 1 atresia: The colon and mesentery remain intact, but the bowel lumen is obstructed by a complete membrane.

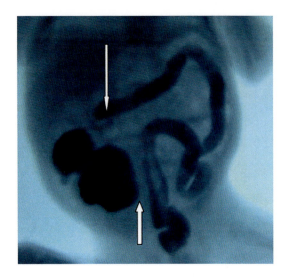

Fig. 23.18 Barium enema showing congenital colonic stenosis. Note the thin film of contrast passing proximally and the dilated right side of the colon (*arrows*)

- Type 2 atresia: The colon is discontinuous, connected by a fibrous cord.
- Type 3 atresia: The colon ends are completely separated, and the mesentery has a gap.
- Colonic stenosis: Characterized by intact bowel with incomplete occlusion.
- The distribution of colonic atresia by site:
  - Ascending colon (28%)
  - Hepatic flexure (3%)
  - Transverse colon (23%)
  - Splenic flexure (25%)
  - Descending and sigmoid (20%)

Investigations

- Ultrasonography may reveal bowel loop distention or polyhydramnios.
- Plain abdominal radiograph: Reveals bowel obstruction with or without a prominent dilated loop and absence of gas in the rectum.
- Contrast enema:
  - This is useful to rule out the presence of other atresias.
  - It reveals a microcolon with a rounded proximal end at the site of atresia.
  - Radiography in congenital colonic stenosis also reveals an obstructive intestinal pattern that may mimic atresia. Contrast enema reveals narrowing of the colon, with limited filling of the dilated proximal colon (Fig. 23.18).

Management

- The initial treatment of newborns with colonic atresia is directed toward resuscitation which include the following:
  - Nasogastric decompression
  - Intravenous fluid resuscitation
  - Intravenous antibiotics

- Intestinal colonic obstruction at any level requires surgical relief.
- The decision to proceed with primary resection and anastomosis or stoma diversion depends on the patient's condition.
- Historically, some authors have advocated resection with primary anastomosis for right colon lesions and colostomy diversion with subsequent reconstruction for left-sided atresia and stenosis.
- The management of colonic atresia is directed at resecting the site of obstruction and establishing intestinal continuity.
- In selected cases (with limited comorbidities and limited associated malformations), this may be performed in one stage (resecting the atretic ends and primary anastomosis).
- If the child has significant comorbidities (severe underlying illness and associated life-threatening malformations may be considered relative contraindications to immediate primary repair), a diverting colostomy just proximal to the site of atresia is done, and reanastomosis to be done at a second operation.
- The association of colonic atresia with Hirschprung's disease is rare. Rectal biopsy (performed either as a suction biopsy prior to surgical correction or at the time of operative correction) should be considered to evaluate for associated Hirschprung's disease.
- In congenital colonic stenosis, one usually finds less difference in the sizes of the proximal and distal limbs, making resection with primary anastomosis the preferred treatment.
- In acquired colonic stenosis following necrotizing enterocolitis, primary excision and anastomosis is the treatment of choice for stable patients without life-threatening comorbidities.

Recommended Reading

Dalla Vecchia LK, Grosfeld JL, West KW, Rescorla FJ, Scherer LR, Engum SA. Intestinal atresia and stenosis: a 25-year experience with 277 cases. *Arch Surg*.1998;133(5):490–6.

Davenport M, Bianchi A, Doig CM, Gough DC. Colonic atresia: current results of treatment. *J R Coll Surg Edinb*. 1990;35(1):25–8.

Piper HG, Alesbury J, Waterford SD, Zurakowski D, Jaksic T. Intestinal atresias: factors affecting clinical outcomes. *J Pediatr Surg*. 2008;43(7):1244–88.

Chapter 24
Intussusception

Introduction

The word "intussusception" comes from the Latin "intus" (within) and "suscipere" (to receive), *i.e.,* "to receive within." Intussusception is the telescoping of one segment of intestine into another adjacent distal segment of the intestine. Most cases of intussusception occur in children between 5 months and 1 year of age. Two-thirds of children with intussusception are younger than 1 year. Although extremely rare, intussusception has been reported in the neonatal period. Intussusception is more common in boys than girls (M:F 3:1). The incidence is approximately one case per 1000–2000 live births.

Etiology

- In infants, the causes of intussusception are not fully known.
- Most cases of intussusception in young children are:
  - Idiopathic.
  - Some viral and bacterial infections may possibly contribute to intussusception in infancy.
  - Intussusception is seen most often in spring and fall, and because of this some theories suggest a possible connection to viruses during these seasons, including upper respiratory infections and gastroenteritis.
  - These infections may cause enlargement of the mesenteric lymph nodes which may act as a leading point to intussusception.

Types of Intussusceptions According to Etiology

- Intussusception is divided into two types according to etiology.
- Idiopathic intussusception:
  - Usually starts at the ileocecal junction and affects infants and toddlers.
  - In this type, there is no apparent leading point as a cause for intussusception.
- Intussusception may be secondary to a lead point:
  - This is seen in approximately 2–12 % of infants and children with intussusception.
  - This is seen most commonly in infants younger than 3 months or older than 5 years of age. The lead points include:

1. Meckel's diverticulum
2. Enlarged mesenteric lymph node
3. Benign or malignant tumors of the mesentery or of the intestine, including:
   - Lymphoma
   - Intestinal polyps
   - Ganglioneuroma
   - Hamartomas associated with Peutz–Jeghers syndrome
4. Mesenteric or duplication cysts
5. Submucosal hematomas, which can occur in patients with Henoch–Schönlein purpura and coagulopathies
6. Ectopic pancreatic and gastric rests
7. Inverted appendiceal stumps
8. Sutures and staples along an anastomosis
9. Intestinal hematomas secondary to abdominal trauma
10. Foreign bodies
11. Intestinal hemangioma
12. Kaposi sarcoma
13. Posttransplantation lymphoproliferative disorders

Types of Intussusception According to Site

- Almost 90% of intussusceptions affect the ileocolic region of the intestine (ileocolic intussusceeption).
- Enteroenteral intussusception (jejunojejunal, jejunoileal, ileoileal):
  - Is rare
  - Occurs in older children or infants less than 3 months of age
  - Usually associated with other medical conditions (Henoch-Schönlein purpura, cystic fibrosis, hematologic dyscrasias)
  - May be secondary to a lead point
  - Occasionally occurs in the postoperative period.

Symptoms and Signs

- The patient is usually chubby and in good general health.
- The illness is often preceded by an upper respiratory tract infection.
- A triad of symptoms including:
  - Vomiting
  - Abdominal pain
  - Passage of blood per rectum (currant jelly stools; Fig. 24.1)
- Usually described but this occurs in only one-third of patients.
- The primary symptom of intussusception is intermittent colicky abdominal pain. The infant intermittently draws the knees up to the chest while crying and in between attacks the child appears calm and relieved.

Fig. 24.1 Red currant jelly stools

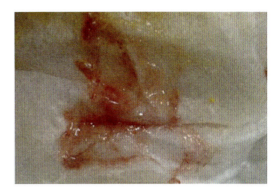

- Most infants will also have episodes of vomiting associated with the pain. This vomiting is usually nonbilious to start with but when intestinal obstruction occurs, it becomes bilious.
- Some infants with time may pass "currant jelly stool." This stool is bloody and mucous.
- As the condition progress, the infant may become weaker and develop additional symptoms, including those associated with shock, such as paleness, lethargy, and fever.
- An abdominal "sausage-shaped" mass (the intussusception itself) may become palpable commonly in the right hypochondrium and a feeling of emptiness in the right lower quadrant (Dance sign). This mass is hard to detect and is best palpated between spasms of colic, when the infant is quiet.
- The mass may be palpable at any site along the colon course and rarely may prolapse through the anal canal.
- Abdominal distention becomes apparent clinically when the obstruction becomes complete.

Diagnosis

- Plain abdominal radiographs reveal signs that suggest intussusception in only 60% of cases. They may be normal early in the course of intussusception.
- As the disease progresses, the earliest radiographic signs include an absence of air in the right lower and upper quadrants and a right upper quadrant soft tissue density which is present in 25–60% of patients.
- These findings are followed by features of small bowel obstruction, with dilatation and air-fluid levels in the small intestines.
- Abdominal ultrasound is the main stay of diagnosing intussusception with an overall sensitivity and specificity of 97.9 and 97.8%, respectively. Ultrasonography should be the first examination in those with suspected intussusception.
- The ultrasonographic signs of intussusception include the target and pseudokidney signs as well as dilated bowel loops (Figs. 24.2 and 24.3).
- The most reliable method to diagnose ileo-ileocolic, ileocolic, or colocolic intussusception is a contrast enema (either barium or air; Fig. 24.4).
- Contrast enema is quick and reliable and has the potential to be therapeutic.
- Absolute contraindications to attempt a nonoperative reduction with a therapeutic enema:
    – The presence of peritonitis
    – Evidence of perforation on plain radiographs

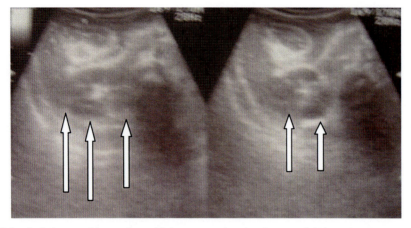

Fig. 24.2 Abdominal ultrasound in a patient with intussusception showing *pseudokidney sign*

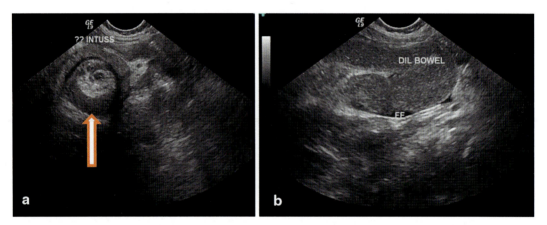

Fig. 24.3 a and **b**, Abdominal ultrasound showing the target sign (*daunt sign*). Note the dilated bowel loops in **b**

Management

- For all children, start intravenous fluid resuscitation, broad-spectrum antibiotics, and nasogastric decompression as soon as possible.
- Nonoperative radiologic reduction is best performed with the pediatric surgeon on standby, because complications (perforation) may develop and require immediate surgery.
- Therapeutic enemas can be hydrostatic, with either barium or water-soluble contrast, or pneumatic, with air insufflation.
- Therapeutic enemas can be performed under fluoroscopic or ultrasonographic guidance (Figs. 24.5 and 24.6).
- When performing a therapeutic enema, the recommended pressure of air insufflation should not exceed 120 cm of water. When using barium or water-soluble contrast, the column of contrast should not exceed 100 cm above the level of the buttocks.
- Traditionally, an attempt was not considered successful until the reducing agent, whether air, barium, or water-soluble contrast, was observed refluxing back into the terminal ileum, but evidence has shown that this is not entirely necessary (Fig. 24.6).

Fig. 24.4 Contrast enema showing intussusception

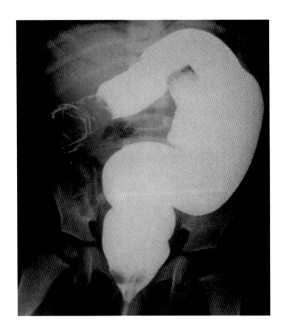

Fig. 24.5 Contrast enema showing intussusception being reduced under fluoroscopic control

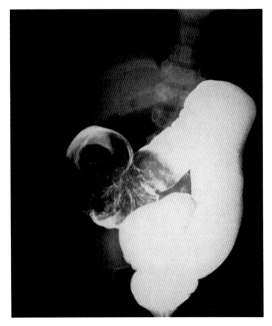

- Most intussusceptions that failed to show reflux into the ileum were due to either an edematous or competent ileocecal valve.
- A patient who becomes asymptomatic after nonoperative reduction that fails to show reflux of the reducing agent into the ileum can safely be observed and, if deemed necessary, a repeat attempt of therapeutic enema can be done.
- The recurrence rate of intussusception after nonoperative reduction is usually <10% but has been reported to be as high as 15%.
- Most intussusceptions recur within 72 h of the initial event; however, recurrences have been reported as long as 36 months later.

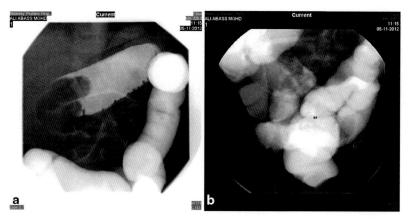

Fig. 24.6 a and **b**, A contrast enema showing intussusception being reduced. Note the reflux of contrast enema into the terminal ileum in **b**

- If the first attempt of nonoperative reduction fails, one or two subsequent attempts can be done within a few minutes to a few hours after the first attempt. The first attempt can reduce the intussusception partially, making the intussusceptum less edematous, with improved venous drainage.
- If repeated attempts are unsuccessful, any progress in pushing back the intussusceptum toward the ileocecal valve is advantageous. This will make the operative approach limited to an incision in the right iliac fossa and makes operative reduction easier.
- Therapeutic enema is of no value in patients with small bowel-to-small bowel intussusception.
- Intussusception in the first month of life is rare. Most of these patients are found to have a surgical lead point; therefore, enemas are rarely successful and are potentially dangerous.
- Once operative reduction was successful a cecopexy is not necessary.
- The risk of recurrence of the intussusception after operative reduction is <5%.
- If manual reduction is not possible or perforation is present, a segmental resection with an end-to-end anastomosis becomes necessary.
- A careful search for any lead points is warranted, especially if the patient is older than 2–3 years.
- Surgical reduction with or without resection becomes necessary in patients:
  - With ileoileal intussusception
  - With failed nonoperative reduction
  - With intussusception in the first month of life
  - With failed manual reduction
  - With perforation
  - With a lead point
- Laparoscopy has become recently one of the favored methods of the treatment of intussusception. It is valuable in reduction of the intussusception, confirmation of radiologic reduction, and detection of lead points.
- Laparoscopy is associated with faster recovery, decreased length of hospital stay, decreased time to full feeds, and lower requirements for analgesia.

Recommended Reading

Saverino BP, Lava C, Lowe LH, Rivard DC. Radiographic findings in the diagnosis of pediatric ileocolic intussusception: comparison to a control population. Pediatr Emerg Care. 2010;26(4):281–4.

Chapter 25
Intestinal Malrotation

Introduction

- Intestinal malrotation is defined as intestinal nonrotation or incomplete rotation around the superior mesenteric artery (Figs. 25.1 and 25.2).
- It involves anomalies of intestinal fixation as well.
- This can occur at a wide range of locations and leads to acute and chronic presentations.
- The most common type found in pediatric patients is incomplete rotation predisposing to midgut volvulus, which can result in short-bowel syndrome or even death.
- In 1936, William E. Ladd wrote the classic article on treatment of malrotation, and his surgical approach (Ladd procedure) remains the cornerstone of practice today.
- The incidence of intestinal malrotation is one in 500 live births.
- The male-to-female ratio is 2:1.
- In infants, the mortality rate ranges from 2 to 24 %.
- As many as 40 % of patients with malrotation present within the 1st week of life.
- This condition is diagnosed in 50 % of patients by age 1 month and is diagnosed in 75 % by age 1 year. The remaining 25 % of patients present after age 1 year and into late adulthood; many are recognized intraoperatively during other procedures or at autopsy.

Embryology

- Malrotation represents a spectrum of anomalies, and understanding the normal embryology of intestinal rotation is important in this regard. This happens in stages and the superior mesenteric artery forms the axis of rotation around which two loops rotate. The duodenojejunal loop begins to rotate superior to the superior mesenteric artery, and the cecocolic loop begins to rotate inferior to the superior mesenteric artery. Both loops make a total of 270°.
- Stage I:
  - Occurs between the 5–10 weeks of gestation.
  - The intestines herniate into the base of the umbilical cord.
  - The duodenojejunal loop begins superior to the superior mesenteric artery at a 90° position and rotates 180° in a counterclockwise direction.
  - At 180°, the loop lies to the right of the superior mesenteric artery and by 270°; it lies beneath the superior mesenteric artery.
  - The cecocolic loop begins beneath the superior mesenteric artery at 270°.

Fig. 25.1 a and **b**, Diagrammatic representation of intestinal volvulus secondary to malrotation. The intestines twist in a clockwise direction around the superior mesenteric artery

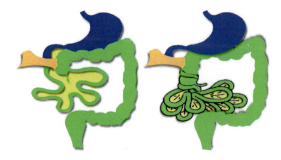

Fig. 25.2 Barium meal and follow-through in a patient with malrotation. Note that the duodenojejunal junction is lying on the right side of the spine and most of the small intestines are lying on the right side

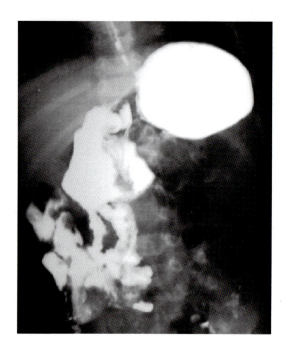

- It rotates 90° in a counterclockwise direction and lies to the left of the superior mesenteric artery at a 0° position.
- Both loops maintain these positions until the bowel returns to the abdominal cavity.
- Also during this stage, the midgut lengthens along the superior mesenteric artery, and, as rotation continues, a very broad pedicle is formed at the base of the mesentery. This broad base protects against midgut volvulus.

- Stage II:

  - Occurs at 10 weeks' gestation, the period when the bowel returns to the abdominal cavity.
  - As the bowel returns to the abdominal cavity, the duodenojejunal loop rotates an additional 90° to lie left of the superior mesenteric artery, the 0° position.
  - The cecocolic loop turns 180° more as it reenters the abdominal cavity. This turn places it to the right of the superior mesenteric artery, a 180° position.

- Stage III:

  - This stage lasts from 11 weeks' gestation until term.
  - During this stage, the cecum descends to the right lower quadrant.
  - Fixation of the mesenteries occurs at this stage.

- Nonrotation:
  - Results from arrest in development at stage I.
  - The duodenojejunal junction does not lie inferior and to the left of the superior mesenteric artery, and the cecum does not lie in the right lower quadrant.
  - The mesentery has a narrow base.
  - This narrow base is prone to clockwise twisting leading to midgut volvulus.
  - The width of the base of the mesentery is different in each patient, and not every patient develops midgut volvulus.
- Incomplete rotation:
  - Results from arrest in development at Stage II.
  - Most likely to result in duodenal obstruction.
  - Typically, the peritoneal bands running from the misplaced cecum to the mesentery compress the third portion of the duodenum leading to extrinsic duodenal obstruction.
  - Depending on how much rotation was completed prior to arrest, the mesenteric base may be narrow and, again, midgut volvulus can occur.
  - Internal herniations may also occur with incomplete rotation if the duodenojejunal loop does not rotate but the cecocolic loop does rotate. This may trap most of the small bowel in the mesentery of the large bowel, creating a right mesocolic (paraduodenal) hernia.
- Incomplete fixation:
  - Failure of the mesentery of the right and left colon and the duodenum to become fixed retroperitoneally leads to the formation of potential hernial pouches.
  - If the descending mesocolon between the inferior mesenteric vein and the posterior parietal attachment remains unfixed, the small intestine may push out through the unsupported area as it migrates to the left upper quadrant. This creates a left mesocolic hernia with possible entrapment and strangulation of the bowel.
  - If the cecum remains unfixed, volvulus of the terminal ileum, cecum, and proximal ascending colon may occur.Malrotation and associated conditions
- Intestinal malrotation is seen in association with the following conditions:
  - Gastroschisis, omphalocele, congenital diaphragmatic hernia, duodenal atresia, jejunoileal atresia, Hirschsprung's disease, gastroesophageal reflux, intussusception, persistent cloaca, anorectal malformations, and extrahepatic anomalies.

Clinical Features

The clinical features of malrotation are variable depending on the age of the patient as well as the type and degree of malrotation. The presentations of malrotation are divided as follows:

- Acute midgut volvulus:
  - This is the most serious presentation of malrotation.
  - Commonly seen in those < 1 year of age.
  - It is characterized by sudden onset of bilious vomiting and commonly abdominal distension.
  - Bleeding per rectum and sometimes hematemesis as a result of bowel vascular compromise.
  - As the symptoms progress, the infant becomes distressed with signs of peritonitis and shock.
  - Midgut volvulus prolongs hospitalization, and the prognosis depends on how much bowel is preserved.

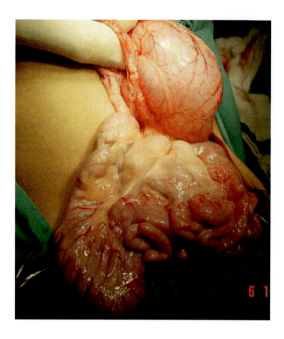

Fig. 25.3 Intraoperative photograph of a child with chronic volvulus

- Chronic midgut volvulus (Fig. 25.3):
  - Chronic midgut volvulus results from intermittent or partial twisting of the bowel.
  - This leads to lymphatic and venous obstruction.
  - The main presenting features are recurrent abdominal pain and malabsorption.
  - Other clinical features include recurrent attacks of diarrhea alternating with constipation, intolerance of solid food, obstructive jaundice, and gastroesophageal reflux.
  - Clinically, the patient appears normal between attacks but during an attack the picture is similar to that of acute midgut volvolus.
  - Chronic midgut volvolus may be complicated by an acute midgut volvulus.
  - Awareness of these clinical features is important to avoid misdiagnosis.

- Acute duodenal obstruction:
  - Malrotation is associated with Ladd bands which can cause compression of the second part of duodenum leading to extrinsic compression.
  - Commonly seen in infants.
  - Patients present with vomiting, which is commonly bile-stained, but may be non bile-stained depending on site of obstruction with respect to the ampulla of Vater.
  - The presence of Ladd bands however does not exclude an intrinsic cause of duodenal obstruction which must be looked for at the time of surgery.

- Chronic duodenal obstruction:
  - The usual presentation is vomiting which is usually bile-stained.
  - The age at diagnosis ranges from infancy to preschool age.
  - Other presenting features include intermittent abdominal pain and failure to thrive.
  - Diagnosis is usually made by history, suspicion, and radiologic studies.

- Internal hernia:
  - Results from herniation of bowels into recesses in the abdominal cavity.
  - They preset chronically with recurrent abdominal pain, vomiting, and constipation.

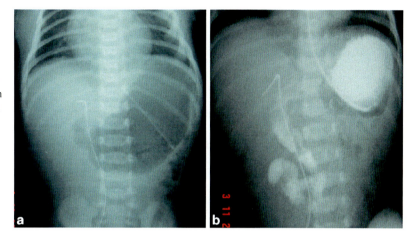

Fig. 25.4 Plain abdominal X-ray (**a**) and upper gastrointestinal contrast study (**b**). Note the dilated stomach and the scanty air distally and position of the duodenojejunal junction on the right side in the second X-ray

- This may progress from an intermittent picture to an acute presentation.
- The diagnosis is made by radiologic studies and index of suspicion but if the bowel is obstructed at the time of presentation, abdominal tenderness and guarding may be present, and a soft globular mass may be palpable the hernia site.

Investigations

The following investigations are important for patients with intestinal malrotation:

- Complete blood count (CBC), arterial, capillary, or venous blood gases, blood urea, creatinine, and electrolytes, urinalysis and urine culture, type and screen, prothrombin time (PT), and activated partial thromboplastin time (aPTT).

Radiological investigations:

- Plain abdominal radiography
  - This may reveal classic pattern for duodenal obstruction (the double-bubble sign) with little gas in the remainder of the intestines (Fig. 25.4).
- Upper gastrointestinal study (Fig. 25.5):
  - This is the study of choice to diagnose malrotation in a stable patient.
  - Normal rotation is present if the duodenal C-loop crosses the midline and the duodenojejunal junction lies to the left of the spine. The small intestines are usually present only in the right side of the abdomen.
  - If the contrast ends abruptly or a corkscrew pattern is seen, midgut volvulus may be present.
  - Contrast studies may not be possible in patients who are actively vomiting or are otherwise unstable and need immediate surgical exploration.
- Lower gastrointestinal study:
  - Contrast enema may be used to identify the location of the cecum.
  - Lower gastrointestinal study can also rule out colonic and ileal atresia obstruction. However, a normally placed cecum does not rule out malrotation.

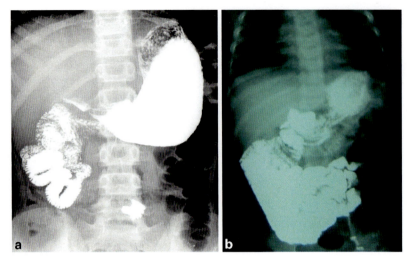

Fig. 25.5 Upper contrast study showing malrotation. Note the position of the duodenojejunal junction on the right side of the spine as well as the position of the small intestines on the right side and upper contrast study showing malrotation with midgut volvulus. Note the position of the duodenojejunal junction and the corkscrew appearance

- Ultrasonography:
  - Ultrasonography has been shown to be very sensitive in detecting neonatal malrotation. This is specially so if water is instilled first by nasogastric tube.
  - The main diagnostic finding is inversion of the superior mesenteric artery and the superior mesenteric vein.
  - Other diagnostic findings include: fixed bowel loops in the midline, duodenal dilation with distal tapering and coiling of the superior mesenteric vein around the superior mesenteric artery.

Management

The management is directed towards preoperative resuscitation, stabilization, and rapid surgical intervention.

- Insert a nasogastric or orogastric tube.
- Keep the patient nil by mouth (NPO).
- Correct intravenous fluids and electrolytes deficits.
- Administer broad-spectrum antibiotics prior to surgery.
- If the patient is unstable, do not delay surgical intervention for further investigations including upper gastrointestinal contrast and laboratory studies.
- Central venous catheter placement: Most patients require long-term intravenous access after surgery for intravenous fluids, antibiotics, and parenteral nutrition. This is especially so if midgut volvulus is present.
- The Ladd procedure remains the cornerstone of surgical treatment for malrotation today (Figs. 25.6, 25.7, and 25.8). This consists of:
  - Reduction of volvulus (if present). Because the volvulus usually twists in a clockwise direction, reduction is accomplished by twisting in a counterclockwise direction.
  - Division of Ladd bands.
  - Division of mesenteric bands including widening of the mesenteric base.
  - Placement of small bowel on the right side and large bowel on the left of the abdomen.
  - Appendectomy: This is important to avoid subsequent diagnostic confusion because of the abnormal position of the appendix when the cecum is placed in the left side of the abdomen.

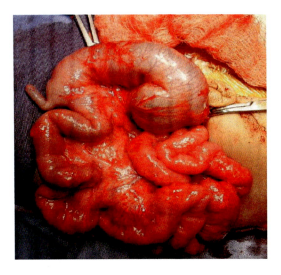

Fig. 25.6 Intraoperative photograph showing malrotation. Note the position of the appendix, colon, and small intestines. Note the mesentery after it was widened

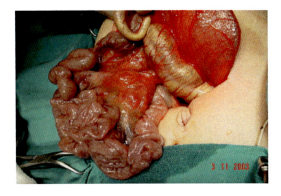

Fig. 25.7 Intraoperative photograph showing malrotation. Note the position of the small intestines on the right side, the colon, and appendix

- Midgut volvulus:
  - The volvulus is reduced.
  - The viability of bowel is checked.
  - When a small localized gangrenous segment is present, this is resected and a primary end-to-end anastomosis is performed.
  - If multiple areas of questionable viability are present, many surgeons choose to leave the areas and perform a second-look operation in 12–24 h if the patient is not showing clinical recovery.
- Duodenal obstruction:
  - In those with duodenal obstruction, all the peritoneal bands crossing the duodenum are divided.
  - If the extrinsic obstruction is due to the abnormally placed cecum, it is mobilized with its mesentery and placed in the left upper quadrant.
  - It is always important after relieving the extrinsic obstruction to check and look that no intrinsic cause for the obstruction exists by passing an NG tube through the duodenum.
- Laparoscopy:
  - With the recent advances in minimal invasive surgery, laparoscopic Ladd procedure has been performed successfully and being reported more frequently in the literature.
  - Currently, it is becoming more accepted as an initial approach to surgical correction of malrotation without midgut volvulus.

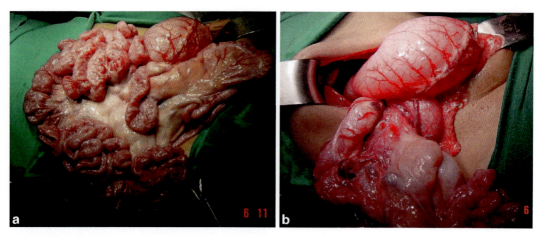

Fig. 25.8 Intraoperative photograph showing malrotation. Note the widened mesentery and the position of all small intestines on the right side and also the venous and lymphatic congestion

Complications

- Short-bowel syndrome:
    - Short-bowel syndrome is the most common complication of midgut volvulus.
    - This results from extensive resection of small bowel because of gangrene.
    - They are at high risk for malabsorption.
    - They require long-term parenteral nutrition.
    - Furthermore, they have more complications from treatment and much longer hospital stays than patients with malrotation and no volvulus.
- Infection:
    - Wound infections and sepsis can occur in the immediate postoperative period, requiring extended treatment with intravenous antibiotics.
    - Infection because of long-term central venous catheters.
    - Translocation of enteric bacteria and superimposed candidal infection further complicate the hospital course.
- Postsurgical complications:
    - Adhesive small-bowel obstruction.
    - Recurrent volvulus.
    - Persistent gastrointestinal symptoms including: constipation, intractable diarrhea, chronic abdominal pain, vomiting, and feeding difficulties.

Recommended Reading

Draus JM Jr, Foley DS, Bond SJ. Laparoscopic Ladd procedure: a minimally invasive approach to malrotation without midgut volvulus. Am Surg. 2007;73(7):693–6.
Palanivelu C, Rangarajan M, Shetty AR, Jani K. Intestinal malrotation with midgut volvulus presenting as acute abdomen in children: value of diagnostic and therapeutic laparoscopy. J Laparoendosc Adv Surg Tech A. 2007;17(4):490–2.
Spigland N, Brandt ML, Yazbeck S. Malrotation presenting beyond the neonatal period. J Pediatr Surg. 1990;25(11): 1139–42.
Stanfill AB, Pearl RH, Kalvakuri K, Wallace LJ, Vegunta RK. Laparoscopic Ladd's procedure: treatment of choice for midgut malrotation in infants and children. J Laparoendosc Adv Surg Tech A. 2010;20:369–72.

Chapter 26
Meckel's Diverticulum

Introduction

- A Meckel's diverticulum is a true congenital diverticulum consisting of all three layers of the bowel wall with mucosa, submucosa, and muscularis propria.
- It is a vestigial remnant of the omphalomesenteric duct (also called the vitelline duct).
- It is the most frequent malformation of the gastrointestinal tract (Fig. 26.1)
- It is present in approximately 2 % of the population.
- It was first described by Fabricius Hildanus in the sixteenth century and later named after Johann Friedrich Meckel, who described its embryological origin in 1809.
- Meckel's diverticulum may harbor abnormal tissues including jejunum, duodenal mucosa, or Brunner glands (2 % of ectopic cases).
- Heterotopic rests of gastric mucosa and pancreatic tissue are seen in 60 and 6 % of cases respectively.
- The prevalence of Meckel's diverticulum in males is three to five times higher than in females.
- The majority of Meckel's diverticulum are asymptomatic and only 2 % of cases are symptomatic.
- Meckel's diverticulum is located in the distal ileum, usually within about 60–100 cm (2 ft) of the ileocecal valve.
- It is typically 3–5 cm long, runs antimesenterically, and has its own blood supply.
- The rule of 2s for Meckel's diverticulum:
  - 2 % of the population.
  - 2 ft from the ileocecal valve.
  - 2 in. (in length).
  - 2 % are symptomatic.
  - 2 types of common ectopic tissue (gastric and pancreatic).
  - 2 years is the most common age at clinical presentation.
  - 2 times more boys are affected.
- Meckel's diverticulum can also present in an indirect hernia, typically on the right side, where it is known as a "Littré Hernia."
- Furthermore, it can be attached to the umbilical region by the vitelline ligament, with the possibility of vitelline cysts, or even a patent vitelline canal forming a vitelline fistula when the umbilical cord is cut. Torsion of intestine around the intestinal stalk may also occur, leading to obstruction, ischemia, and necrosis.

Fig. 26.1 Diagrammatic representation of Meckel's diverticulum. It is a true diverticulum composed of all the three layers and lies on the antimesenteric border of the intestines

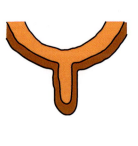

Fig. 26.2 Diagrammatic representation of Meckel's diverticulum

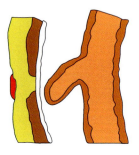

Fig. 26.3 Diagrammatic representation of an omphalomesenteric fibrous band attached to the site of Meckel's diverticulum on the intestines side and site of umbilicus

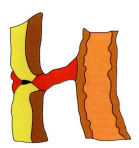

Embryology

- Embryologically, the omphalomesenteric duct (omphaloenteric duct, vitelline duct, or yolk stalk) connects the embryonic midgut to the yolk sac ventrally, providing nutrients to the midgut during embryonic development.
- Subsequently, the vitelline duct narrows progressively and disappears between the 5th and 8th weeks of gestation.
- Sometimes, the proximal part of vitelline duct fails to regress and involute, and remains as a remnant of variable length forming Meckel's diverticulum (Fig. 26.2).
- Meckel's diverticulum lies on the antimesenteric border of the ileum and extends into the umbilical cord of the embryo.
- The left and right vitelline arteries originate from the primitive dorsal aorta, and travel with the omphaloenteric duct. The right branch becomes the superior mesenteric artery that supplies a terminal branch to Meckel's diverticulum, while the left involutes.
- Other possible omphaloenteric duct anomalies include:
    - An omphalomesentric ligament/fibrous band (Fig. 26.3).
    - An omphalomesenteric fistula (Fig. 26.4).
    - An omphalomesentric cyst (Fig. 26.5).
    - A persistent vitelline artery running along the fibrous cord which connects the ileum to the umbilicus.

Symptoms

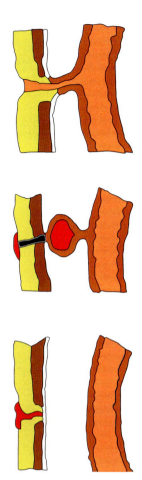

Fig. 26.4 Diagrammatic representation of an omphalomesenteric fistula. Note the communication between the intestines and umbilicus

Fig. 26.5 Diagrammatic representation of an omphalomesenteric cyst. The cyst is attached to the site of Meckel's diverticulum on one side and the umbilicus on the other side

Fig. 26.6 Diagrammatic representation of an umbilical sinus

- An umbilical sinus (Fig. 26.6).
- Meckel's diverticulum may also contain heterotropic tissues as follows:
  - Gastric mucosa (60%).
  - Pancreatic tissue (6%).
  - Both pancreatic tissue and gastric mucosa (5%).
  - Jejunal mucosa (2%).
  - Brunner tissue (2%).
  - Both gastric and duodenal mucosa (2%).
  - Rarely, colonic, rectal, endometrial, and hepatobiliary tissues have been noted.

Symptoms

- The majority of people with Meckel's diverticulum are asymptomatic.
- Meckel's diverticulum is most frequently diagnosed as an incidental finding when a laparotomy or laparoscopy is performed for other abdominal conditions.
- The lifetime risk for a person with Meckel's diverticulum to develop complications is about 4–6%.
- Meckel's diverticulum becomes symptomatic as a result of complications.

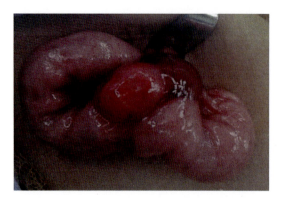

Fig. 26.7 An intraoperative photograph of a patient with bleeding Meckel's diverticulum. Note the ectopic tissue at the site of Meckel's diverticulum

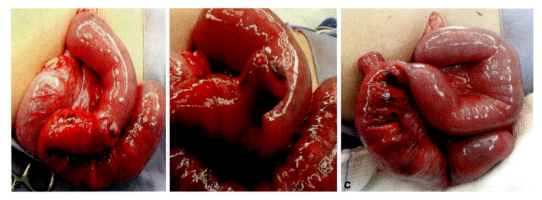

Fig. 26.8 a–c An intraoperative photograph showing Meckel's diverticulum as a lead point causing intussusception, which is being reduced

- This is estimated to occur in as many as 4–16 % of patients.
- Complications include:
  - Obstruction (25–35 %)
  - Ectopic tissue causing bleeding or intussusception (Figs. 26.7 and 26.8)

Volvolus

1. Intussusception.
2. Inflammation (diverticulitis) (10–20 %).
3. Hemorrhage (20–30 %).
4. Umbilical fistula (10 %).
5. Other umbilical anomalies (1 %).

- If symptoms do occur, they typically appear before the age of 2 years.
- The most common presenting symptom is painless rectal bleeding followed by intestinal obstruction, volvulus, and intussusception.
- Most of the time, bleeding occurs without warning and stops spontaneously.
- Occasionally, Meckel's diverticulitis may present with all the features of acute appendicitis.
- Hemorrhage:

Fig. 26.9 A clinical photograph of a resected Meckel's diverticulum that was opened. Note the ectopic gastric tissue causing ulceration and bleeding

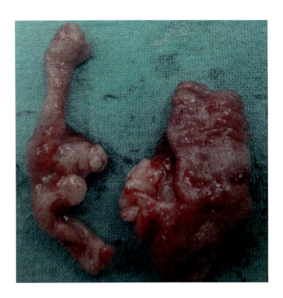

- May be caused by ectopic gastric or pancreatic mucosa (Fig. 26.9).
- Secretion of gastric acid or alkaline pancreatic fluid from the ectopic tissue leads to ulceration in the adjacent ileal mucosa (peptic or pancreatic ulcer).
- This will lead to pain, bleeding, or perforation of the bowel at the diverticulum.
- Mechanical stimulation may also cause erosion and ulceration.
- Acute gastrointestinal bleeding may be self-limiting but chronic bleeding may lead to iron deficiency anemia.

- Diverticulitis:
  - Inflammation of Meckel's diverticulum can mimic symptoms of acute appendicitis.
  - Perforation of the inflamed diverticulum can result in peritonitis.
  - Diverticulitis can also cause adhesions, leading to intestinal obstruction.
  - Meckel's diverticulum is less prone to inflammation than the appendix because most diverticula have a wide mouth, have very little lymphoid tissue, and are self-emptying.

- A mesodiverticular band:
  - A mesodiverticular band attached to Meckel's diverticulum tip can lead to torsion causing inflammation and ischemia.

- Perforation of Meckel's diverticulum can also be caused by trauma or ingested foreign material (e.g. fish/chicken bone) that become lodged in the diverticulum.
- Intestinal obstruction:
  - Luminal obstruction due to tumors, enterolith, foreign body, leading to stasis or bacterial infection with subsequent adhesions and obstruction.
  - The vitelline vessel remnant that connects the diverticulum to the umbilicus may form a fibrous or twisting band (volvulus), trapping the small intestine and causing obstruction.
  - Incarceration: when a Meckel's diverticulum is constricted in an inguinal hernia, forming a Littré hernia that obstructs the intestine.
  - Tumors: Direct spread of an adenocarcinoma arising in the diverticulum may lead to obstruction.
  - The diverticulum itself or tumor within it may cause intussusception.

Fig. 26.10 Diagrammatic representation showing prolapse of intestinal loops through a persistent vitelline duct fistula at the umbilicus

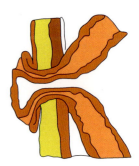

- Stones (lithiasis) that are rarely formed in Meckel's diverticulum can extrude into the terminal ileum, leading to obstruction or induce local inflammation and intussusception.
- Obstruction can be the result of various mechanisms.
  ○ Omphalomesenteric band (most frequent cause).
  ○ Internal hernia through vitelline duct remnants.
  ○ Volvulus occurring around vitelline duct remnants.
  ○ T-shaped prolapse of both efferent and afferent loops of intestine through a persistent vitelline duct fistula at the umbilicus (Fig. 26.10).
  ○ Intussusception: when Meckel's diverticulum itself acts as a lead point for an ileocolic or ileoileal intussusception.
• Meckel's diverticulum rarely present in the neonatal period but there are reports of Meckel's diverticulum presenting as perforation, intussusception, segmental ileal dilation, and ileal volvulus in newborns.

Diagnosis

• According to Mayo, "Meckel's Diverticulum is frequently suspected, often looked for, and seldom found."
• Preoperative diagnosis of Meckel's diverticulum is difficult, especially if the presenting symptom is not GI bleeding.
• Routine laboratory tests including complete blood count (CBC), electrolytes, blood urea nitrogen (BUN), creatinine, and coagulation screen, blood grouping, and cross matching are necessary to manage a patient with GI bleeding.
• When a patient has GI bleeding suggestive of Meckel's diverticulum, a technetium-99 m (99mTc) pertechnetate scan, also called Meckel's scan, is the investigation of choice.
• This scan detects gastric mucosa which is displayed as a spot on the scan distant from the stomach itself.
• In children, a Meckel's scan has a sensitivity of 80–90 %, a specificity of 95 %, and an accuracy of 90 %.
• A bleeding scan can be performed to identify the source if the patient is bleeding at a rate of 0.1 ml/min or more.
• Other tests such as colonoscopy and screenings for bleeding disorders should be performed.
• Angiography can assist in determining the location and severity of bleeding but this is an invasive procedure.
• Barium studies have largely been replaced by other imaging techniques
• In asymptomatic patients, Meckel's diverticulum is often diagnosed as an incidental finding during laparoscopy or laparotomy.

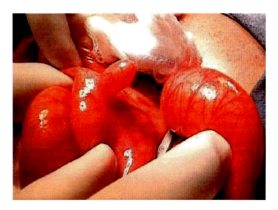

Fig. 26.11 An intraoperative clinical photograph showing Meckel's diverticulum which is short and with a wide neck

- Ultrasonography has been used in some cases of Meckel's diverticulum.
- Capsule endoscopy has been successfully used to identify Meckel's diverticulum in young children.

Treatment

- Most symptomatic patients with Meckel's diverticulum are acutely ill and it is important to establish an intravenous (IV) line, start IV fluids, and keep the patient nothing by mouth. Obtain the necessary investigations and arrange for blood grouping and cross match.
- If significant bleeding occurs, transfuse packed red blood cells.
- A patient who presents with intestinal obstruction should also have a nasogastric tube for gastric decompression.
- Treatment of Meckel's diverticulum is surgical excision.
- Excision is carried out by performing a wedge resection of adjacent ileum and anastomosis, with the use of a stapling device. Adjacent ileum is included in the resection because ulcers frequently develop in the adjacent part of the ileum.
- Successful resection of a Meckel's diverticulum, even in children and infants, can also be accomplished laparoscopically.
- Asymptomatic Meckel's diverticulum:
  - Management of Meckel's diverticulum in asymptomatic patients is controversial.
  - Some recommend looking for Meckel's diverticulum in every case of appendicectomy/laparotomy done for acute abdomen and if found, Meckel's diverticulectomy or resection should be performed to avoid secondary complications arising from it.
  - This is supported by the fact that Meckel's diverticulectomy is a simple operation, and managing a complication of Meckel's diverticulum is associated with high morbidity and mortality rates.
  - Others feel the only exception to universal excision is if the diverticulum has a wide neck or so short that stapled excision cannot be performed.
  - This practice was questioned when a large series described an overall 4.2% likelihood of complications in Meckel's diverticulum and a decreasing risk with increasing age.
  - The general consensus for removing an asymptomatic Meckel's diverticulum discovered at laparotomy or laparoscopy is:
    - If it has a narrow neck (Fig. 26.11).
    - If it contains visible ectopic tissue.

Recommended Reading

Pepper VK, Stanfill AB, Pearl RH. Diagnosis and management of pediatric appendicitis, intussusception, and meckel diverticulum. Surg Clin North Am. 2012;92(3):505–26.

Tauro LF, Martis JJ, Menezes LT, Shenoy HD. Clinical profile and surgical outcome of Meckel's diverticulum. J Indian Med Assoc. 2011;109:489–90.

Chapter 27
Meconium Ileus

Introduction

- Meconium ileus is a common cause of neonatal distal small-bowel (the terminal ileum) obstruction. It is the third most common cause of neonatal bowel obstruction after atresia and malrotation.
- It accounts for up to 30 % of neonatal small-bowel obstructions.
- Meconium ileus is caused by abnormally tenacious meconium.
- It is seen commonly in neonates with cystic fibrosis.
- About 10–20 % of infants with cystic fibrosis present with meconium ileus at birth, but it may be associated more rarely with other conditions such as:
  - Pancreatic aplasia
  - Pancreatic duct obstruction
  - Decreased intestinal motility with no apparent abnormality
- In cystic fibrosis, the meconium is thick and viscous, due to the pancreatic enzyme deficiencies and abnormal chloride secretion in the intestine.
- Meconium ileus may be the first clinical manifestation of cystic fibrosis.

Etiology

- Meconium ileus associated with cystic fibrosis is a manifestation of intestinal and pancreatic dysfunction that results in the accumulation of viscid, sticky, and inspissated intraluminal meconium that adheres to the intestinal mucosa.
- Obstruction occurs at the level of the terminal ileum.
- Meconium ileus is an early manifestation of cystic fibrosis which is an autosomal recessive disease.
- This results from mutation of the cystic fibrosis transmembrane conductance regulator (CFTR) gene.
- The CFTR gene is located on the long (q) arm of chromosome 7 at position 31.2.
- The CFTR gene provides instructions for making a protein called the cystic fibrosis transmembrane conductance regulator.
- This protein functions as a channel across the membrane of cells that produce mucus, sweat, saliva, tears, and digestive enzymes.

- The channel transports chloride ions into and out of cells.
- The transport of chloride ions helps control the movement of water in tissues, which is necessary for the production of thin, freely flowing mucus.
- The CFTR protein also regulates the function of other channels, such as those that transport sodium ions across cell membranes. These channels are necessary for the normal function of organs such as the lungs and pancreas.
- As a result, cells that line the passageways of the lungs, pancreas, and other organs produce mucus that is abnormally thick and sticky. The abnormal mucus obstructs the airways and glands, leading to the characteristic signs and symptoms of cystic fibrosis.
- Fetal achylia.
- Fetal pancreatic fibrosis.
- In association with bilateral renal dysplasia, fetal pancreatic fibrosis, meconium ileus, and situs inversus totalis.
- Pancreatic aplasia (pancreas agenesis).

Clinical Presentation

- Clinically, the neonate may have abdominal distension, failure to pass meconium, and bilious vomiting (Fig. 27.1).
- Meconium ileus is divided into simple or complicated.
- Simple meconium ileus: There is simple obstruction of the terminal ileum. The distal small bowel (terminal ileum) contains inspissated, thick viscous meconium, and proximal to this the ileum is distended while the colon is small and unused (microcolon).
- Complicated meconium ileus: can be associated with:
    - Volvulus
    - Bowel gangrene
    - Perforation
    - Intestinal atresia
    - Pseudocyst formation
    - Perforation
    - Meconium peritonitis
- Volvulus occurs due to the distended loops of terminal ileum and can lead to vascular compromise and bowel gangrene.
- Perforation can occur and causes meconium peritonitis. This is generally a sterile, chemical peritonitis that causes irritation of the peritoneal surfaces. With healing, calcifications can take place.

Differential Diagnosis

- Meconium plug syndrome, ileal atresia, colonic atresia, intestinal pseudo-obstruction, and Hirschsprung's disease

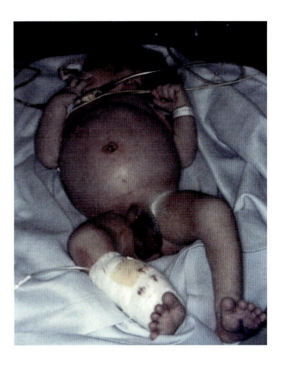

Fig. 27.1 A clinical photograph showing a newborn with abdominal distension secondary to meconium ileus

Investigations

- Plain abdominal radiographs: These are usually nonspecific and show multiple dilated loops of small bowel. The thick meconium has a ground-glass appearance and when mixed with air gives the intestinal contents a granular soap-bubble appearance (Fig. 27.2).
- The soap-bubble appearance may be seen also in Hirschsprung's disease, ileal or colonic atresia, or meconium plug syndrome.
- Air-fluid levels may be seen in the dilated small bowel. The presence of air-fluid levels should raise the possibility of associated intestinal atresia (Fig. 27.3).
- The presence of calcifications on abdominal radiographs is suggestive of meconium peritonitis. This is seen as scattered amorphous or curvilinear calcifications. The calcifications can also be associated with formation of adhesions and subsequent bowel obstruction.
- Contrast enema: Typically show a microcolon (unused small colon). The contrast enema should reflux into the terminal ileum, which is filled with pellets of meconium and establishes the diagnosis. Contrast enema can be diagnostic and therapeutic. In the absence of contrast reflux into the terminal ileum, surgery may be required to confirm the diagnosis (Fig. 27.4).

Treatment and Outcome

- The treatment of meconium ileus is divided into two types:
- Nonoperative:
  - This is the treatment of choice and consists of gastrograffin (meglumine diatrizoate) enemas.
  - Gastrograffin is a hyperosmolar aqueous solution which draws fluid into the bowel and softens and loosens the meconium, and it is important to adequately hydrate the infant prior to the enema.

Fig. 27.2 Plain abdominal radiograph showing dilated bowel loops

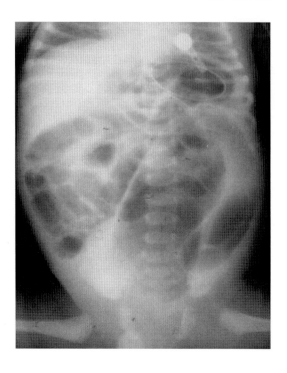

Fig. 27.3 Abdominal radiograph showing dilated bowel loops with air-fluid levels

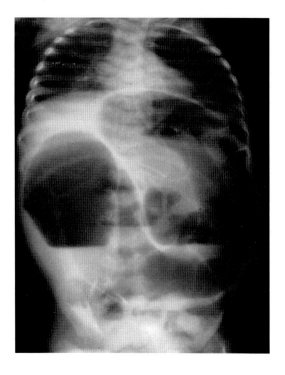

Fig. 27.4 Contrast enema showing small unused colon indicative of proximal small-bowel obstruction

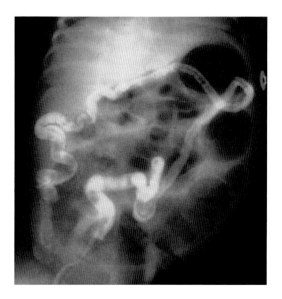

- Nonoperative therapy (therapeutic enemas) is effective in 40–60% of simple meconium ileus.
- The risk of perforation is approximately 3%.
- These enemas can be repeated at regular 12-h intervals until all meconium is evacuated.
- Patients with meconium ileus should be evaluated for cystic fibrosis.
- Pancreatic enzyme replacement and other measures specific to treatment of cystic fibrosis may be required.
- Surgery is reserved for those who fail nonoperative management.

- Surgical therapy (Fig. 27.5):
    - This is reserved for:
        - Patients with simple meconium ileus in whom nonoperative treatment fails
        - Those with complicated meconium ileus
    - The therapeutic options include:
        - Enterostomy with irrigation
        - Resection with anastomosis
        - Resection with ileostomy (Mikulicz, Bishop-Koop, and Santulli)
        - T-tube enterostomy with irrigation

- Postoperative management includes:
    - 10% N-acetylcysteine orally and through the ileostomy if present
    - Oral feedings (pregestimil)
    - Pancreatic enzyme replacement
    - Prophylactic pulmonary therapy

- Long-term prognosis depends on the degree of severity and progression of cystic fibrosis pulmonary complications:
    - Overall survival rates 80–90%.
    - 20% develop meconium ileus equivalent later in life.
    - Small risk of adhesive mechanical small-bowel obstructions later in life.

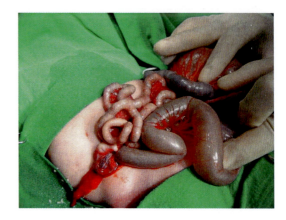

Fig. 27.5 Intraoperative clinical photograph showing meconium ileus. Note the dilated proximal bowel and the collapsed terminal ileum full of inspissated intraluminal meconium

Recommended Reading

Carlyle BE, Borowitz DS, Glick PL. A review of pathophysiology and management of fetuses and neonates with meconium ileus for the pediatric surgeon. J Pediatr Surg. 2012;47(4):772–81.

Jawaheer J, Khalil B, Plummer T, Bianchi A, Morecroft J, Rakoczy G, et al. Primary resection and anastomosis for complicated meconium ileus: a safe procedure? Pediatr Surg Int. 2007;23(11):1091–3.

Karimi A, Gorter RR, Sleeboom C, Kneepkens CM, Heij HA. Issues in the management of simple and complex meconium ileus. Pediatr Surg Int. 2011;27(9):963–8.

Chapter 28
Meconium Plug Syndrome

Introduction

- Meconium plug syndrome was first reported by Clatworthy in 1956.
- He described a syndrome of colonic obstruction because of inspissated meconium.
- Meconium plug syndrome is also called functional immaturity of the colon.
- Meconium plug syndrome is the most common form of functional bowel obstruction in the newborn, with an incidence of 1/500 newborns.
- Meconium plug syndrome is a transient disorder characterized by a delayed passage (>24–48 h) of meconium and intestinal dilatation.
- In general, meconium plug syndrome is observed in premature newborns that are otherwise normal.
- Cystic fibrosis and Hirschsprung's disease may be associated with meconium plug syndrome and should be excluded.

Etiology

- The exact cause of meconium plug syndrome is not known.
- The abnormality is due to functional immaturity of the colon in the newborn.

Associated Conditions

- Prematurity: Meconium obstruction in prematures is a distinct entity. It occurs in premature infants who develop obstructive symptoms several days after having passed meconium initially.
- Maternal diabetes has been associated with functional colonic obstruction.
- Generally, infants with meconium plug syndrome have normal bowel function after passing meconium but there is an association with Hirschsprung's disease (10–30 %) and cystic fibrosis (30–40 %).

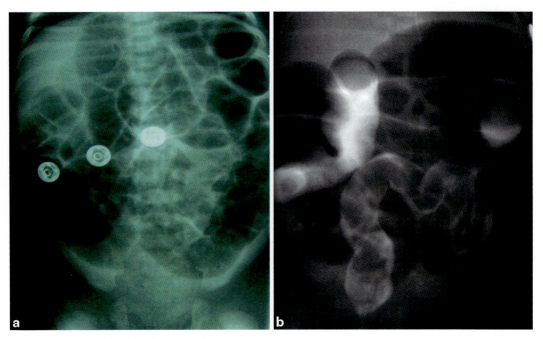

Fig. 28.1 a and **b** Plain abdominal x-ray showing dilated bowel loops with absent gas in the rectum. Gastrograffin contrast enema showing meconium plug syndrome

Clinical Features

- Meconium plug syndrome is a transient form of distal colonic obstruction caused by inspissated and dehydrated meconium.
- The impacted meconium leads to:
  - Failure to pass meconium
  - Abdominal distension
  - Vomiting

Differential Diagnosis

This includes:

- Hirschprung's disease, neuronal intestinal dysplasia, visceral neuropathies, meconium ileus, small left colon syndrome, and megacystis-microcolon-hypoperistalsis syndrome.

Diagnosis, Treatment, and Outcome

- Plain abdominal x-ray: The initial radiograph demonstrates numerous moderately distended loops of bowel with the absence of rectal gas which suggests a low gastrointestinal tract obstruction (Fig. 28.1a).

- Contrast enema: Gastrografin is a hypertonic solution containing both wetting and detergent agents. However, it is associated with complications secondary to hyperosmolarity which can lead to dehydration (Fig. 28.1b).
- When meconium plug syndrome is suspected, water-soluble contrast is used not only as a diagnostic tool but also to provide therapeutic benefits in helping to expel the meconium plugs from the colon and relieve the obstruction.
- Contrast enema usually shows a moderately dilated colon filled with radiolucent material (the meconium plug that produces a double-contrast effect).
- Contrast enema usually eliminates congenital small bowel obstruction and rare colon abnormalities.
- Following contrast enema, there may be a prompt passage of large meconium plugs with a fairly prompt resolution of the obstruction. The obstruction is often more severe and may require repeated contrast enema to relieve the obstruction.
- Infants with apparent meconium plug syndrome should be evaluated for Hirschsprung's disease (rectal-suction biopsy) when the findings persist after one to two enemas.
- Infants with meconium plug syndrome require subsequent testing for cystic fibrosis.

Recommended Reading

Burge DM, Drewett M. Meconium plug obstruction. Pediatr Surg Int. 2004;20(2):108–10.
Clatworthy HW Jr, Howard WH, Lloyd J. The meconium plug syndrome. Surgery. 1956;39(1):131–42.
Fuchs JR, Langer JC. Long-term outcome after neonatal meconium obstruction. Pediatrics. 1998;101(4):E7.

Chapter 29
Small Left Colon Syndrome

Introduction

- Neonatal small left colon syndrome is an uncommon cause of neonatal intestinal obstruction.
- In 1974, Davis coined the term small left colon syndrome. He described 20 infants with colonic obstruction not caused by a meconium plug or Hirschsprung's disease.
- Neonatal small left colon syndrome is characterized by an abrupt colonic caliber transition at or near the splenic flexure (Fig. 29.1).
- In the past, neonatal small left colon syndrome was included in the spectrum of obstructive conditions referred to as meconium plug syndrome.
- There is a strong association between neonatal small left colon syndrome and maternal gestational diabetes mellitus.

Etiology

- The exact etiology of neonatal small left colon syndrome is not known.
- Several theories have been proposed, including neural, humoral, and drug-induced etiologies.
- A frequent association of neonatal small left colon syndrome with maternal gestational diabetes mellitus has been reported.
- Maternal gestational diabetes mellitus induces neonatal hypoglycemia which affects intestinal motility via activation of the autonomic nervous system and glucagon release.
- Glucagon release is known to decrease motility in the left colon.
- Neonatal hypoglycemia also stimulates the sympathetic and parasympathetic autonomic nervous system.
- Parasympathetic stimulation results in increased motility in its area of distribution, which ends at the splenic flexure, whereas sympathetic stimulation results in diminished motility.
- The combined effect of glucagon release with sympathetic and parasympathetic stimulation results in an overall diminution in intestinal motility, with a functional obstruction in the colon beyond the splenic flexure.
- In 1974, Davis et al. reported the association of neonatal small left colon syndrome with abnormalities of intestinal neurohistology. Their initial report described increased numbers of immature small ganglion cells in the myenteric plexus (in both the narrowed and dilated parts of the colon) in patients with neonatal small left colon syndrome. They compared the histology from patients with small left colon syndrome with that of control subjects, including infants of dia-

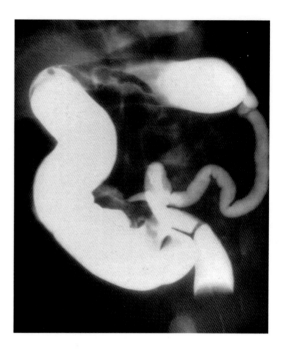

Fig. 29.1 Water-soluble enema showing small left colon syndrome

betic mothers without colon changes, premature infants, and term infants. They concluded that the hypercellularity observed in the specimens from patients with neonatal small left colon syndrome most closely resembled the histology observed in the colons of premature infants.
- Neonatal small left colon syndrome could be a form of intestinal neuronal dysplasia with an increase in the number of acetylcholinesterase (AChE)-stained fibers in the mucosa and increased submucosal ganglia or large ganglia. These changes are also observed with prematurity, and because most infants with neonatal small left colon syndrome in these reports were premature, it is difficult to conclude on these findings.
- Maternal drugs used during the third trimester can cross the placenta and affect the fetus. This was observed in infants born to mothers using psychotropic drugs with known anticholinergic effects. This as well as the hypermagnesemia (in infants born to eclamptic mothers treated with magnesium sulfate) can also cause hypomotility.
- Stress (eclampsia) may mediate the same changes through similar mechanisms.

Clinical Features

- Most patients with neonatal small left colon syndrome are born at or near term and are of normal birth weight.
- Approximately 50% have a history of maternal diabetes mellitus, and other maternal comorbidities (usually eclampsia), which contribute to neonatal stress.
- Failure to pass meconium within the first 24 h of life.
- Abdominal distension.
- Bilious vomiting.
- A small number of infants develop progressive distension leading to perforation, typically in the cecum, within the first 24–36 h of life.

Investigations

- Complete blood count and differential, C-reactive protein, coagulation profiles, and blood cultures.
- Measure serum levels of glucose, calcium, and magnesium in infants of mothers with diabetes mellitus or eclampsia.
- Blood grouping and crossmatching.
- Abdominal x-rays: This usually shows features of intestinal obstruction. Pneumoperitoneum which may result from a cecal perforation must be excluded.
- A water-soluble contrast enema: The diagnosis of neonatal small left colon syndrome on contrast enema examination is based on the following:

    1. Proximal dilation of the colon
    2. An abrupt cone-shaped caliber transition at or just distal to the splenic flexure
    3. A constricted, small and smooth contoured descending and sigmoid colon with a slightly larger caliber rectum (Fig. 29.2)

- The differential diagnosis includes meconium plug syndrome and Hirschsprung's disease.
- Hirschsprung's disease with a splenic flexure transition zone is clinically and radiologically indistinguishable from neonatal small left colon syndrome.
- The diagnosis of neonatal small left colon syndrome is not definitive until Hirschsprung's disease has been excluded and all infants must have a suction rectal biopsy performed to exclude aganglionosis.

Treatment

- Intravenous fluids.
- Nasogastric decompression.
- Intravenous antibiotics (if clinically indicated).
- Once plain abdominal radiographs have revealed a distal obstruction without pneumoperitoneum, the infant should undergo a water-soluble contrast enema.
- The contrast enema is not only diagnostic but also therapeutic. The vast majority of infants experience spontaneous passage of meconium after the enema and their abdominal distension resolves. Most infants completely respond to contrast enema decompression and are able to progress quite rapidly to full enteral feedings.
- Surgery is reserved for infants with intestinal perforation or for those in whom obstruction is refractory or recurrent, despite appropriate conservative measures.
- The type of surgery depends on the patient's general condition, availability of a pathologist for frozen suction, and the presence or absence of perforation.
- If the infant's condition is stable and a pathologist is available, seromuscular biopsies from the distal colon, the transition zone, and proximally should be performed and a stoma created in ganglionic bowel.
- In the rare case of intestinal perforation, a formal stoma or exteriorization of the perforation should be performed.
- Close follow-up during the first 2 weeks of life is important in these patients as they are liable to develop delayed complications in the form of recurrent or persistent obstruction or delayed perforation.

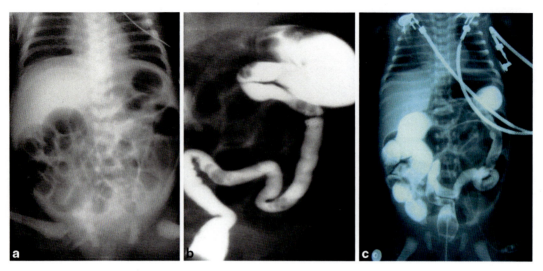

Fig. 29.2 a–c Plain abdominal x-ray showing dilated bowel loops and absence of air distally. Water-soluble enemas showing features of neonatal small left colon syndrome. Note the dilated proximal colon, transition zone, and slightly dilated rectum

Recommended Reading

Ellis H, Kumar R, Kostyrka B. Neonatal small left colon syndrome in the offspring of diabetic mothers-an analysis of 105 children. J Pediatr Surg. 2009;44(12):2343–6.

Falterman CG, Richardson CJ. Small left colon syndrome associated with maternal ingestion of psychotropic drugs. J Pediatr. 1980;97(2):308–10.

Kanto WP Jr, Morales V, Parrish R. Antenatal intestinal perforation and meconium peritonitis associated with the neonatal small left colon syndrome. South Med J. 1979;72(7):894–5.

Rangecroft L. Neonatal small left colon syndrome. Arch Dis Child. 1979;54(8):635.

Chapter 30
Congenital Rectal Stenosis and Atresia

Introduction

- Congenital rectal atresia is an extremely rare malformation.
- It is characterized by a normally placed anus and well-developed sphincter muscles.
- Congenital rectal atresia constitutes 1–2 % of all anorectal malformations.
- The anal canal is normal and the anus appears normal; however, there is obstruction usually 1–2 cm proximal to the dentate line.
- Its incidence is low worldwide.
- It is much more common in males, with a male-to-female ratio of 7:1.
- The largest series of congenital rectal atresia was reported by Dorairajan from the southern part of India (state of Tamil Nadu) where it constitutes about 14 % of all anorectal malformations. He reported 147 cases of congenital rectal atresia. The reason for this high incidence of congenital rectal atresia in that part of the world is not known.
- There is no well-established surgical technique to treat congenital rectal atresia, and several operative procedures were described.

Classification

- Congenital rectal atresia is considered a rare variant of anorectal malformations but there are different types depending on the classification used.
- Dorairajan classified congenital rectal atresia into four grades, depending on the distance between the proximal rectum and distal anorectum:
    - Grade 1: Rectal atresia with a short gap between each end. This is the commonest variety.
    - Grade 2: Rectal atresia with a long gap.
    - Grade 3: Membranous septal type.
    - Grade 4: Rectal stenosis (Fig. 30.1).
- Gupta and Sharma classified congenital rectal atresia into five types:
    - Type I: Rectal stenosis
    - Type II: Rectal atresia with a septal defect
    - Type III: Rectal atresia with a fibrous cord between the two atretic ends
    - Type IV: Rectal atresia with a gap
    - Type V: Multiple rectal atresia with stenosis (A) or without stenosis (B)

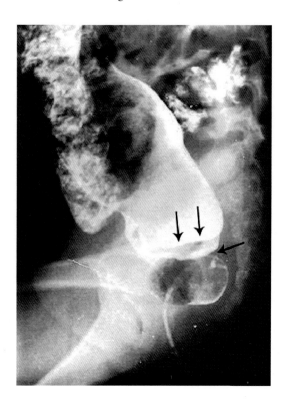

Fig. 30.1 A lateral photograph of a barium enema showing congenital rectal stenosis marked by *arrows*

Clinical Features

- Congenital rectal atresia in contrast to anorectal malformations is characterized by:
  - A normal-looking anus.
  - The anal canal and lower rectum are surrounded by a normally developed sphincter and hence a good functional postoperative outcome is expected.
- Unlike other anorectal malformations, congenital rectal atresia usually has no associated fistula communication with the urogenital system.
- Congenital rectal atresia commonly is an isolated malformation and without any other additional congenital anomalies.

Diagnosis

- The diagnosis of congenital rectal atresia is clinical.
- Patients usually present in the neonatal period with failure to pass meconium and abdominal distension (Fig. 30.2).
- Clinically, there is a normal-looking anus.
- Failure to pass a thermometer confirms the diagnosis.
- Abdominal X-ray shows dilated bowel loops with no gas distally and an invertogram shows stoppage of the air in the distal rectum (Fig. 30.3).

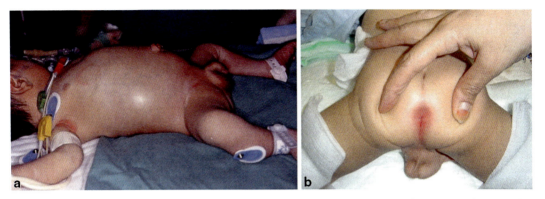

Fig. 30.2 Clinical photograph showing abdominal distension and a normal-looking anus in a patient with congenital rectal atresia

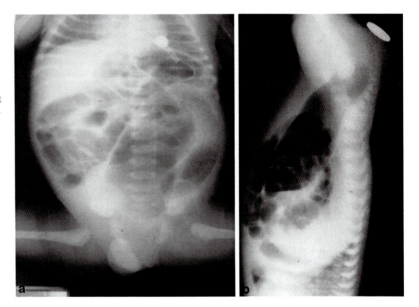

Fig. 30.3 Abdominal X-ray in a patient with congenital rectal atresia. Note the dilated bowel loops and absent gas distally in the pelvis (**a**) and an invertogram of a patient with congenital rectal atresia (**b**). Note the distance from the anal site and the gas in the distal rectum

- Once the diagnosis is suspected clinically, it can be confirmed by contrast study through the anal opening (Fig. 30.4).

Treatment

- The initial management is supportive with a nasogastric or orogastric tube, intravenous (IV) fluids, and IV antibiotics.
- The initial management is a sigmoid colostomy to decompress the abdominal distension and divert the stools.
- The distance from the anal verge can be confirmed subsequently by a contrast study through the colostomy and a marker in the anal opening.

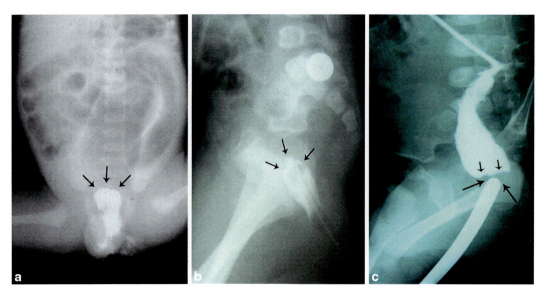

Fig. 30.4 A contrast study through the anal opening in a patient with congenital rectal atresia. **a** Note the site of the atresia marked with the *arrow*. **b** The lateral view shows the site of obstruction. The catheter is clearly seen pushing the site of atresia and contrast study through the colostomy. **c** A small dilator is passed through the anal opening to measure the distance between the two walls

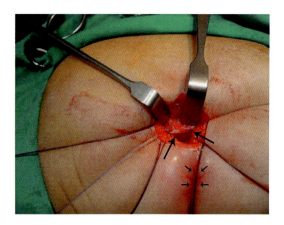

Fig. 30.5 An intraoperative photograph of a patient with congenital rectal atresia approached through a posterior sagittal incision. Note the site of rectal atresia marked by *large arrows*. Note also the extent of the incision to avoid division of the muscle complex. The site of normal anus is marked by *small arrows*

- The definitive treatment of congenital rectal atresia is controversial and several operative procedures have been described.
- These include:
  - Simple perforation of the membrane.
  - Transanal end-to-end rectorectal anastomosis.
  - Mucosal proctectomy and coloanal anastomosis.
  - Posterior sagittal anorectoplasty (Fig. 30.5).
  - Duhamel pull-through.
  - Laparoscopic and transanal approach.
  - Resection of rectal stenosis secondary to a membrane can be done using end-to-end anastomosis (EEA; Fig. 30.6).

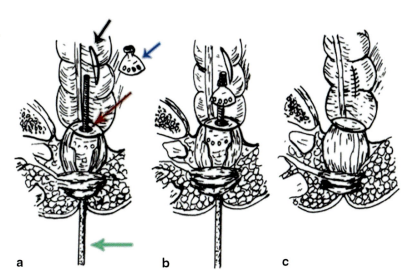

Fig. 30.6 Diagrammatic representation of the operative treatment of congenital rectal stenosis using EEA which is marked by the *green arrow*. The site of congenital rectal stenosis is marked by the *red arrow*, the anvil of the EEA is marked with a *blue arrow*, and the site of the colotomy is marked with a *black arrow*

- Since the anal canal and lower rectum are usually well developed and are surrounded by a normal sphincter, the long-term prognosis of these patients is excellent in term of bowel control and continence.
- Patients with congenital rectal atresia have a normally well-developed sphincteric muscle complex, and every attempt should be made to preserve it.
- Dividing the muscle complex is unnecessary to repair congenital rectal atresia and should be avoided.

Recommended Reading

Gupta DK, Sharma S. Rectal atresia and rectal ectasia. In: Hohlschneider AM, Hustson JM, editors. Anorectal malformations in children. Embryology, diagnosis, surgical treatment, follow-up. Berlin: Springer; 2006. p. 223–30.

Upadhyaya P. Rectal atresia: transanal, end-to-end, rectorectal anastomosis: a simplified, rational approach to management. J Pediatr Surg. 1990;25:535–37.

Chapter 31
Necrotizing Enterocolitis

Introduction

- Necrotizing enterocolitis (NEC) is an acute inflammatory condition characterized by variable degrees of damage to the intestines ranging from mucosal injury to full-thickness necrosis and perforation.
- NEC is the most common and serious gastrointestinal disorder occurring in neonates and typically affects premature infants but it can also be observed in term and near-term babies (Fig. 31.1).

Incidence

- The incidence of NEC is variable but generally affects 1–3 per 2000–4000 live births or between 1 and 5 % of neonatal intensive care unit admissions.
- The condition is typically seen in premature infants with an incidence of 30 per 1000 live births for extremely low-birth-weight neonates and 7–10 % of infants who weigh < 1500 g.
- Currently, NEC is occurring in more neonates, possibly because of the higher incidence and survival of premature and low-birth-weight neonates.
- NEC sometimes seems to occur in "epidemics," affecting several infants in the same nursery.

Etiology

- The exact etiology of NEC is unknown.
- NEC usually occurs within the first 2–3 weeks of life.
- Term infants, however develop NEC much earlier, with the average age of onset within the first week of life or, sometimes, within the first 1–2 days of life.
- The etiology is multifactorial.
- An ischemic or toxic event that causes damage to the immature gastrointestinal mucosa and loss of mucosal integrity has been proposed to precede NEC development.
- Conditions that compromise the intestinal circulation include:
  - Polycythemia/hyperviscosity
  - Birth asphyxia

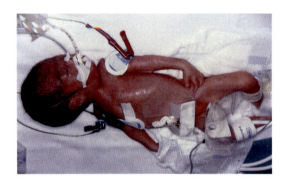

Fig. 31.1 Clinical photograph of a premature infant who is typically susceptible to NEC

- Exchange blood transfusion
- Severe congenital heart disease

• An infectious agent has been suspected, as cluster outbreaks in neonatal intensive care units have been seen.

- Gram-positive and gram-negative bacteria, fungi, and viruses have all been isolated from affected infants; however, many infants have negative cultures.
- Infectious organisms are thought to play a key role in the development of NEC.
- Positive blood cultures are found in 30% of patients; the most commonly identified organisms are *Escherichia coli* and *Klebsiella pneumoniae*. Other organisms include Proteus mirabilis, Staphylococcus aureus, S. epidermidis, Enterococcus species, Clostridium perfringens, and Pseudomonas aeruginosa.

• There are several risk factors for developing NEC. These include:

1. Premature neonates (less than 34 weeks' gestation)
2. Those of low birth weight (< 5 lb; 2.3 kg)
3. Enteral formula feeding
4. A difficult delivery and lowered oxygen levels during labor
5. Mechanical ventilation
6. Umbilical artery catheterization
7. Patent ductus arteriosus
8. *Premature rupture of membranes*
9. Patients treated with indomethacin to close PDA
10. *Polycythemia/hyperviscosity and exchange blood transfusion*

Clinical Features

• NEC most commonly affects the terminal ileum and the proximal ascending colon.
• However, varying degrees of NEC can affect any segment of the small intestine or colon.
• The near entire bowel may be also involved (NEC totalis) and may be irreversibly damaged.
• NEC represents a significant clinical problem and the clinical features are variable depending on the severity and extent of bowel involvement. Symptoms may come on slowly or suddenly.
• The classic clinical triad consists of:

- Abdominal distension
- Bloody stools
- Pneumatosis intestinalis

- The clinical presentation of NEC however includes nonspecific symptoms such as vomiting, diarrhea, feeding intolerance, and high gastric residuals following feedings.
- With disease progression, abdominal tenderness, abdominal wall edema, erythema, or palpable bowel loops indicating a fixed and dilated loop of bowel may develop.
- Systemic signs, such as apnea, bradycardia, lethargy, labile body temperature, hypoglycemia, and shock, are indicators of physiologic instability.
- The Bell system is the staging system most commonly used to describe NEC.

Bell stage I suspected NEC:

Stage IA characterized by the following:

- Mild, nonspecific systemic signs such as apnea, bradycardia, and temperature instability.
- Mild intestinal signs such as increased gastric residuals and mild abdominal distention.
- Radiographic findings can be normal or can show some mild nonspecific distention.

Stage IB diagnosis is the same as stage IA, with the addition of grossly bloody stool.

Bell stage II definite disease:

Stage IIA characterized by the following:

- Patient is mildly ill.
- Diagnostic signs include the mild systemic signs present in stage IA.
- Intestinal signs include all of the signs present in stage I, with the addition of absent bowel sounds and abdominal tenderness.
- Radiographic findings show ileus and/or pneumatosis intestinalis.

This diagnosis is sometimes referred to as "medical" NEC as surgical intervention is not needed to successfully treat the patient.

Stage IIB characterized by the following:

- Patient is moderately ill.
- Diagnosis requires all of stage I signs plus the systemic signs of moderate illness, such as mild metabolic acidosis and mild thrombocytopenia.
- Abdominal examination reveals definite tenderness, erythema, and/or right lower quadrant mass.
- Radiographs show portal venous gas with or without ascites.

Bell stage III advanced disease:

This stage represents advanced, severe NEC that has a high likelihood of surgical intervention.

Stage IIIA characterized by the following:

- Patient has severe NEC with an intact bowel.
- Diagnosis requires all of the above conditions, with the addition of hypotension, bradycardia, respiratory failure, severe metabolic acidosis, coagulopathy, and/or neutropenia.
- Abdominal examination shows marked distention with signs of generalized peritonitis.
- Radiographic examination reveals definitive evidence of ascites.

Stage IIIB designation is reserved for the severely ill infant with perforated bowel on radiographs in addition to the findings for stage IIIA.

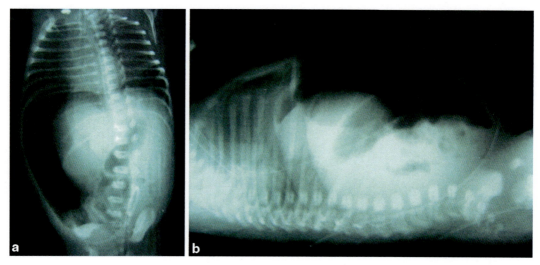

Fig. 31.2 An anteroposterior (*AP*) abdominal radiograph (**a**) and a left lateral decubitus radiograph (**b**) in a patient with NEC and pneumoperitoneum

Fig. 31.3 Abdominal radiograph showing thickened dilated bowel loops in a patient with NEC

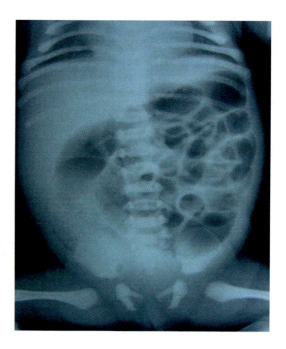

Diagnosis

- Various clinical, laboratory and radiographic signs and symptoms are used to make the diagnosis of NEC.
- The mainstay of diagnostic imaging is abdominal radiography.
- An anteroposterior (AP) abdominal radiograph and a left lateral decubitus radiograph are essential for evaluating any baby with suspected NEC (Fig. 31.2). These radiographs are repeated at 6-hour or greater intervals, depending on severity of presentation and clinical course. This is to assess disease progression.

Diagnosis

Fig. 31.4 a and **b** Abdominal radiographs in a patient with NEC showing pneumatosis intestinalis

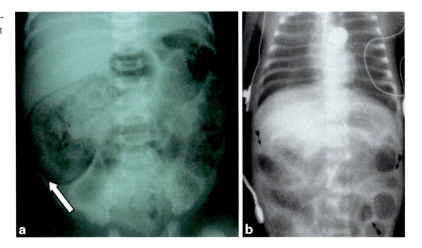

Fig. 31.5 a and **b** Abdominal x-ray showing portal venous air in a patient with NEC

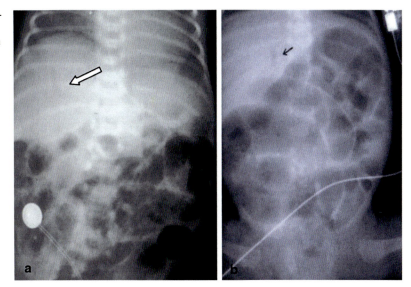

- Radiographic signs of NEC include:
    1. Dilated thickened bowel loops (Fig. 31.3).
    2. Paucity of gas.
    3. A "fixed and dilated bowel loop" that persists over several examinations.
    4. Pneumatosis intestinalis. This is the pathognomic radiological sign of NEC. It appears as characteristic train-track lucency within the bowel wall. The extent of pneumatosis intestinalis does not correlated with the severity of NEC (Fig. 31.4).
    5. Portal venous gas. Portal gas appears as linear, branching areas of decreased density over the liver shadow and represents air in the portal venous system (Fig. 31.5). Its presence is considered to be a poor prognostic sign. Portal gas is much more dramatically observed on ultrasonography.
    6. Pneumoperitoneum either in the form of free air or sometimes in the form of a large pocket of air overlying liver and the ligamentum teres known as a "football sign" (Fig. 31.6).

Fig. 31.6 a and **b** Abdominal x-ray showing pneumoperitenum (*football sign*) in a patient with NEC

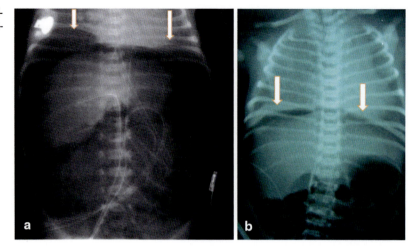

Fig. 31.7 Clinical photograph of a patient with NEC who had stomas. Note the central line catheter

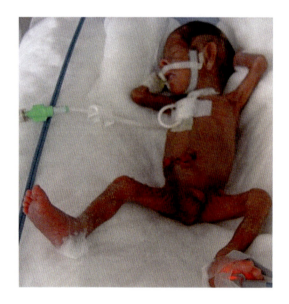

Treatment

The treatment of NEC is generally supportive, nonoperative and consists of:

1. N.P.O.
2. Nasogastric decompression.
3. Fluid replacement to correct electrolyte abnormalities and third space losses.
4. Support for blood pressure.
5. Parenteral nutrition. Many of these babies have difficult intravenous (IV) access. Therefore, the need for prolonged parenteral nutrition frequently requires placing central venous catheters (Fig. 31.7).
6. Prompt antibiotic therapy. Antibiotic coverage consists of ampicillin, gentamicin, and either clindamycin or metronidazole. The specific regimen used should be tailored to the most common nosocomial organisms found in the particular NICU. This may be changed depending on the results of blood culture.

Treatment

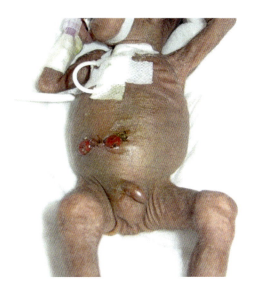

Fig. 31.8 Clinical photograph in a patient with NEC who had surgery. Note the two stomas on either side of the wound and a central line for prolonged parenteral nutrition

7. If the baby is rapidly deteriorating, with apnea and/or signs of impending circulatory and respiratory collapse, airway control and mechanical ventilation is indicated.

Indications for Surgery

- Surgical intervention is needed in <25 % of infants with NEC.
- The average mortality is 30–40 %, even higher in severe cases.
- With improved supportive intensive care, including ventilatory management, anesthetic techniques, and total parenteral nutrition, the survival of infants with NEC has steadily improved.
- The principle indication for operative intervention in NEC is perforated or necrotic intestines. The absolute indication for operative intervention is pneumoperitoneum.
- Other relative indications for operative intervention are:

    1. Clinical:
        - Erythema of the abdominal wall
        - Clinical deterioration
        - Signs of peritonitis
        - Hemodynamic instability

    2. Radiological:
        - Gas in the portal vein
        - Persistent fixed bowel loops
        - Ascites

    3. Laboratory:
        - Positive paracentesis (at least 0.5 mL of brownish fluid that contains bacteria on Gram staining)
        - Worsening and intractable acidosis
        - Persistent thrombocytopenia
        - Rising leukocytosis or worsening leucopenia

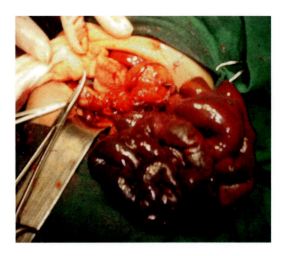

Fig. 31.9 Clinical photograph showing NEC (NEC totalis)

- The type and extent of surgery however depends on the severity of NEC and the general condition of the patient.
- In general, the principle of surgery for NEC is to resect only perforated and unquestionably necrotic intestine and to make every effort to preserve the ileocecal valve.
- If the viability of remaining bowel is significantly questionable, a second-look operation can be performed in 24–48 h to assess the viability of the remaining intestines.
- The necrotic area of the bowel is resected; a proximal stoma and distal mucus fistula are created. The enterostomy and mucus fistula are brought out at opposite ends of the incision (Fig. 31.8).
- Primary anastomosis is not generally advocated, because of the risk of ischemia at the anastomosis, leading to increased incidence of leakage, stricture, fistula, or breakdown.
- However, intestinal resection with primary anastomosis may be safely performed in select cases (patients with a clearly demarcated necrotic segment of bowel with normal-appearing residual intestine, good general condition with no evidence of sepsis, coagulopathy, or physiologic compromise).
- Neonates who are extremely ill and unable to tolerate surgery may be treated initially by means of peritoneal drainage.
    - A right lower quadrant incision is made at the bedside under local anesthesia, and a Penrose drain is inserted.
    - The procedure is intended as a temporary form of treatment till the patient's general condition improves and a formal laparotomy is carried out.
    - Some infants, however, survive with this procedure alone and do not require subsequent laparotomy.
- NEC totalis is considered when <25% of the intestinal length is found to be viable at the time of operation (Fig. 31.9).
- If multiple segments of intestines are affected because of necrosis or perforation, the individual segments of affected intestine are resected, and multiple ostomies are created. However, a number of other surgical options have been proposed. A single proximal stoma may be created and the distal bowel segments anastomosed in continuity, thus avoiding multiple stomas.
- A technique of patch, drain, and wait, which involves transverse, single-layer repair of bowel perforations (patch); placement of two Penrose drains in the lower quadrants (drain), and initiation of long-term parenteral nutrition (wait); however, this technique is not widely advocated.

- Vaughn described a technique of clip and drop-back. The unquestionably necrotic segments of intestine are resected and the transected ends are stapled closed. A second-look operation is performed in 48–72 h when the clips are removed, and reanastomosis is performed without any ostomies.
- All patients who have any remaining large intestine after an initial operation for NEC must have an enema to identify any areas of stricture before the stomas are closed. If any such areas are present, they are resected at the time of enterostomy closure.

Long-term Complications

- Of those patients who survive, 50% develop a long-term complication.
- Prolonged parenteral nutrition may be associated with cholestasis and direct hyperbilirubinemia. This condition resolves gradually following initiation of enteral feeds.
- The two most common complications are intestinal stricture and short gut syndrome.
- Intestinal strictures occur in 9–36% of survivors most commonly in the colon, but ileum and jejunum may be involved.
- Short bowel syndrome occurs in 9% of those who undergo surgery and require extensive small bowel resection.
- Neurodevelopment delay.
- Psychomotor retardation.

Recommended Reading

Grosfeld JL, Cheu H, Schlatter M, West KW, Rescorla FJ. Changing trends in necrotizing enterocolitis. Experience with 302 cases in two decades. Ann Surg. 1991;214(3):300–7.

Rees C, Hall N, Eaton S, Pierro A. Surgical strategies for necrotisingenterocolitis: a survey of practice in the United Kingdom. Arch Dis Child Fetal Neonatal Ed. 2005;90:F152–5.

Chapter 32
Hirschprung's Disease (Congenital Aganglionic Megacolon)

Introduction

- Hirschprung's disease (HD) is a developmental disorder caused by the failure of ganglion cells to migrate cephalocaudally through the neural crest during weeks 4–12 of gestation.
- This will result in an absence of ganglion cells in a varying length of the colon and functional colonic obstruction.
- The aganglionic segment usually begins at the anorectal region and extends proximally.
- Short-segment HD is the most common and affects the rectosigmoid region of the colon.
- Long-segment HD extends past this region and rarely can affect the entire colon (total colonic HD).
- Extremely rare, both the small and large intestines are involved (total intestinal aganglionosis).

Incidence

- The first report of HD dates back to 1691, however, the disease is named after Harald Hirschsprung, the Danish physician who first described two infants who died of this disorder in 1888.
- The incidence of HD is 1 in 5000 live births and has a male-to-female predominance of 4:1; however, in long-segment HD (total colonic) this is not the case with a male-to-female ratio approaching 1:1.
- No racial predilection exists for HD.

Pathophysiology

- Embryologically, the ganglion cells are derived from the neural crest. They migrate from cranial to caudal to reach the distal part of the rectum.
- Arrest or failure of migration results in lack of intramural ganglionic cells (Fig. 32.1):

  1. Submucosa level (Meissner's plexus)
  2. Myenteric level (Auerbach's Plexus)

- The lack of these ganglion cells leads to failure of the distal colon to relax which results in progressive functional constipation.
- The disease can affect varying lengths of bowel segment.
- In 75% of cases, the rectosigmoid area is involved.

Fig. 32.1 Rectal biopsy showing ganglion cells

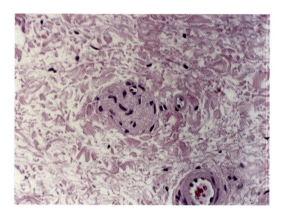

- In 15–20 %, the aganglionosis extends variably to the rest of the colon.
- In the most severe cases (5–10 %), the entire colon is affected. This condition is known as total colonic aganglionosis, or TCA.
- In extremely rare cases, the entire intestinal tract (< 1 %) can be affected (total intestinal aganglionosis).
- Patients with HD are prone to develop enterocolitis.

Etiology

- The exact cause of HD is not known and several factors have been incriminated.
- It is multifactorial, and can be familial or develop spontaneously.
- The most accepted theory is that HD is due to a defect in the craniocaudal migration of enteric ganglia which are derived from the neural crest cells that occur during the first 12 weeks of gestation.
- It is more common in boys than girls (male to female ratio: 3:1 or 4:1).
- Family history in 3–7 % of cases.
- There is increased risk for HD with affected sibling.

  1. Boys with sibling affected: 3–5 %.
  2. Girls with sibling affected: 1 %.
  3. The risk is substantially higher (12–30 %) in siblings of children with total colonic HD.

- Eight genomes have been associated with HD. The predominantly affected gene is Ret-proto oncogene on chromosome 10q11.2 which affects 50 % of familial and 20 % of sporadic cases.
- HD is associated with other chromosomal abnormalities and syndromes such as trisomy 21 and multiple endocrine neoplasia IIa (MEN IIa).
- Environmental factors, intrauterine intestinal ischemia, and infectious etiology have also been incriminated.

Symptoms and Signs

- Signs and symptoms of HD may vary with the severity of the condition.
- Symptoms range from early presentation with neonatal intestinal obstruction to chronic progressive constipation in older children.

Symptoms and Signs

Fig. 32.2 Clinical photograph of a patient with HD showing abdominal distension

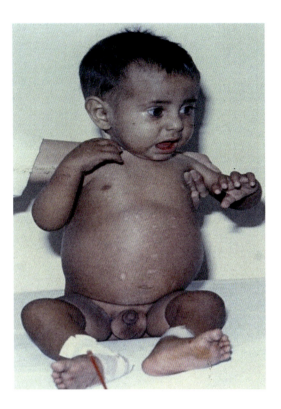

- Approximately 80% of patients present in the first few months of life with constipation, poor feeding, and abdominal distension (Fig. 32.2).
- Up to 90% of infants with Hirschsprung's disease fail to pass meconium in the first 24 h of life.
- Signs and symptoms of neonatal presentation may include:
  - Failure to pass meconium within the first or second day of life
  - Poor feeding
  - Bilious vomiting
  - Infrequent, explosive bowel movements
  - Progressive abdominal distension
  - Poor weight gain
  - Enterocolitis-associated diarrhea

- HD at other times may not be apparent until the baby becomes a teenager or rarely an adult.
- Symptoms in older children include:
  - Chronic progressive constipation
  - Fecal impaction
  - Absence of soiling or overflow incontinence
  - Malnutrition
  - Failure to thrive
  - Abdominal distension

- Patients may present with enterocolitis, a serious infection with diarrhea, fever and vomiting, and sometimes a dangerous dilatation of the colon.

Enterocolitis

- Enterocolitis is a serious infection that accounts for significant morbidity and mortality in patients with Hirschsprung's disease.
- Occurs in 10–30% of infants with Hirschsprung's disease.
- It may occur in both the aganglionic and ganglionic segments of intestines and so it is seen both preoperatively and postoperatively.
- Infants should continue to be monitored closely for enterocolitis many years after corrective surgery because the infection has been reported to occur up to 10 years postoperatively.
- However, most postoperative enterocolitis cases occur within the first 2 years of pull-through.
- Contrast enemas should be avoided in patients with enterocolitis because of the risk of perforation.
- Symptoms of enterocolitis in patients with Hirschsprung's disease include:
  - Abdominal distention
  - Foul-smelling, watery diarrhea
  - Lethargy, fever, vomiting, and poor feeding
- Enterocolitis should be treated aggressively as it may lead to shock and death.
- Treatment includes:
  - Nothing by mouth.
  - Rectal irrigation several times a day.
  - Antibiotics.
  - Oral metronidazole (Flagyl) can be used alone with rectal irrigation in patients with mild enterocolitis.
  - More severe cases should be treated with intravenous broad-spectrum antibiotics and rectal irrigation.
  - If there is no response, a diversion colostomy may become necessary.

Associated Anomalies

- Approximately 20% of infants with HD will have one or more associated abnormality involving the neurological, cardiovascular, urological, or gastrointestinal system.
- Down's syndrome (trisomy 21) is the most common chromosomal abnormality associated with the disease, accounting for approximately 10% of patients.
- Hirschsprung's disease has been found to be associated with the following syndromes and general anomalies:

1. Down's syndrome
2. Neurocristopathy syndromes
3. Waardenburg–Shah syndrome
4. Yemenite deaf–blind syndrome
5. Piebaldism
6. Goldberg–Shprintzen syndrome
7. Multiple endocrine neoplasia type II
8. Congenital central hypoventilation syndrome (Ondine's Curse)

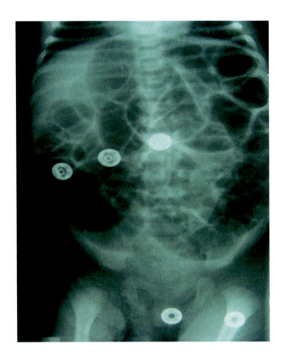

Fig. 32.3 Abdominal x-ray in a patient with HD. Note the dilated bowel loops and absent distal air

- Associated anomalies include:
  - Bladder diveticulum, congenital deafness, cryptorchidism, hydrocephalus, imperforate anus, Meckel's diverticulum, neuroblastoma, renal agenesis, ventricular septal defect, pheochromocytoma, and meningomyelocele

Diagnosis

1. Abdominal x-ray:
    - Colonic distension with gas and feces
    - Absent air in the distal bowel
    - Air–fluid levels
    - Air in the bowel wall suggests enterocolitis (Fig. 32.3)

2. Barium enema:
    - This should be done without bowel preparation to avoid loss of the transitional zone.
    - The first enema that a neonate with suspected HD receives should be a contrast enema.
    - A narrowed distal colon with proximal colonic dilation is the classic finding of Hirschsprung's disease (Figs. 32.4 and 32.5a).
    - The barium may also be retained in the proximal colon for more than 24 h (Fig. 32.5b).
    - However, findings in neonates (babies aged <1 mo) are difficult to interpret and will fail to demonstrate this transition zone in approximately 25% of the cases.

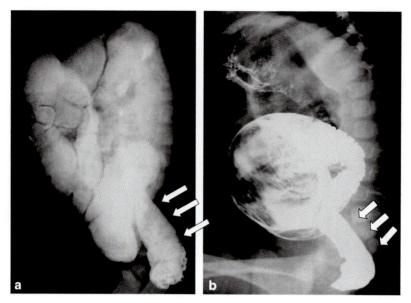

Fig. 32.4 Barium enema in a patient with HD. Note the collapsed aganglionic distal colon (**a**, *arrows*) and proximal colonic dilatation (**b**, *arrows*)

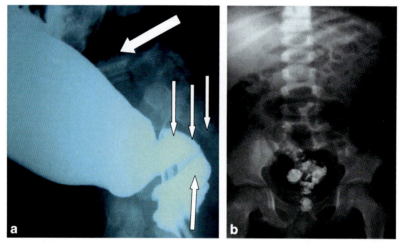

Fig. 32.5 Barium enema in a patient with HD. **a** Note the collapsed aganglionic segment (*large arrow*), transition zone (*three arrows*), and (*single arrow*) dilated proximal colon. **b** Abdominal x-ray in a patient with HD. Note the retained barium in colon more than 24 h following barium enema

3. Anorectal manometry:
   - Normally, there is relaxation reflex of the internal sphincter after distension of the rectal lumen.
   - This normal inhibitory reflex is absent in patients with Hirschsprung's disease.
   - Anorectal manometry is useful but there are false positive and false negative results and because of this it is not commonly used to diagnose HD.
   - Anorectal manometry however is valuable to diagnose ultra short segment HD.

4. Rectal biopsy:
   - The diagnosis of HD can be confirmed with a rectal biopsy, which should show absence of Meissner, Auerbach's ganglion plexuses and marked hypertrophy of nerve trunks.
   - The biopsy site should at least be 0.6 in. (1.5 cm) above the dentate line because the distal rectum normally does not have ganglion cells.
   - The definitive diagnosis of Hirschsprung's disease is confirmed by a full-thickness rectal biopsy. This however requires general anesthesia.
   - More recently, simple suction rectal biopsy has been used to obtain tissue for histological examination. This is obtained via a simple biopsy gun which sucks the rectal mucosa and submucosa, and a self-contained cylindrical knife cuts off the tissue.
   - The advantage of the suction biopsy is that it can be easily performed without the need for a general anesthesia. However, samples obtained by suction biopsies are considerably more difficult to pathologically diagnose Hirschsprung's disease than samples obtained by a full-thickness biopsy.
   - The diagnosis can be improved with the use of acetylcholinesterase staining, which intensely stains the hypertrophied nerve fibers throughout the lamina propria and muscularis propria.
   - More recently, immunohistochemistry with calretinin has also been used for histological examination of aganglionic bowel which might be more accurate than acetylcholinesterase in detecting aganglionosis.

Treatment

- Traditionally, the treatment of HD includes creating a diverting colostomy at the time of diagnosis, and once the child grows and weighs more than 10 kg, the definitive pull-through procedure is performed.
- However, with better understanding of the disease, advances in surgical techniques and safer anesthesia, a primary pull-through procedure without a diverting colostomy is increasingly being performed.
- Contraindications to a one-stage procedure include massively dilated proximal bowel, severe enterocolitis, perforation, malnutrition, and inability to accurately determine the transition zone by frozen section.
- For those who are first treated with a diverting colostomy, the colostomy is placed just above the transition zone (Fig. 32.6).
- The presence of ganglion cells at the colostomy site must be confirmed by a frozen-section biopsy. Either a loop or end colostomy is performed based on the surgeon's preference.
- The pull-through procedure usually is performed 4–6 months after performing a colostomy.
- There are several pull-through techniques. The three most commonly performed pull-through operations are the Swenson, Duhamel, and Soave procedures.
  1. The Swenson procedure
     - The Swenson procedure was the original pull-through procedure used to treat Hirschsprung's disease. It was described in 1948.
     - The aganglionic segment is resected and a colo-anal anastomosis is performed.
  2. The Duhamel procedure
     - The Duhamel procedure was first described in 1956.
     - The proximal ganglionic colon is brought through the retrorectal space and an end-to-side anastomosis is performed between the pulled-through colon and the rectum.
     - The septum between the two walls is divided using an endo-GIA stapler and the opening in the divided rectum is closed.

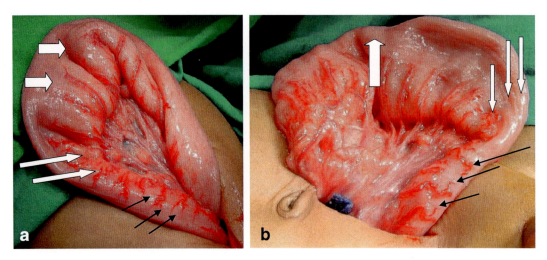

Fig. 32.6 a and **b** An intraoperative photograph showing a collapsed distal colon (black arrows), a transition zone (thin white arrows), and a dilated proximal colon (thick white arrows). If an initial colostomy is planned, it should be placed just proximal to the transition zone

3. The Soave procedure
   - The Soave procedure was introduced in the 1960s.
   - It consists of removing the mucosa and submucosa of the rectum and preserving the muscular cuff of the colon.
   - The ganglionic colon is then pulled through the aganglionic muscular cuff of the rectum. No formal anastomosis is performed and relies on adhesions between the pull-through colon and the surrounding aganglionic rectum.
   - The procedure was modified by Boley to include a primary anastomosis between the pulled-through colon and the anus.

Laparoscopic Approach to the Surgical Treatment of Hirschsprung's Disease

- This was first described in 1999 by Keith Georgeson.
- The transition zone is first identified laparoscopically.
- The ganglionic segment is confirmed by frozen section.
- The colon and rectum are mobilized. A transanal mucosal dissection is performed, followed by a trans-anal pull-through and an anastomosis is performed between the pulled-through ganglionic colon and anus.
- Subsequently, laparoscopic Duhamel pull-through was also found to be feasible and safe in children.

Transanal Pull-through

- In this, no intra-abdominal dissection and the whole procedure is performed transanally.
- The transition zone is identified and anastomosis is performed between the ganglionic portion of the colon and the anus similar to the laparoscopic approach.

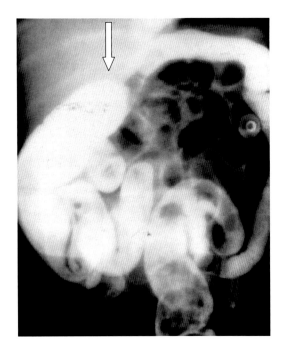

Fig. 32.7 Barium enema in a patient with long segment HD. The aganglionic segment extended up to the hepatic flexure (arrow)

- The advantages of this approach include no intraperitoneal dissection, on abdominal scars, minimal analgesia, and shortened hospital stay.
- The outcome is similar to the single open stage pull-through procedure.
- There is however a significantly higher rate of incontinence with the transanal approach. This is reduced with laparoscopic assisted pull-through which avoids excessive stretching of the sphincters.

Anorectal Myomectomy

- For children with ultrashort-segment Hirschsprung's disease, a 1-cm-wide strip of posterior midline rectal wall is removed.
- The procedure removes an extramucosal rectal wall strip beginning immediately proximal to the dentate line and extending to the normal ganglionic rectum proximally.
- The mucosa and submucosa are preserved and closed.

Long-segment Hirschsprung's Disease

- Patients with total colonic HD require modified pull-through procedures (Fig. 32.7).
- This includes a side-to-side anastomosis of the ganglionic small bowel to a short segment of the aganglionic colon.
- This is to preserve the absorptive surface area and allow for proper growth and nutritional support.
- The possibility of stem cell transplantation into the aganglionic gut and the reactivation of dormant stem cells in the gut to regenerate the enteric nervous system are being actively investigated.

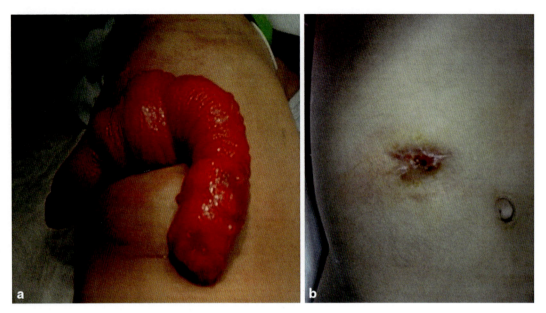

Fig. 32.8 Clinical photograph showing prolapsed colostomy (**a**) and colostomy stenosis (**b**)

Neuronal Intestinal Dysplasia

- Neuronal intestinal dysplasia is one of the causes of constipation in infants and children.
- It is a distinct histopatologic entity and usually presents as long-standing constipation after pull-through operation in patients with HD.
- It is found in 0.3–40% of suction rectal biopsies performed but the incidence in association with HD 10–20%.
- The diagnosis is usually established by increased acetylcholine esterase staining and increase in the ganglion cell number (larger ganglia with more than seven nerve cells/ganglia).
- This results in decrease in intestinal motility.
- The diagnosis of neuronal intestinal dysplasia is usually not made until the patient develops defecation problem after a definitive pull-through procedure.
- The medical treatment is usually the first line of therapy in the form of enemas and cathartics.
- If there is no response to conservative treatment for 6 months, internal sphincter myectomy is the procedure of choice.

Complications and Outcome

- In general, the complications following definitive surgical procedures are:
    1. Anastomotic leakage and stricture formation (5–15%).
    2. Intestinal obstruction (5%).
    3. Pelvic abscess (5%).
    4. Wound infection and wound dehiscence (10%).
    5. Incomplete resection requiring reoperation (5%).
    6. Patients with two-staged operations may also develop colostomy complications such as skin excoriation, prolapse, or stenosis (Fig. 32.8).

- Later complications associated with Hirschsprung's disease include:
  1. Enterocolitis
  2. Continued obstructive symptoms
  3. Incontinence (1%)
  4. Chronic constipation (10–15%)

- The long-term outcome after definitive repair of Hirschsprung's disease is difficult to determine.
- In general, more than 80% of patients with Hirschsprung disease have satisfactory outcomes.
- Many patients however may have disturbances of bowel function for several years before developing normal continence and normal bowel function.
- Patients with Down's syndrome (trisomy 21) tend to have poorer clinical outcomes.

Recommended Reading

Puri P, Shinkai T. Pathogenesis of Hirschsprung's disease and its variants: recent progress. Semin Pediatr Surg. 2004;13:18–24.

Swenson O. My early experience with Hirschsprung's disease. J Pediatr Surg. 1989;24:839–44.

Chapter 33
Congenital Segmental Dilatation of the Intestines

Introduction

- Congenital segmental dilatation (CSD) is defined as a localized dilatation that is limited to a segment of the small or large intestines and an abrupt transition between the normal and dilated intestines (Fig. 33.1).
- It is a very rare condition of unknown etiology and in all the neuronal enteric plexus is normal in the affected segment, proximally and distally.
- Most cases are asymptomatic, discovered during exploration for other conditions namely:
  - Omphalocele.
  - Bowel atresia.
  - Anorectal malformations.
  - But there are reports of CSD causing intestinal obstruction, perforation, or bleeding (Fig. 33.2).
- CSD can affect any part of the intestines from the duodenum to the rectum, with the ileum being the most commonly affected site.
- Within the colon, the rectosigmoid region is the most affected site.
- The presentation of CSD of the rectosigmoid colon is usually chronic constipation with abdominal distension and in the majority it is treated as functional constipation or the diagnosis is confused with Hirschsprung's disease (Fig. 33.3).
- Swenson and Rathauser were the first to describe CSD in 1959. They described three cases affecting the colon.

Etiology

- The etiology of CSD is unknown and several theories have been proposed to explain its pathogenesis.
- Irving and Lister proposed an extrinsic intrauterine intestinal compression such as an umbilical ring, vitelline vessels, or omphalomesenteric band.
- This theory may explain the occurrence of CSD in association with omphalocele, but it does not however explain its occurrence in the other parts of intestines, especially the rectosigmoid colon.
- Mathe et al. on the other hand proposed a primitive neuromuscular dysfunction of the bowel, but this does not explain the selective occurrence of segmental dilatation.
- Heller et al. suggested a disturbance during splitting of the notochord from the endoderm as an etiology for segmental dilatation.

Fig. 33.1 Barium enema showing congenital segmental dilatation of the rectosigmoid colon. Note the dilated segment and abrupt transition to a normal colon marked by the *arrow*

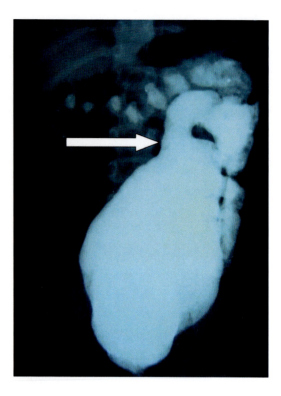

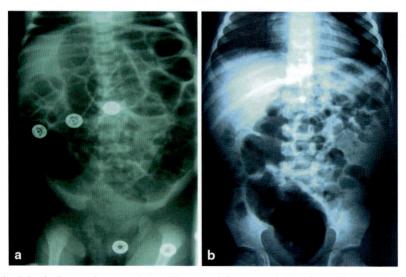

Fig. 33.2 Plain abdominal x-rays in two patients with congenital segmental dilatation of the rectosigmoid colon. The first one **a** showed features of neonatal intestinal obstruction while the other had constipation and abdominal distension. Note the air in the dilated segment of the rectosigmoid colon in the second film (**b**)

Sites 233

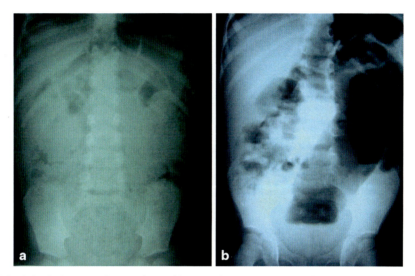

Fig. 33.3 Plain abdominal x-rays of two patients with congenital segmental dilatation of the rectosigmoid colon showing chronic constipation in the first one (**a**) and an air-fluid level in the second one (**b**). This is in the dilated segment of the rectosigmoid colon

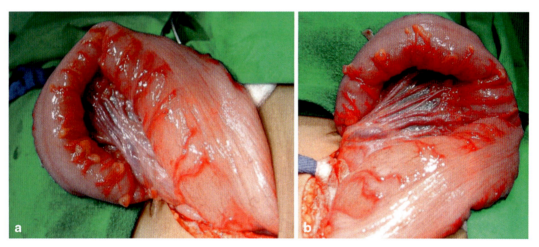

Fig. 33.4 Intraoperative photograph of congenital segmental dilatation of the colon. Note the transition from the dilated segment to a normal colon marked by an *arrow* (**a**). Note also the thick wall and dilated blood vessels (**b**)

- A notable feature is the presence of abundant, dilated, and tortuous serosal and mesenteric blood vessels which may suggest a vascular role in its etiology (Fig. 33.4).

Sites

- CSD can affect any part of the intestines from the duodenum to the rectum with the ileum being the commonest affected site in the small intestines and the rectosigmoid colon in the large intestines.
- CSD of the rectosigmoid colon should be included in the differential diagnosis of chronic constipation in infants and children and physicians caring for these patients must be aware of this as it is a curable condition.

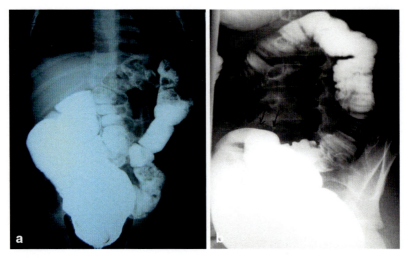

Fig. 33.5 a and **b** Barium enemas showing congenital segmental dilatation of the rectosigmoid colon

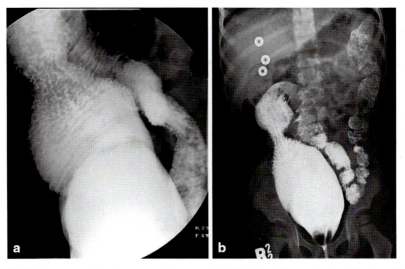

Fig. 33.6 a and **b** Barium enema showing congenital segmental dilatation of the rectosigmoid colon. Note the dilated segment in the post-evacuation second film (**b**)

Diagnosis

- Whereas contrast studies may not be helpful in the diagnosis of CSD affecting the small intestines, barium enema is a useful investigation to diagnose CSD of the colon and should form part of the diagnostic evaluation of these children (Figs. 33.5 and 33.6).
- Children who present with chronic constipation and abdominal distension should have barium enema as part of their evaluation.
- Barium enema is also useful in differentiating CSD from simple Hirschsprung's disease and functional constipation, demonstrating a localized dilation of the rectosigmoid colon with an abrupt transition to a normal colon proximally.

- Clinically, CSD of the rectosigmoid colon can resemble Hirschsprung's disease and radiologically it may be confused with ultra-short-segment Hirschsprung's disease.
- Normal distensibility of the distal bowel on radiological examination and relaxation of the internal sphincter on manometric examination will exclude even the short-segment Hirschsprung's disease, but the final differentiation between these two conditions is via a rectal biopsy.
- The surgical treatment of CSD of the rectosigmoid colon is a modified Duhamel's pull-through.
- The majority of the dilated segment should be resected as well as anterior reduction by excising part of the anterior wall of the remaining part of the dilated segment in an elliptical fashion. With this technique, the majority of the dilated segment will be excised.
- An alternative technique is a low anterior resection with an end-to-end anastomosis. This however requires extensive pelvic dissection with the danger of injuring surrounding structures.
- CSD affecting other parts of the gastrointestinal tract should be resected with an end-to-end anastomosis.

Recommended Reading

Ben Brahim M, Belghith M, Mekki M, Jouini R, Sahnoun L, Maazoun K, et al. Segmental dilatation of the intestine. J Pediatr Surg. 2006;41:1130–3.

Irving IM, Lister J. Segmental dilatation of the ileum. J Pediatr Surg. 1977;12:103–12.

Mathé JC, Khirallah S, Phat Vuoung N, et al. Dilatation segmentaire du grele a revelation neonatale. Nouv Press Med. 1982;11:265–6.

Swenson O, Rathauser F. Segmental dilatation of the colon: a new entity. Am J Surg. 1959;97:734–8.

Yadav KJ, Singh G, Budhiraja S. Congenital segmental dilatation of intestine. Indian J Pediatr. 1996;63:561–3.

Chapter 34
Megacystis Microcolon Intestinal Hypoperistalsis Syndrome

Introduction

- Megacystis microcolon intestinal hypoperistalsis syndrome (MMIHS) is a very rare congenital condition of unknown etiology.
- It is characterized by abdominal distension caused by a markedly distended, nonobstructed urinary bladder, microcolon, and intestinal hypoperistalsis with functional intestinal obstruction (Figs. 34.1 and 34.2).
- MMIHS was first described by Berdon et al. in 1976.
- MMIHS usually has a fatal prognosis and in most of the cases infants die within the early months of their lives; nevertheless, there are some case reports of long-term survival.

Etiology

- The exact etiology of MMIHS is not known.
- The most commonly accepted etiology is that MMIHS is a form of visceral myopathy.
- It is a rare congenital anomaly inherited as an autosomal recessive that predominantly affects females (4:1 ratio).
- Histological studies suggest that the predominant intestinal manifestation is smooth muscle myopathy.
- Molecular observations have linked the disease to the neuronal nicotinic acetylcholine receptor (ηAChR), namely the absence of a functional α3 subunit of the ηAChR, a de novo deletion of the proximal long arm of chromosome 15 (15q11.2).
- Histological evaluation revealed an appropriate light microscopic appearance of both the circular and longitudinal layers of the small bowel muscularis propria.
- Immunohistochemical staining for smooth muscle actin, however, was selectively absent in the circular layer, demonstrating isolated absence in a unique and previously undescribed pattern. These observations raise the possibility that the proximal long arm of chromosome 15 (15q11) may be of clinical significance in MMIHS.

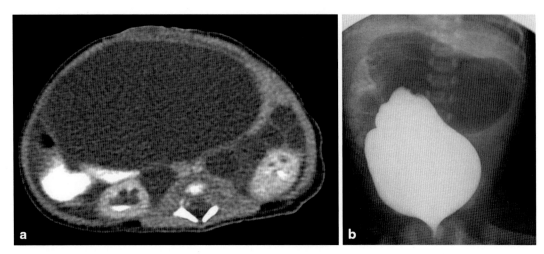

Fig. 34.1 Abdominal computed tomography (CT) scan showing markedly dilated urinary bladder (**a**) and micturating cystourethrogram (**b**) showing a markedly dilated urinary bladder. There was no evidence of vesicoureteric reflux

Fig. 34.2 Barium enema showing small unused microcolon

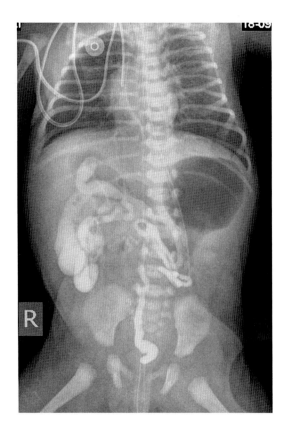

Clinical Features

Fig. 34.3 Intraoperative photograph showing a markedly dilated urinary bladder

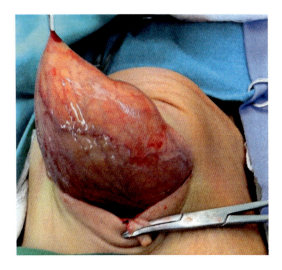

Fig. 34.4 Barium swallow and meal showing dilated esophagus, stomach, and upper part of the small intestines

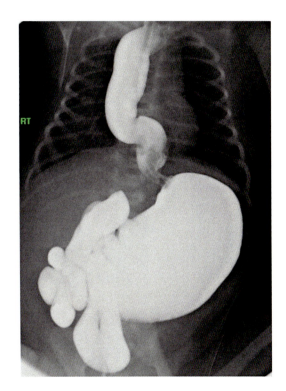

Clinical Features

- The main manifestation of MMIHS is intestinal obstruction in newborns, with other associated abnormalities.
- MMIHS is characterized by the presence of:
    - A markedly distended urinary bladder without distal urinary tract obstruction (Fig. 34.3)
    - Microcolon
    - Decreased or absent intestinal peristalsis

Fig. 34.5 A clinical photograph showing the two stomas. The proximal stoma never functioned

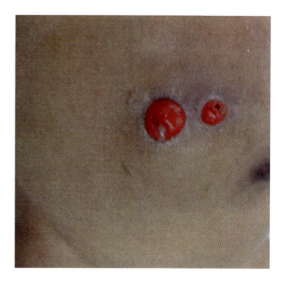

Other reported anomalies include malrotation, short bowel, segmental stenosis of small bowel, dilated proximal small bowel, dilated esophagus and stomach (Fig. 34.4), bilateral streak gonads, and bilateral duplicated urinary system.

Treatment

- There is no definite cure for MMIHS and the majority of patients die within the first year of life.
- The small intestines are usually decompressed with an ileostomy.
- A vesicostomy to decompress the distended urinary bladder may also be added (Fig. 34.5).
- The most frequent cause of death was overwhelming sepsis followed by malnutrition and multiple organ failure.
- There are however reports of long-term survivors and these patients are on total parenteral nutrition which is known to ultimately cause liver failure.
- Several attempts at multiorgan transplantation or combined liver and intestinal transplant in infants with MMIHS have been met with success.
- Currently, multivisceral transplantation is the only accepted treatment modality for these patients.

Recommended Reading

Gosemann JH, Puri P. Megacystis microcolon intestinal hypoperistalsis syndrome: systematic review of outcome. Pediatr Surg Int. 2011;1041–6.
Mantan M, Singhal KK, Sethi GR, Aggarwal SK. Megacystis, microcolon, intestinal hypoperistalsis syndrome and bilateral streak gonads. Indian J Nephrol. 2011;21(3):212–4.
Puri P, Shinkai M. Megacystis microcolon intestinal hypoperistalsis syndrome. Semin Pediatr Surg. 2005;14(1):58–63.

Chapter 35
Perianal Abscess and Fistula-in-Ano

Introduction

- A fistula is an abnormal tract connecting two epithelial-lined surfaces.
- In fistula-in-ano, the communication is usually between the anal canal and the perineal skin.
- As a clinical entity, fistula-in-ano has been well recognized from ancient times.
- Hippocrates (460 BC) used a seton to cure fistula-in-ano.
- In 1337, John Anderne was the first to surgically treat a fistula-in-ano.
- Fistula-in-ano in infants and children is a poorly understood condition.
- Generally, fistula-in-ano is more common in boys than in girls and it has been reported that fistula-in-ano in infants occurs exclusively in males.
- Ninety-five percent of fistula-in-ano cases occur in infants younger than 1 year (Fig. 35.1a).
- It is considered generally that fistulae-in-ano are a consequence of an underlying perianal infection.
- Up to 85 % of children with perianal abscess may progress to form a fistula (Fig. 35.1b).
- Perianal abscesses and fistulae-in-ano in neonates are different conditions than those found in older children and adults. They have certain characteristics including:
  - Much more common in males.
  - Occur in the majority in infants younger than 1 year of age.
  - Can be bilateral or have multiple tracts (Fig. 35.2).
  - The majority are of low type and complex fistulae are rare.
  - Low incidence of recurrence.
- Older children presenting with perianal abscesses or fistulas tend to have a higher incidence of underlying conditions such as inflammatory bowel disease, tuberculosis, or leukemia.

Classification

- Congenital type.
- Acquired type. This is secondary to:
  - A perianal abscess
  - Tuberculosis
  - Inflammatory bowel disease (Crohn's disease and ulcerative colitis)
  - Immunosuppression and leukemia
- In the congenital form, the fistulous tract may appear spontaneously or present initially as a perianal abscess.

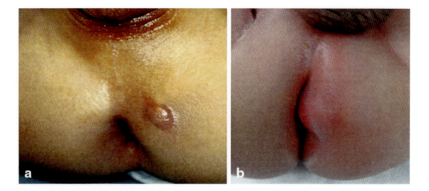

Fig. 35.1 A clinical photograph showing fistula-in-ano in an infant. Note the discharging opening near the anus in (**a**) and a perianal abscess in (**b**)

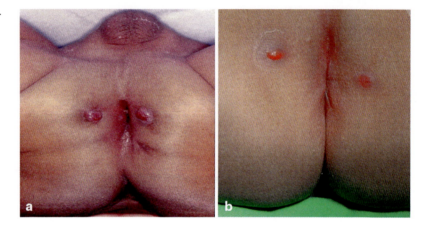

Fig. 35.2 a and **b** A clinical photograph showing bilateral fistula-in-ano in an infant

- In the congenital form, the fistulous tract is usually lined with stratified squamous epithelium, columnar epithelium, or both.
- The acquired form manifests with repeated perianal abscesses and has an inflamed fibrous tract lined by granulation tissue with no epithelial lining upon microscopic examination.
- Perianal abscesses in male infants usually grow enteric organisms (*E. coli, coliforms, pseudomonas, proteus,* etc.) while female infants with perianal abscess usually grow *Staphylococcus aureus*. This is of importance as the majority of male infants who present with perianal abscess will subsequently develop fistula-in-ano which is not the case in female infants.

Etiology

- The exact etiology of fistula-in-ano is not known and several factors have been suggested.
- Fistula-in-ano in an otherwise healthy neonate is suspected to originate as anal cryptitis, which progresses to form a perianal abscess.
- Hormonal imbalance:
  - It has been postulated that androgen excess or androgen–estrogen imbalance may cause the formation of abnormal crypts of Morgagni with a predisposition to cryptitis and abscess formation.

Etiology

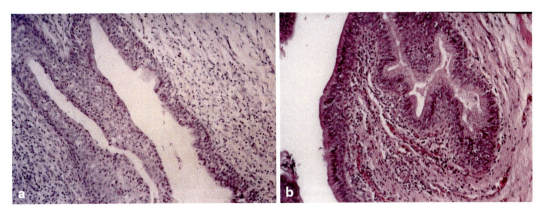

Fig. 35.3 a and **b** Histological pictures of a resected fistula-in-ano showing the fistula tracts lined by stratified squamous epithelium, columnar epithelium, or both

- Androgen excess: This may stimulate the sebaceous glands, resulting in secondary infection with perianal abscess formation and fistulae.
- Abnormal crypts of Morgagni:
  - Although the etiology of abnormal crypt formation remains unknown, it has been shown that the crypts of infants with fistulas tend to be deeper (3–10 mm) than crypts seen in normal infants (1–2 mm).
  - Deep crypts of Morgagni facilitate the trapping of bacteria, which cause cryptitis that leads to perianal abscess formation and fistulae.
- Abnormal anal glands.
- Congenital theory: Fistula-in-ano in infants and children is suggested to be congenital in origin. This is supported by the following:
  - Early occurrence in infants and sometimes in newborns. More than 96% of cases occur in infants younger than 1 year.
  - The occurrence of fistula-in-ano as an initial manifestation rather than a consequence of a perianal abscess.
  - The bilateral and sometimes multiple fistulae (Fig. 35.2).
  - The fistulous tract is lined with stratified squamous epithelium, columnar epithelium, or both in the majority rather than the normal granulation tissue (Fig. 35.3).
  - The growth of enteric organisms in infants with perianal abscess.
- Acquired fistula-in-ano:
  - The usual presentation involves a recurrent perianal abscess.
  - Perianal abscess is regarded as a precursor to fistula-in-ano.
  - More than 95% of patients with perianal abscesses that lead to fistula-in-ano are boys younger than 1 year.
  - Perianal abscesses are seen in 22% of girls with fistula-in-ano, 68% of whom present after the age of 2 years.

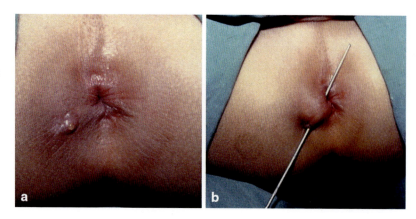

Fig. 35.4 a and **b** Clinical photographs showing fistula-in-ano. Note the probe in the fistula tract (**b**). Note that the fistula is of the low type

Clinical features

- The usual presentation is that of a perianal abscess or a discharging opening in the perianal region.
- Examination of the perineum may reveal an external opening of the fistula, with an outpouching of granulation tissue or purulent discharge.
- The fistula may appear as a perianal abscess.
- An internal opening may be felt as a nodule on the wall of the anal canal.
- The opening is invariably single but can be bilateral or multiple.
- Probing the fistula should be done with the patient under anesthesia to avoid creating false passages.

Treatment

- Fistulotomy is the treatment of choice for fistula-in-ano. Unfortunately, fistulotomy can result in recurrence.
- Fistulectomy is a more extensive treatment with low very recurrence rates.
- Several series have shown good results for the treatment of fistula-in-ano with early fistulotomy or fistulectomy.
- Although antibiotics may serve an important adjuvant role for immunocompromised patients with perianal abscesses, their use in healthy neonates may be avoided with no adverse effects.
- The nonoperative management of fistula-in-ano in healthy infants appears to be safe and effective.
- Although the advantages of a nonoperative management are the avoidance of general anesthesia and surgical intervention, the risks of general anesthesia in this patient group are extremely low and the surgical technique is simple and the results are excellent.
- Fistulectomy (Figs. 35.4 and 35.5):
    - With the patient under anesthesia, the fistula tract is:
        - Probed.
        - Dissected from all sides by means of sharp dissection with scissors or diathermy from the external opening to the internal opening.
        - This dissection is facilitated with the use of the probe till it is completely excised.
        - The cavity left behind is allowed to heal by secondary intention.

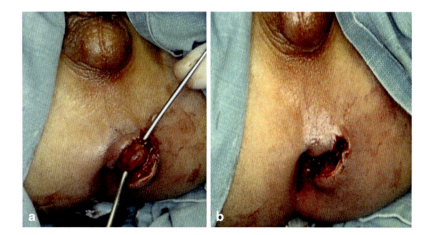

Fig. 35.5 a and **b** Clinical photographs showing fistulectomy

- Fistulotomy:
  - With the patient under anesthesia, the fistula tract is:
    ○ Probed.
    ○ The probe is passed from the external opening and taken out from the internal opening.
    ○ The whole fistula tract is then laid open over the probe.
    ○ The wound is allowed to heal by secondary intention.
- Treatment of high fistula-in-ano:
  - A supralevator (pelvirectal) fistula may be secondary to local disease. If a traumatic fistula perforates the rectal ampulla, colostomy is usually needed.
  - A transsphincteric fistula usually starts as an intersphincteric tract with a secondary tract in the ischiorectal fossa extending up to the levator axis. Treatment is directed toward the lower part of the tract, as healing of the upper tract may occur. If this does not take place, colostomy is required.
  - An intersphincteric fistula primarily starts as an abscess of the anal gland and extends upward and downward between the internal and external sphincters. Patients may have an opening into rectum above the anorectal ring. Treatment consists of laying open the tract by dividing only a small segment of the internal sphincter.
  - The use of seton, including medicated seton (kshara sutra):
    ○ A seton is a surgical thread often used to treat fistula-in-ano.
    ○ The seton can be silk, cotton, or any other suture material.
    ○ It may also be coated with medications.

Recommended Reading

Al-Salem AH, Qaisaruddin S, Qureshi SS. Perianal abscess and fistula-in-ano in infancy and childhood: a clinicopathological study. Pediatr Pathol Lab Med. 1996;16:755–4.

Fitzgerald RJ, Harding B, Ryan W. Fistula-in-ano in childhood: a congenital etiology. J Pediatr Surg. 1985;20:80–1.

Chapter 36
Gastroschisis

Introduction

- Gastroschisis is a congenital defect in the anterior abdominal wall through which the abdominal contents freely protrude outside.
- There is no overlying sac and the size of the defect is variable but usually <4 cm in diameter.
- The abdominal wall defect is located at the junction of the umbilicus and normal skin, and is almost always to the right side of the umbilicus (Fig. 36.1).
- Omphalocele on the other hand is a congenital birth defect through the umbilical cord and the contents remain enclosed in a sac of visceral peritoneum. With omphalocele, the defect is usually much larger than in gastroschisis.
- Gastroschisis is a relatively uncommon condition. It occurs in approximately 1 out of every 5000 live births. It has been reported that the incidence of gastroschisis has increased in recent years.
- Gastroschisis is usually inherited in an autosomal recessive manner. It may begin as a sporadic mutation, can be associated with nongenetic congenital disorders, but has also been observed to be autosomal dominant.
- During the 4th week of development, the lateral body folds move ventrally and fuse in the midline to form the anterior body wall. Incomplete fusion results in a defect that allows abdominal viscera to protrude through the abdominal wall. The bowel typically herniates through a defect to the right of the umbilicus.
- The malformation is slightly more frequent in males than females.
- The frequency of gastroschisis is associated with young maternal age and low number of gestations.

Etiology

- The exact etiology of gastroschisis is not known.
- It is associated with younger maternal age and almost never occurs in mothers over 30 years of age.
- The following factors have been incriminated as possible etiological factors:
    - The use of salicylates
    - Maternal cigarette smoking
    - Maternal alcohol and drug use

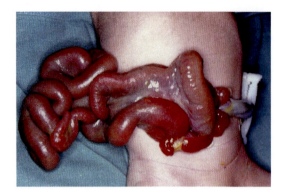

Fig. 36.1 A clinical photograph showing gastroschisis. Note the site of the herniated intestines to the right of the umbilicus

- Several embryological hypotheses have been proposed as contributing factors for gastroschisis. These include:
  1. Failure of mesoderm to form in the body wall
  2. Rupture of the amnion around the umbilical ring with subsequent herniation of bowel
  3. Abnormal involution of the right umbilical vein leading to weakening of the body wall and gut herniation
  4. Disruption of the right vitelline (yolk sac) artery with subsequent body wall damage and gut herniation
  5. Abnormal folding of the body wall which results in a ventral body wall defect through which the gut herniates
  6. Failure to incorporate the yolk sac and related vitelline structures into the yolk sac

Diagnosis

- The diagnosis of gastroschisis is commonly made antenatally by a routine ultrasound examination.
- Rarely, polyhydramnios may prompt an antenatal ultrasound examination.
- The herniated bowel in gastroschisis is bathed by amniotic fluid and both maternal serum and amniotic fluid alpha-fetoprotein (AFP) levels are elevated. This should be evaluated by an abdominal ultrasound.
- Maternal abdominal ultrasound usually shows the herniated bowel and perhaps the liver floating in the amniotic fluid.
- Plans should be made for careful delivery and immediate management after birth.
- Ultrasound may also reveal intrauterine growth retardation which occurs in 38–77 % of fetuses with gastroschisis.
- This is usually secondary to nutrient loss through exposed intestines.
- Approximately 48 % of infants with gastroschisis are small for their gestational age.

Examination

- Clinically, the appearance of bowel may range from almost normal-to-thick-walled inflamed intestines forming a mass (Fig. 36.2).
- Atresia or necrosis of intestines may be present. These have been associated with defects that have a small diameter (Fig. 36.3).

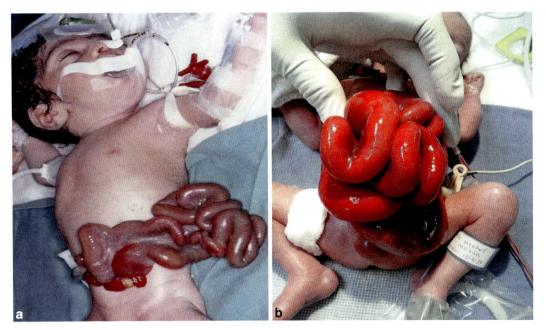

Fig. 36.2 Clinical photographs showing gastroschisis. Note the normal looking intestines in the first (**a**) and congested edematous intestines in the other (**b**)

Associated Anomalies

- Gastroschisis is not commonly associated with any other birth defects except intestinal atresia.
- This occurs in 10 % of cases and includes:
  - Gastrointestinal anomalies, central nervous system anomalies, cardiovascular anomalies, musculoskeletal malformations, and genitourinary anomalies.
- Polyhydramnios and fetal bowel dilatation on antenatal ultrasound are associated with intestinal atresia.

Management and Outcome

- Newborns with gastroschisis are prone to develop:
  - Hypothermia
  - Dehydration
  - Sepsis
  - Hypoglycemia
  - Add to this, prematurity and low birth weight
- Fluids and electrolytes need to be corrected and heat losses must be minimized.
- Gastroschisis is associated with significant ongoing fluid losses which must be corrected. This is done with an intravenous (IV) fluid bolus (20 ml/kg ringer lactate solution or normal saline), followed by 10 % dextrose/0.25 normal saline solution at two to three times the baby's maintenance fluid rate. This will also help compensate for postoperative third-space loses.

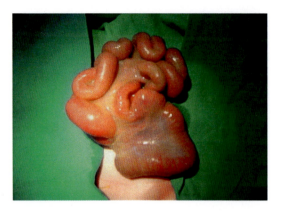

Fig. 36.3 A clinical photograph showing gastroschisis with associated intestinal atresia

- The baby should be placed under a warmer.
- The exposed intestines should be covered with a moist warm pad and the eviscerated intestines should be situated on top of the baby's abdomen to avoid traction upon the bowel mesentery.
- A urinary catheter should be inserted to monitor urine output and assess the efficacy of fluid resuscitation.
- Reduction of the herniated viscera is facilitated by evacuating meconium from the sigmoid colon; this can be easily accomplished during the operative procedure.
- Broad-spectrum antibiotics are administered to prevent contamination of the peritoneal cavity.
- It is not uncommon for infants with gastroschisis to require ventilatory support and total parenteral nutrition for a period of time after surgery.
- A central venous line is placed intraoperatively to provide parenteral nutrition.
- These patients may require prolonged parenteral nutrition because of intestinal dysmotility and malabsorption. The extent of intestinal dysfunction depends on the magnitude of the inflammatory and ischemic injury caused by the exposure of the intestines to the amniotic fluid and compression of the herniated intestinal mesentery by the abdominal wall defect (Fig. 36.4).
- The recent advances in surgical techniques, intensive care management, and total parenteral nutrition for neonates have increased the survival rate of those with gastroschisis to 90%.
- Cesarean section delivery is performed in many mothers of fetuses with gastroschisis, although this does not convey any advantage over vaginal delivery.
- Surgical reduction of herniated intestines and repair should be performed within the 1st day after delivery to avoid further thickening and dilatation of bowel and infection.
- The general procedure for gastroschisis repair is to simply reduce the herniated bowel back into the abdominal cavity. This can be tried in the neonatal intensive care unit once the baby is intubated, ventilated, and sedated. This is also known as ward reduction.
- The factors that preclude ward reduction include:
  - Poor bowel condition
  - Bowel/mesentery attached to the defect
  - Gross viscera-abdominal disproportion
  - Narrow defect diameter
  - Deteriorating metabolic acidosis
- If ward reduction is not feasible, reduction and repair should be done in the operation room. The intestine is returned to the abdominal cavity and the abdominal wall defect is closed during the first procedure (primary repair).
- An excessively tight closure of the abdominal wall defect should be avoided as it may impede splanchnic blood flow and result in intestinal ischemia or necrosis.

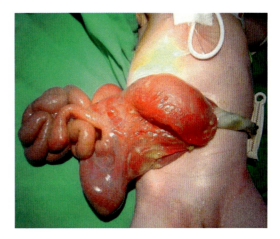

Fig. 36.4 A clinical photograph showing gastroschisis. Note the central line for parenteral nutrition and the dilated edematous proximal intestines

- In addition, tight closure of the abdominal cavity impedes venous return to the heart, which compromises cardiac output and decreases renal blood flow and urine output.
- Diminished mesenteric blood flow compounds the risk of necrotizing enterocolitis because the intestine of these infants is immature immunologically and the dysmotility leads to stagnation and bacterial overgrowth.
- The intra-abdominal pressure can be measured by connecting a manometer to a Foley catheter or a nasogastric tube. The central venous pressure, intravesical pressure, and the intragastric pressure should not exceed 20 cm H_2O to avoid development of the abdominal compartment syndrome.
- Prenatal exposure of the fetal intestines to the amniotic fluid can be associated with bowel dilation and inflammation, thus making primary repair unfeasible. If the amount of bowel outside the abdomen is large or dilated or if the baby's condition is unstable, a staged repair is performed over an average of 5–10 days (staged repair).
- Upon admission to the neonatal intensive care unit, the herniated intestines are placed in a protective "silo," then slowly compressing the silo to push the herniated intestine into the abdominal cavity. This allows for the bowel to return to its intended location without further traumatizing the infant's viscera with undue internal pressure. The bowel is then slowly and gently pushed back down into the abdomen over the course of a few days. The infant is then taken to the operating room where the silo is removed and the defect in the abdomen is closed surgically.
- Correction of an associated intestinal atresia is best delayed until several weeks after closure of the abdominal cavity. Treatment of associated intestinal atresia is also variable depending on how much healthy the bowel is including:
  – Primary anastomosis
  – Delayed anastomosis
  – Stoma formation followed by anastomosis
- The main cause for lengthy recovery periods in patients with gastroschisis is the time taken for the infants' bowel function to return to normal.
- The mortality rate of gastroschisis is about 10–15%.
- Long-term morbidity from gastroschisis is related to intestinal dysfunction and gastroesophageal reflux. Intestinal dysfunction may take as long as 4–6 weeks to resolve. Until then, infants are supported with total parenteral nutrition.

Recommended Reading

Ghionzoli M, James CP, David AL, Shah D, Tan AW, Iskaros J, Drake DP, Curry JI, Kiely EM, Cross K, Eaton S, De Coppi P, Pierro A. Gastroschisis with intestinal atresia—predictive value of antenatal diagnosis and outcome of postnatal treatment. J Pediatr Surg. 2012;47(2):322–8.

Kassa AM, Lilja HE. Predictors of postnatal outcome in neonates with gastroschisis. J Pediatr Surg. 2011;46(11):2108–14.

Ledbetter DJ. Gastroschisis and omphalocele. Surg Clin North Am. 2006;86:249–60.

Chapter 37
Omphalocele

Introduction

- The term "*omphalocele*" comes from the Greek words "*omphalos*" meaning "umbilicus" and "*cele*" meaning "cavity."
- Omphalocele, also known as exomphalos, is an abdominal wall defect in which the intestines, liver, and occasionally other organs remain outside of the abdomen in a sac (Figs. 37.1 and 37.2).
- The incidence of omphalocele is variable but generally occurs in 2.5/10,000 births. Small omphaloceles on the other hand occur with a rate of 1 case in 5000 live births. Large omphaloceles occur with a rate of 1 case in 10,000 live births.
- The mean size of omphalocele defect is 2.5–5 cm (4–12 cm).
- Omphalocele is classified into two types: minor and major.
- Minor omphalocele: There is protrusion of a small portion of the intestine only and the size of the defect is <5 cm in diameter.
- Major omphalocele: There is protrusion of the intestines, liver, and other organs and the diameter of the defect is >5 cm.
- The omphalocele sac is ruptured in 10–20% of cases. This may occur in utero or during delivery (Fig. 37.2b).

Etiology

- The exact etiology of omphalocele is not known.
- Various theories have been postulated; these include:
  - Failure of the bowel to return into the abdomen by 10–12 weeks
  - Failure of lateral mesodermal body folds to migrate centrally
  - Persistence of the body stalk beyond 12 weeks' gestation
  - A defect in the development of the muscles of the abdominal wall.

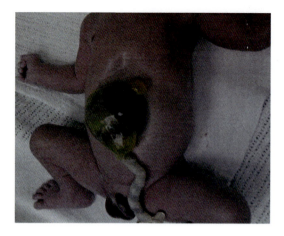

Fig. 37.1 Clinical photograph showing omphalocele. Note the location of the omphalocele in the center of the umbilical cord

Diagnosis

- Omphalocele is usually detected antenatally during routine ultrasonographic evaluation.
- An omphalocele is diagnosed when an anterior midline abdominal mass is demonstrated on fetal ultrasonic evaluation.
- The mass consists of abdominal contents that have herniated through a midline central defect at the base of the umbilical cord insertion. The mass usually has a smooth surface and contains abdominal viscera, usually the liver, intestines, and stomach.
- Diagnostic amniocentesis is indicated when an omphalocele is demonstrated on antenatal ultrasound evaluation. This is to detect associated chromosomal abnormalities.
- The finding of an omphalocele should prompt a detailed ultrasonographic evaluation to detect associated anomalies.
- Fetal echocardiography and karyotyping should also be performed.

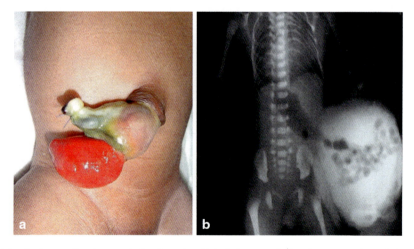

Fig. 37.2 Abdominal x-ray showing omphalocele and a clinical photograph showing ruptured omphalocele

Fig. 37.3 Clinical photograph showing ruptured omphalocele with ruptured Meckel's diverticulum

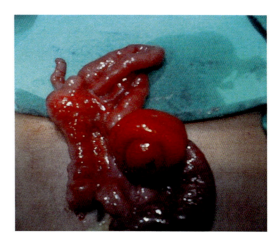

Associated Anomalies

- Omphaloceles are associated with other anomalies in 70–80 % of the cases.
- The most common associated abnormalities are (Figs. 37.3, 37.4 and 37.5):
    - Congenital heart disease (25 %): Most commonly ventricular septal defect, atrial septal defect, and tetralogy of Fallot.
    - Central nervous system anomalies, congenital diaphragmatic hernia, renal anomalies, and skeletal abnormalities.
    - Gastrointestinal abnormalities including midgut volvolus, malrotation, Meckel's diverticulum, anorectal malformations, and intestinal and colonic atresia.

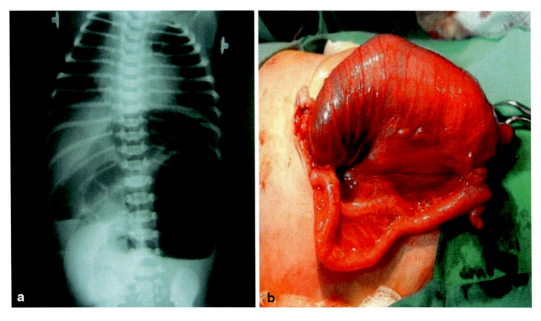

Fig. 37.4 Plain abdominal x-ray showing features of intestinal obstruction in a patient with omphalocele (**a**) and a clinical photograph showing intestinal atresia in a patient with omphalocele (**b**)

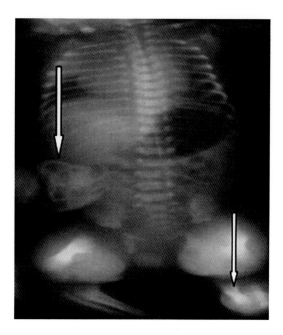

Fig. 37.5 Plain x-ray showing skeletal malformations in a patient with omphalocele

- Approximately 30–40% of patients with an omphalocele have an abnormal karyotype, most commonly Trisomy 13, Trisomy 18, Trisomy 21, and Turner syndrome.
- Some infants with omphalocele have an association with Beckwith–Wiedemann syndrome (i.e., exomphalos, macroglossia, and gigantism). They have coarse, rounded facial features, hyperplasia of the pancreatic islet cells with hypoglycemia, visceromegaly, and genitourinary abnormalities.
- Neurologic disorders, renal anomalies, and bladder extrophy.
- Omphalocele may be associated with pentalogy of Cantrell (epigastric omphalocele; cleft sternum; anterior diaphragmatic hernia, Morgagni; absent pericardium; and cardiac defects, ectopia cordis and ventricular septal defects).

Management and Outcome

- The size of the omphalocele determines the mode of delivery as well as the postnatal treatment.
- The degree of liver herniation into the sac determines the type of omphalocele treatment.
- While fetuses with omphaloceles are often delivered by cesarean section, there are a number of studies demonstrating no significant difference between vaginal and cesarean delivery with regard to infant mortality and acute or long-term outcome.
- If the omphalocele is small and does not involve the liver, a vaginal delivery might be possible.
- After birth, the exposed organs are returned to the abdominal cavity and the hernia is closed via surgery. Closure of a small or moderate-sized omphalocele is accomplished without difficulty.
- A giant omphalocele usually requires a Cesarean delivery to avoid membrane rupture and liver trauma.
- With a large omphalocele, dystocia may occur and result in injury to the liver.
- Herniation of the fetal liver is frequently associated with a small abdominal size and pulmonary hypoplasia, two factors that can complicate the postnatal course.

Surgical Management

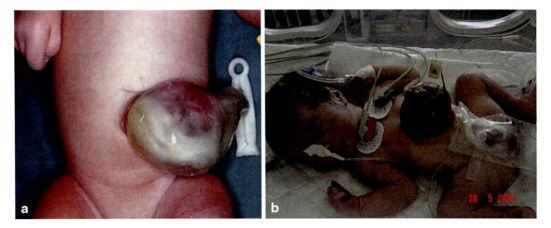

Fig. 37.6 **a** and **b** Clinical photographs showing omphalocele minor and major

Fig. 37.7 A clinical photograph showing omphalocele major in a premature with chromosomal abnormalities

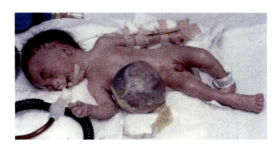

- Treatment for infants with an omphalocele depends on a number of factors, including (Figs. 37.6 and 37.7):

  1. The size of the omphalocele
  2. The presence of other birth defects or chromosomal abnormalities
  3. The baby's gestational age

Surgical Management

- If the omphalocele is small (omphalocele minor), usually it is treated with surgery soon after birth. The contents are reduced and the defect is closed primarily (Fig. 37.8).
- If the omphalocele is large (omphalocele major), the repair might be done in stages. The exposed organs should be covered by nonadherent dressing and slowly, over time, the organs will be moved back into the abdomen. When all the organs have been put back in the abdomen, the opening is closed surgically.
- The baby should be carefully examined to detect any associated anomalies, such as Beckwith–Wiedemann syndrome, chromosomal abnormalities, congenital heart disease, or any other associated malformations.
- Intravenous fluids are administered and the omphalocele sac is covered with a nonadherent dressing.
- The infant's temperature should be preserved.
- Prophylactic antibiotics are given preoperatively.
- Closure of giant omphaloceles containing the liver is always challenging. The options include (Figs. 37.9 and 37.10):

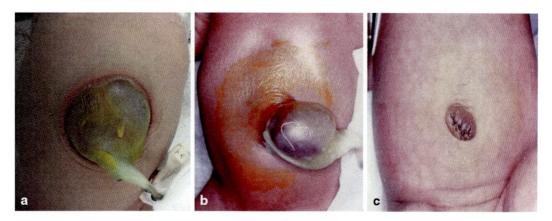

Fig. 37.8 a–c A clinical photograph showing omphalocele minor closed primarily

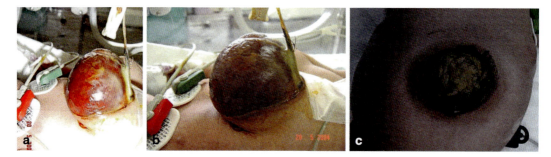

Fig. 37.9 Clinical photograph showing a large omphalocele containing the liver (**a**) and being reduced gradually (**b**) and after being reduced completely (**c**)

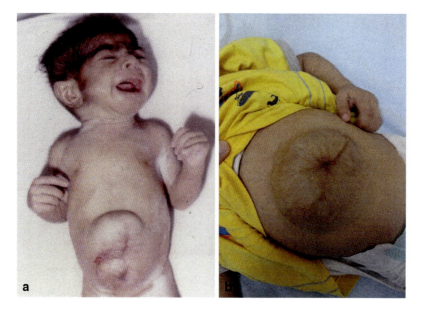

Fig. 37.10 a and b A clinical photograph showing an incisional hernia following closure of a large omphalocele

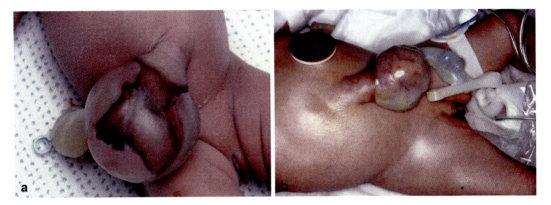

Fig. 37.11 a and **b** A clinical photograph showing hernia of the umbilical cord. Note the skin covering the umbilicus. Note also the skin attached to the sac. Note the size of the defect in **b** and the skin covering the umbilical side of the defect

- Short-term silo reduction (2 weeks)
- Followed by closure with a mesh
- Long-term silo reduction (2–6 weeks)
- Staged closure
- Skin flap closure
- Repair the incisional hernia at 6–12 months of age

- The severity of the associated anomalies determines the prognosis.
- The mortality rate is 80% when severe associated anomalies are present, and it increases to 100% when chromosomal and cardiovascular abnormalities are present.
- The perinatal mortality in fetuses with omphaloceles is between 25 and 75% and is invariably related to the associated malformations or karyotype abnormalities.
- Infants with isolated omphaloceles have a relatively good prognosis, with a survival rate as high as 90%.

Hernia of the Umbilical Cord

- This is a defect in the anterior abdominal wall through the umbilical cord that is:
    - Usually <4 cm in diameter.
    - The umbilical cord is normally covered with skin (Fig. 37.11).

Recommended Reading

Ledbetter DJ. Gastroschisis and omphalocele. Surg Clin North Am. 2006;86:249–60.
Stoll C, Alembik Y, Dott B, Roth MP. Omphalocele and gastroschisis and associated malformations. Am J Med Genet A. 2008;146A(10):1280–5.

Chapter 38
The Spleen

Introduction

- The spleen is considered part of the lymphatic system.
- It is the largest lymphoid tissue of human body, accounting for 25 % of total lymphocytes.
- The spleen, in healthy adult humans, is approximately 11 cm (4.3 in.) in length. It usually weighs between 150 g (5.3 oz) and 200 g (7.1 oz).
- The role of $1 \times 3 \times 5 \times 7 \times 9 \times 11$, an easy way to remember the anatomy of the spleen. The spleen is 1" by 3" by 5", weighs approximately 7 oz, and lies between the 9th and 11th ribs on the left side.

Embryology

- The spleen is unique with respect to its development within the gut. While most of the gut viscera are endodermally derived (with the exception of the neural-crest derived suprarenal gland), the spleen is derived from mesenchymal tissue.
- Specifically, the spleen forms within and from the dorsal mesentery. However, it still shares the same blood supply—the celiac trunk—as the foregut organs.
- The spleen appears about the fifth week as a localized thickening of the mesoderm in the dorsal mesogastrium above the tail of the pancreas. With the change in position of the stomach, the spleen is carried to the left, and comes to lie behind the stomach and in contact with the left kidney. The part of the dorsal mesogastrium which intervened between the spleen and the greater curvature of the stomach forms the gastrosplenic ligament.
- The spleen is made of two parts:
  - The red pulp
  - The white pulp separated by marginal zone

Functions of the Spleen

- Red pulp:
  - Made up of thin-walled venous sinusoids which are lined by special endothelial cells with a discontinuous wall allowing the passage of red blood cells (RBCs) between the sinuses and cords.
  - The sinuses are separated by splenic cords (cords of Billroth) which contain macrophages.

1. Filters RBCs and ingests old RBC, damaged RBC such as sickle cells or spherocytes, antibody coated RBC.
2. Remove Heinz bodies or other RBC inclusions such as Howell–Jolly bodies.

- White pulp:
  - Made up of sheaths of lymphoid cells around arteries (periarteriolar lymphatic sheath).
  - These are composed of T cells and lymphoid follicles (B cells); traps antigens for processing.
    1. Responsible for the active immune response through humoral and cell-mediated pathways.

Other Functions of the Spleen

- Production of opsonins, properdin, and tuftsin
- Creation of RBCs:
  - While the bone marrow is the primary site of hematopoiesis in the adult, the spleen has important hematopoietic functions up until the fifth month of gestation.
  - After birth, erythropoietic functions cease, except in some hematologic disorders.
  - As a major lymphoid organ and a central player in the reticuloendothelial system, the spleen retains the ability to produce lymphocytes and, as such, remains a hematopoietic organ.
- Storage of RBCs, lymphocytes, and other formed elements
  - The RBCs can be released when needed. In humans, up to a cup (236.5 ml) of RBCs can be held in the spleen and released in cases of hypovolemia.
  - It can store platelets in case of an emergency.
  - Up to a quarter of lymphocytes can be stored in the spleen at any one time.

Splenectomy is Associated with

- An increase in blood leukocytes.
- An increase in platelets. The postsplenectomy platelet count may rise to abnormally high levels (thrombocytosis), leading to an increased risk of potentially fatal clot formation.
- Splenectomy patients typically have Howell–Jolly bodies and less commonly Heinz bodies in their blood smears. Heinz bodies are usually found in cases of G6PD (Glucose-6-Phosphate Dehydrogenase) and chronic liver disease.
- Diminished responsiveness to some vaccines.
- Increased susceptibility to infections by bacteria and protozoa; in particular, there is an increased risk of postsplenectomy sepsis from polysaccharide encapsulated bacteria such as pneumococci.

Pathological Conditions of the Spleen

Splenomegaly

Splenomegaly is enlargement of the spleen (Fig. 38.1).

- A number of infections and diseases can contribute to splenomegaly. These include:
  - Viral infections, such as infectious mononucleosis

Fig. 38.1 Clinical photograph showing a child with splenomegaly

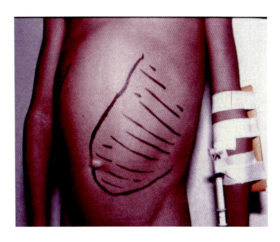

Fig. 38.2 Intraoperative photograph showing massive splenomegaly

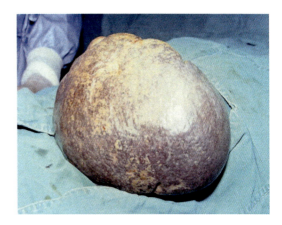

- Bacterial infections, such as syphilis or subacute bacterial endocarditis
- Parasitic infections, such as malaria
- Cirrhosis and other diseases affecting the liver
- Various types of hemolytic anemia—a condition characterized by premature destruction of RBCs
- Blood cancers, such as leukemia, and lymphomas, such as Hodgkin's disease
- Metabolic disorders, such as Gaucher's disease and Niemann–Pick disease
- Pressure on the veins in the spleen or liver (liver cirrhosis) or thrombosis in these veins (portal vein thrombosis)

Massive Splenomegaly

- This describes a spleen that weighs more than 1000 g (Fig. 38.2).
- Causes: chronic myeloid leukemia, Gaucher's disease, hairy cell leukemia, marginal zone B cell lymphoma, myelofibrosis, plasmacytoma, and prolymphocytic leukemia.

Splenic Rupture

- Splenic rupture is due to blunt trauma, penetrating trauma, or abdominal surgery.
- Only rarely ruptures occur spontaneously (associated with infectious mononucleosis, malaria, typhoid fever, leukemia/lymphoma, other tumors, subacute bacterial endocarditis, peliosis lienis, acute splenitis, and pregnancy).

Splenosis

- Splenosis is a condition where foci of splenic tissue undergo autotransplantation, most often following trauma or splenectomy.
- Displaced tissue fragments can implant on well-vascularized surfaces in the abdominal cavity, or, if the diaphragmatic barrier is broken, the thorax.
- The spleen can regenerate through various mechanisms. Autotransplantation of splenic tissue after traumatic disruption of the splenic capsule is well recognized. Splenic tissue can lodge anywhere in the peritoneal cavity following traumatic disruption and regenerates under favorable conditions.
- The incidence of splenic regeneration correlates with the severity of splenic injury. Patients requiring a splenectomy for trauma tend to be those with the greatest splenic damage and dissipation of splenic tissue, which favors autotransplantation.
- They are supplied by newly formed arteries that penetrate the capsule.

Accessory Spleen

- An accessory spleen (*supernumerary spleen, splenule, or splenunculus*) is a small nodule of splenic tissue found apart from the main spleen.
- Accessory spleens are found in approximately 10% of the population and in 20–30% of autopsies.
- Accessory spleens are typically around 1 cm in diameter but may reach up to 4 cm.
- They form either by the result of developmental anomalies or trauma.
- Accessory spleens resemble normal spleen macroscopically and microscopically.
- They may be found anywhere:
    - Along the splenic vessels
    - In the gastrosplenic ligament
    - In the splenorenal ligament
    - In the walls of the stomach or intestines
    - In the pancreatic tail
    - In the greater omentum, the mesentery or the gonads and their path of descent (Fig. 38.3)
- An accessory spleen derives its blood supply from branches of the splenic artery.
- The presence of spleniculi is important to document or find in patients at the time of splenectomy for hematologic diseases specially patients with idiopathic thrombocytopenic purpura (ITP).
- These accessory spleens can enlarge following splenectomy and be the source of recurrent symptoms in those operated on for hematological disorders (Fig. 38.4).

Pathological Conditions of the Spleen

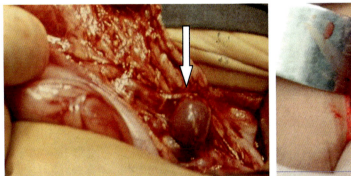
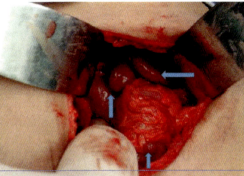

Fig. 38.3 Intraoperative photograph showing a spleniculi and intraoperative photograph showing multiple accessory spleens

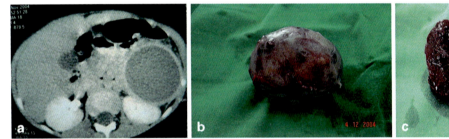

Fig. 38.4 a CT scan of the abdomen showing an enlarged spleniculi in a patient with congenital asplenia. This spleniculi enlarged and became ischemic causing abdominal pain. **b** and **c**, A clinical photograph showing an enlarged spleniculi that was removed. Note that macroscopically it resembles a normal spleen

Asplenia (Congenital Absence of Spleen)

- Congenital absence of the spleen is very rare.
- It is associated with other malformations including:
  - Cardiac malformations (80%, usually involving atrioventricular endocardial cushion and ventricular outflow tract)
  - Situs inversus
  - Anomalies of blood vessels, lung, and abdominal viscera

Hepatolienal Fusion

This is a very rare condition in which there is fusion of liver and spleen.

Polysplenia

Polysplenia is the presence of multiple spleens. This is commonly associated with extrahepatic biliary atresia (Fig. 38.5).

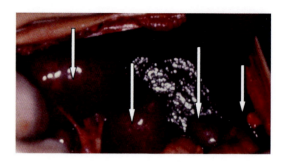

Fig. 38.5 Intraoperative photograph in a patient with biliary atresia and polysplenia

Splenogonadal Fusion

- Splenogonadal fusion is a rare congenital anomaly in which ectopic splenic tissue unites with a gonad and can result in one or more accessory spleens along a path from the abdomen into the pelvis or scrotum.
- Splenogonadal fusion is divided into two types: continuous or discontinuous.
- Continuous: The spleen is connected to ectopic splenic mass by cord of splenic and/or fibrous tissue that is connected to the gonad.
- Discontinuous: There is no connection between the spleen and ectopic splenic mass which unites with a gonad.
- Ninety percent occurs in males and usually on the left sided.
- Twenty percent of continuous types are associated with other congenital defects, including:

  – Peromelus (fetus with malformed limbs), micrognathia, testicular ectopia, inguinal hernia

- Diagnosis: Technetium Tc 99 m sulfur colloid scans is diagnostic.
- Treatment: Surgical excision of ectopic splenic tissue to prevent testicular atrophy, torsion, or infarction and preserve fertility.

Splenorenal Fusion

- Splenorenal fusion is very rare.
- It may be due to splenosis after splenic trauma or splenectomy.
- Less commonly, it may be a developmental anomaly resulting in fusion of splenic and renal tissue.
- It may present as a renal mass or rarely with symptoms of hypersplenism.

Wandering Spleen

- Wandering spleen is most commonly diagnosed in young children as well as women between the ages of 20 and 40.
- It is very rare and <0.5% of all splenectomies are performed for wandering spleen.
- Wandering spleen is due to congenital loss or weakness of ligamentous attachment of the spleen to surrounding structures. Normally, these help to keep the spleen located in the left upper part of the abdomen.
- Clinical features include:

  – Enlargement in the size of the spleen.
  – A change from the spleen's original position to another location, usually in either in other parts of the abdomen or into the pelvis.

Pathological Conditions of the Spleen

- This ability of the spleen to move to another location is commonly attributed to the spleen's pedicle being abnormally long.
- It may be found incidentally.
- It may cause constipation.
- It may cause numerous spleen-related diseases such as hypersplenism, thrombocytopenia, and lymphoma.
- Rarely, torsion of the wandering spleen can also result in abdominal pain or swelling.

- The diagnosis can be confirmed by imaging techniques such as:
  - Abdominal ultrasonography
  - Magnetic resonance imaging
  - Abdominal computed tomography (CT) scan

- The usual treatment is:
  - Splenopexy (fixation of the spleen).
  - If there is torsion with ischemia after unwinding the spleen through detorsion, then splenectomy can be performed.

Splenic Cysts

- Echinococcal cysts (hydatid cyst): These are usually seen in the liver and occasionally in spleen.
- Epithelial cysts:
  - Usually seen in children or young adults.
  - They can be solitary or multiple.
  - May be associated with accessory spleen.
  - Called "epithelioid" if lined by squamous epithelium.
  - Their origin is unknown; may be derived from metaplasia in mesothelial cysts.
  - Often large in size and require splenectomy.
  - Grossly they have a glistening inner surface with marked trabeculation.
  - Microscopically they are lined by squamous, columnar, cuboidal or mesothelial-like epithelium, and no skin adnexae. Rarely are they mucinous associated with pseudomyxoma peritonei. They stain positively for carcinoembryonic antigen (CEA), CA19-9.

- Mesothelial cysts:
  - Also called solitary splenic lymphangioma.
  - May be due to trauma.
  - Microscopically they are subcapsular, multicystic, and may resemble lymphangioma.
  - They stain positive for keratin, HBME-1, and negative for factor VIII–related antigen, CD31, CD34.

- Pseudocyst:
  - They account for 75% of nonparasitic splenic cysts.
  - Usually due to trauma.
  - Some may be epithelial cysts with denuded epithelial lining.
  - Usually solitary and asymptomatic.
  - Their wall is composed of dense fibrous tissue without an epithelial lining and often calcified. Often contains blood and necrotic debris.
  - Their rupture may cause massive hemoperitoneum.

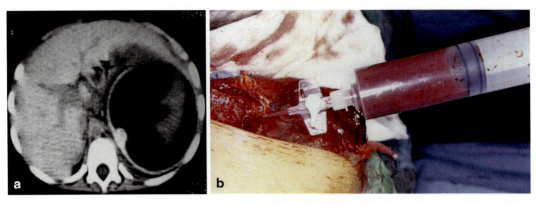

Fig. 38.6 a Abdominal CT scan showing a large splenic abscess in a child with splenic abscess, and **b** pus being aspirated

Splenic Abscess

- Splenic abscess is rare accounting for 0.14–0.7% of necropsy specimens.
- Several factors have been described to predispose to splenic abscess, but sepsis is the commonest predisposing factor in the majority of the cases, with infective endocarditis being the commonest.
- A variety of organisms can cause splenic abscess including staphylococci, Streptococci, and gram-negative bacilli.
- Although abdominal ultrasound is diagnostic, CT scan is more valuable as it allows more accurate anatomical localization of site and size of the abscess (Fig. 38.6a).
- In the past, total splenectomy was the treatment of choice for splenic abscess. To obviate overwhelming postsplenectomy sepsis, splenic preservation was advocated even in those with splenic abscess.
- A variety of procedures have been proposed including:
  - Partial splenectomy
  - CT-guided percutaneous catheter drainage
  - Noninterventional treatment of splenic abscess with antibiotics (Fig. 38.6b)

Massive Splenic Infarction

- Splenic infarctions are common in patients with sickle-cell anemia but these are usually small and repetitive and secondary to vasoocclusion leading to autosplenectomy (Fig. 38.7).
- Massive splenic infarction (splenic infarction involving more than 50% of the spleen size) is very rare and has been reported both in hematological and nonhematological diseases.
- These include:
  - Evans syndrome, subacute bacterial endocarditis, polycythaemia vera, paroxysmal nocturnal hemoglobinuria, Hb SC disease, Hb S-beta-thalassemia
- Splenic infarction is a well-documented complication of hemoglobinopathies. Among these at greatest risk of developing splenic infarction are:
  - Sickle-cell hemoglobin C disease, sickle-cell-beta-thalassemia, sickle-cell trait, sickle-cell anemia

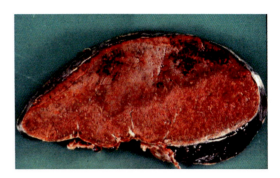

Fig. 38.7 Clinical photograph showing a cut surface of the spleen in a patient with sickle-cell anemia. Note the multiple small infarcts

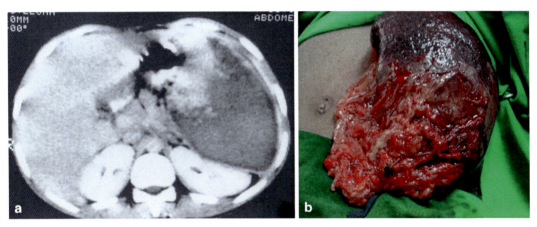

Fig. 38.8 a Abdominal CT scan showing massive splenic infarction in a child with sickle-cell anemia. **b** Intraoperative photograph showing a massive splenic infarction in a child with sickle-cell anemia. Note the adherent omentum to the site of infarction

- The precipitating factor in them is usually high altitude induced hypoxia typically in unpressurized airplanes but has been reported to occur at mountain altitudes of 5000–7000 ft above sea level. This promotes sickling by metabolic effects such as acidosis, hypoxia, and dehydration.
- Although splenic infarction has been reported in patients with sickle-cell trait at high altitude, there have also been reported cases of splenic infarction not related to high altitude exposure.
- The presentation of massive splenic infarction is variable but the majority present with:
  - Sudden onset of severe pain in the left upper quadrant of the abdomen.
  - This may be associated with nausea, vomiting, fever, and chills.
  - Clinically, there is tender splenomegaly.
- Although ultrasound is the main noninvasive investigation, CT scan is more valuable. It accurately outlines the site and size of splenic infarction and help in differentiating this from other conditions (Figs. 38.8 and 38.9).
- Treatment of splenic infarction should be supportive and directed toward correcting any predisposing conditions, intravenous fluids, blood transfusion where necessary, and analgesia. This however warrants close follow-up of these patients as they are liable to develop complications including:
  - Splenic rupture, hemorrhage, splenic abscess, pseudocyst formation

Fig. 38.9 Clinical photograph of a resected spleen from a child with massive splenic infarction

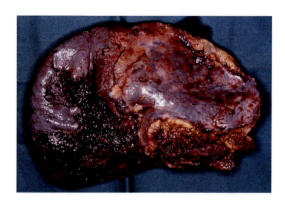

Congestive Splenomegaly

This is caused by portal hypertension, which may be due to:

- Prehepatic: Thrombosis of splenic veins, portal vein thrombosis or stenosis, congestive heart failure
- Hepatic: liver cirrhosis
- Posthepatic: Budd–Chiari syndrome (thrombosis of hepatic veins)

Immunizations and Splenectomy

- As splenectomy causes an increased risk of sepsis due to encapsulated organisms (such as *S. pneumoniae* and *Haemophilus influenzae*), the patient especially children should receive immunization prior to splenectomy. These vaccines are:
  - Pneumococcal vaccine
  - Meningococcal vaccines
  - Haemophilus influenza type b vaccine
- These vaccines should be given at least 2 weeks prior to splenectomy.
- If splenectomy is done for an emergency reason, these vaccines can be given postoperatively.
- Children who undergo splenectomy should also receive prophylactic antibiotics for a minimum of 2 years depending on their age at the time of splenectomy. This is in the form of penicillin prophylaxis either orally or intramuscularly.
- This is because overwhelming postsplenectomy sepsis is commonly seen within the first 2 years postsplenectomy.

Partial Splenectomy

- Splenectomy is usually done through an open incision (upper midline or left upper transverse) but currently and with the recent advances in minimal invasive surgery, laparoscopy is the preferred procedure in cases where the spleen is not too large and when the procedure is elective.
- Total splenectomy should however be avoided whenever possible, because there are severe consequences of an asplenia.

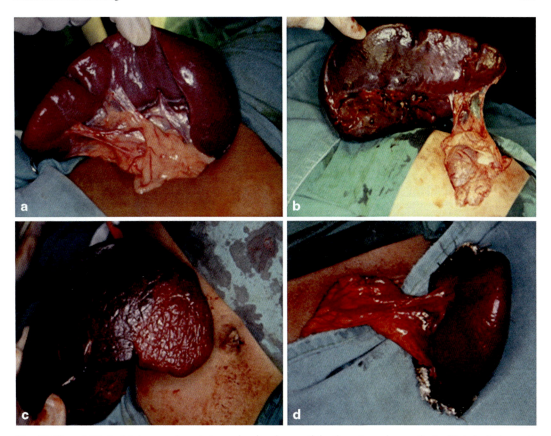

Fig. 38.10 a–d Clinical intraoperative photographs showing partial splenectomy in a patient with beta thalassemia major

- Whilst vaccination and antibiotics provide good protection against the risks of asplenia, this is not 100% effective and not always available especially in poorer countries. Add to this the poor compliance of patients specially children in taking these antibiotics.
- Thus, partial splenectomy or partial arterial embolization of the spleen has been advocated. Much of the spleen's protective roles can be maintained if a small amount of spleen can be left behind (up to one-third of the size of the normal spleen). Where clinically appropriate, attempts are now often made to perform either surgical subtotal (partial) splenectomy, or partial splenic embolization (Fig. 38.10).
- However, as it may take some time for the preserved splenic tissue to provide the full protection, it has been advised that preoperative vaccination still be given to these patients.

Recommended Reading

Al-Salem AH. Splenic complications of sickle cell anemia and the role of splenectomy. ISRN Hematol. 2011;2011:864257.

Corcione F, Pirozzi F, Aragiusto G, Galante F, Sciuto A. Laparoscopic splenectomy: experience of a single center in a series of 300 cases. Surg Endosc. 2012;26:2870–6.

Montenovo MI, Ahad S, Oelschlager BK. Laparoscopic splenopexy for wandering spleen: case report and review of the literature. Surg Laparosc Endosc Percutan Tech. 2010;20(5):e182.

Papparella A, Nino F, Coppola S, Donniacono D, Parmeggiani P. Laparoscopy in the diagnosis and management of splenogonadal fusion: case report. Eur J Pediatr Surg. 2011;21(3):203–4.

Chapter 39
Splenogonadal Fusion

Introduction

- Splenogonadal fusion is a very rare congenital malformation.
- It is characterized by fusion of the spleen and gonad.
- The first case of splenogonadal fusion was described by Bostroem in 1883.

Classification

- There are two types of splenogonadal fusion:
    - Continuous
    - Discontinuous

- The continuous form occurs when the normally located spleen is attached to the gonad by a discrete cord that may be:
    - Totally made up of splenic tissue
    - Made up of multiple connected beads of splenic tissue
    - A cord made up of fibrous tissue

- In the discontinuous type, the splenic tissue is attached to the gonad and completely separated from the normal spleen. This is considered a rare variant of an accessory spleen.
- Both types occur with equal frequency and the discontinuous type may be discovered incidentally during:
    - Herniotomy
    - Orchidopexy
    - Or present as a scrotal swelling

- Thirty-seven percent of the reported patients had an orchiectomy because of suspicion of a testicular tumor.

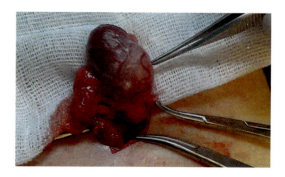

Fig. 39.1 Intraoperative photograph showing discontinuous splenogonadal fusion

Etiology

- The exact etiology of splenogonadal fusion is not known.
- Embryologically, the testis starts to descend from its initial embryological position between the dorsal mesogastrium and the mesonephros at around the 8th week of intrauterine life. This occurs at the time of splenic development.
- Splenogonadal fusion is thought to result from partial fusion of splenic and gonadal tissues in the 4th to 8th weeks of intra-uterine life.
- Subsequent descent of the gonad during the 8th to 10th weeks of gestation results in the descent of a part of the developing spleen along with it.
- In the discontinuous type, there is complete detachment from the normal spleen while in the continuous type there is attachment to the normal spleen by a cord-like structure. This cord can be made up of splenic tissue or be totally fibrotic. Occasionally, there are multiple nodules along this cord which represent foci of splenic tissue that got detached and developed separately.
- This however does not fully explain the occasional occurrence of right-sided splenogonadal fusion.

Clinical Features

- Splenogonadal fusion is commonly asymptomatic, discovered incidentally during routine herniotomy or orchidopexy (Fig. 39.1).
- Many of these cases however go unnoticed or discovered at autopsy.
- In the pediatric age group, these patients commonly present with a scrotal swelling and may rarely present with an acute scrotal pain as a result of torsion or involvement of splenic tissue with other pathological conditions such as mumps, malaria, leukemia, trauma, and infectious mononucleosis.
- The left side is far more commonly affected than the right in 98% of the cases.
- It is more common in males with an M to F ratio of 16:1.
- This however may not be true as the ovary is not easily accessible and since the majority of these cases are asymptomatic, the incidence of splenogonadal fusion in females may be underestimated.

Associated Anomalies

- Not uncommonly, splenogonadal fusion is associated with other anomalies or discovered during the evaluation of these associated anomalies.

- This is more so with the continuous type which is known to be associated with other associated anomalies in as much as 30% of the cases.
- These anomalies include:
  - Peromelia which is categorized as a separate syndrome (splenogonadal fusion limb syndrome)
  - Micrognathia, congenital heart disease, microgastria, cleft palate, craniocynostosis, osteogenesis imperfecta, spina bifida, congenital diaphragmatic hernia, and anorectal anomalies
- There is also an association between splenogonadal fusion and testicular malignancy.
- In the literature, there are about seven reported cases of splenogonadal fusion and testicular malignancy but in all of these cases the malignancy developed in adults with undescended testes or following orchidopexy for undescended testes.
- This may represent an association rather than an increased risk in this subset group of patients as patients with undescended testes have a well-known increased risk of malignancy.

Treatment

- If suspected preoperatively, the diagnosis of splenogonadal fusion can be confirmed by a ^{99m}Tc-sulphur colloid scan.
- Treatment is surgical excision and every attempt should be made to preserve the gonad at the time of dissection and excision which should not be difficult since true fusion with the gonad is rare.

Recommended Reading

Gouw AS, Elema JD, Bink-Boelkens MT, De Jongh JH, ten Kate LP. The spectrum of splenogonadal fusion. Case report and review of 84 reported cases. Eur J Pediatr. 1985;144:316–23.

Chapter 40
Cholelithiasis and Choledocholithiasis

Introduction

- Cholelithiasis is more common in adults and remains relatively rare in children; however, the incidence of cholelithiasis in children is rising (Fig. 40.1).
- The increasing incidence of cholelithiasis in children is attributed to:
  - Increased use of ultrasonography with increased detection rate
  - The growing obesity in children
- The incidence of cholelithiasis in children ranges from 0.15 to 0.22 %.
- The different types of gallstones in children differ from those in adults, with cholesterol stones being the most common type in adults and pigment stones being the most common type in children.
- The distribution of the different types of gallstones in children is as follows:
  - Black pigment stones (48 %)
  - Cholesterol stones (21 %)
  - Calcium carbonate stones (24 %)
  - Protein-dominant stones (5 %)
  - Brown pigment stones (3 %)
- Black pigment stones:
  - These make up 48 % of gallstones in children.
  - They are formed when bile becomes supersaturated with calcium bilirubinate, the calcium salt of unconjugated bilirubin.
  - Black pigment stones are commonly formed in hemolytic disorders (sickle-cell anemia, thalassemia, hemolytic anemia) and can also develop in children receiving parenteral nutrition.
- Calcium carbonate stones:
  - They are more common in children than in adults
  - They account for 24 % of gallstones in children
- Cholesterol stones:
  - They are formed from cholesterol supersaturation of bile

Fig. 40.1 Intraoperative picture showing an open gallbladder with stones

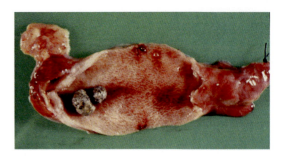

- They are composed of 70–100% cholesterol with an admixture of protein, bilirubin, and carbonate
- They account for most gallstones in adults but make up only about 21% of stones in children
- Brown pigment stones:
  - These are rare, accounting for only 3% of gallstones in children
  - They form in the presence of biliary stasis and bacterial infection
  - They are composed of calcium bilirubinate and the calcium salts of fatty acids
  - They develop more often in the bile ducts than in the gallbladder
- Protein-dominant stones:
  - They make up about 5% of gallstones in children
- Cholelithiasis in children has various predisposing factors:
  - Hemolytic anemias including sickle-cell anemia and thalassemia, hepatobiliary disease, obesity, prolonged parenteral nutrition, abdominal surgery with ileal resection, and sepsis.
  - Other less prominent risk factors include: acute renal failure, prolonged fasting, low-calorie diets, rapid weight loss, the use of certain medications, primarily ceftriaxone.
- Prior to puberty, the sex ratio of cholelithiasis in children appears to be equal. However, after puberty, the frequency of cholelithiasis is significantly greater in females than in males with ratio of 4:1 female predominance.
- The frequency of cholelithiasis in children with sickle-cell anemia is high and increases with age, occurring in approximately 50% of patients by age 20 years.

Etiology

- There are several factors that contribute to the development of gallstones in children, and depending on the cause, gallstones are divided into:
  - Hemolytic gallstones (20–30%):

Sickle-cell disease, hereditary spherocytosis, and thalassemia major

  - Nonhemolytic gallstones (40–50%):

Total parenteral nutrition (TPN), prolonged fasting, ileal disease (like Crohn's disease) or ileal resection, prematurity, furosemide and ceftriaxone therapy, cardiopulmonary bypass, congenital biliary malformations, chronic liver disease, cystic fibrosis, teenage pregnancy, and obesity

  - Idiopathic gallstones (30–40%)

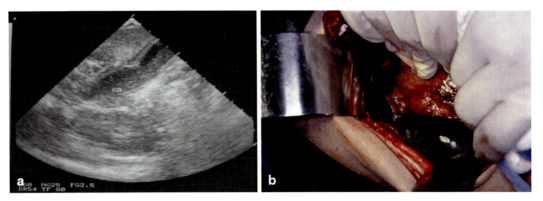

Fig. 40.2 An abdominal ultrasound showing acute cholecystitis with thickened gallbladder wall and intraoperative photograph showing acute cholecystitis

- A unique group of patients are those with chronic hemolytic disease.
- In this group, cholelithiasis is usually not seen before the age of 5 years and the incidence increases with age.
    - In sickle-cell anemia, the prevalence of gallstones was reported to be 10–15% in children under 10 years of age, it increases to 40% in those aged 10–18 years, and 50% in adults.
    - The prevalence of gallstones in hereditary spherocytosis is 10–20% and increases to 40% in adults.
    - In thalassemia, the prevalence of gallstones is 10–15%. With improved survival of thalassemia patients, higher prevalence of gallstones (50%) has been reported.

Complications

- Gallstones in children are asymptomatic, an incidental finding in 30–40% of children.
- Commonly, they cause nonspecific, intermittent abdominal pain or colicky right upper quadrant abdominal pain.
- Cholelithiasis can however cause serious complications including:
    - Acute cholecystitis (Fig. 40.2)
    - Ascending cholangitis
    - Choledocholithiasis
    - Obstructive jaundice with or without cholangitis
    - Gallstone ileus
    - Biliary hepatitis
    - Biliary pancreatitis

Investigations

- Abdominal ultrasonography is the study of choice in patients with cholelithiasis (Fig. 40.3).
- Plain abdominal X-ray may show radiopaque gallstones (Fig. 40.3c).
- Laboratory tests should include a complete blood count, liver function tests, amylase, urinalysis, direct and indirect bilirubin, and alkaline phosphatase.

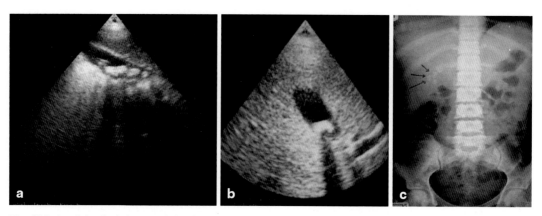

Fig. 40.3 An abdominal ultrasound showing multiple and single gallstones and plain abdominal X-ray showing radiopaque gallstones

- In children with suspected hepatobiliary complications, magnetic resonance cholangiopancreatography (MRCP) or endoscopic retrograde cholangiopancreatography (ERCP) can help delineate the anatomy of the extrahepatic and intrahepatic biliary tract and identify the presence of bile ductal stones. MRCP is a noninvasive and valuable investigation for the evaluation of choledocholithiasis.
- ERCP is valuable as a diagnostic tool and also therapeutic by removing stones from the bile ducts or decompressing the biliary tract. This is especially so prior to cholecystectomy and also postcholecystectomy in those with residual choledocholithiasis (Fig. 40.4).

Treatment

- Laparoscopic cholecystectomy is currently the standard treatment of symptomatic cholelithiasis. It has been proven to be safe and effective in children with a low rate of postoperative complications.
- Surgical complications of laparoscopic cholecystectomy include:
  - Common bile duct injury
  - Bile leaks
  - Postcholecystectomy syndrome
- The postcholecystectomy syndrome is reported in about 4.7%.
- Cholecystectomy for asymptomatic gallstones is still controversial.
- Expectant management with periodic clinical and ultrasonographic surveillance for asymptomatic cholelithiasis has been suggested by some authors.
- Others advocate cholecystectomy for asymptomatic gallstones. These young patients are likely to develop gallstones-related complications.
- Laparoscopic cholecystectomy with intraoperative cholangiography is an alternative to ERCP in patients with suspected choledocholithiasis.
- Laparoscopic cholecystectomy has also been demonstrated to be safe and effective in patients with sickle-cell anemia and cholelithiasis or biliary sludge (Fig. 40.5).

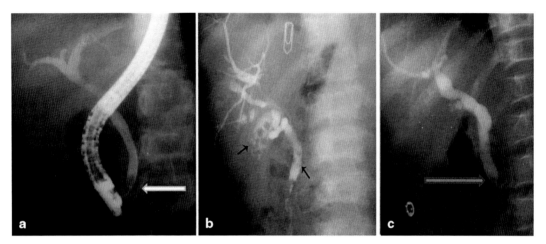

Fig. 40.4 ERCP showing a stone in the lower CBD (**a**), multiple gallstones and CBD stones and ERCP in a child following cholecystectomy (**b**). Note the retained stone in the lower CBD (**c**)

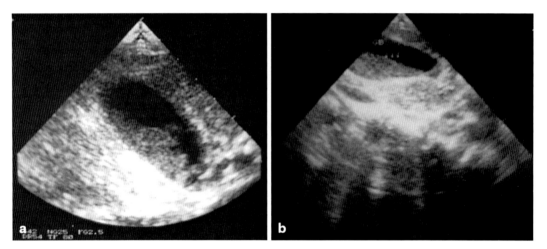

Fig. 40.5 a and **b**, Abdominal ultrasound showing biliary sludge in the gallbladder (*arrows*)

- Elective laparoscopic cholecystectomy should be the standard treatment in children with sickle-cell anemia and cholelithiasis, whether symptomatic or asymptomatic, to prevent the potential complications of gallstones. Add to this the fact that cholecystectomy in these patients should simplify their future management if they present with abdominal crisis, as the possibility of acute cholecystitis is excluded.

Recommended Reading

Siddiqui S, Newbrough S, Alterman D, Anderson A, Kennedy A Jr. Efficacy of laparoscopic cholecystectomy in the pediatric population. J Pediatr Surg. 2008;43(1):109–13.

Wesdorp I, Bosman D, de Graaff A, Aronson D, van der Blij F, Taminiau J. Clinical presentations and predisposing factors of cholelithiasis and sludge in children. J Pediatr Gastroenterol Nutr. 2000;31(4):411–7.

Chapter 41
Choledochal Cyst

Introduction

- Choledochal cyst is a rare congenital anomaly characterized by cystic dilatation of the biliary tract.
- It is rare with an incidence of 1:100,000–150,000.
- Although they may be discovered at any age, 60% are diagnosed before the age of 10 years.
- There is a strong female predilection with an M:F ratio of 1:4.
- There is a greater prevalence of choledochal cyst in East Asia with a much higher incidence as high as 1:1000 in Japan.

Etiology

The exact cause of choledochal cysts is unknown and several theories have been proposed to explain its pathogenesis:

- Congenital malformation.
- Weakness of the wall of the bile duct leading to its dilation.
- Obstruction of the distal common bile duct.
- Combination of distal obstruction and weakness of the wall of bile ducts.
- Reflux of pancreatic enzymes into the common bile duct as a result of an anomaly of the pancreaticobiliary junction (APBJ).
- More than 90% of patients with choledochal cysts have an APBJ with the pancreatic duct joining the common bile duct >1 cm proximal to the ampulla.

Classification

In 1959, Alonso-Lej et al. classified choledochal cyst into three types, which was modified in 1977 by Todani.

- Type I: The most common variety (80–90%) characterized by fusiform dilatation of a portion or entire common bile duct (CBD) with normal intrahepatic duct (Fig. 41.1a). It is subdivided into three types:
    - IA: Fusiform dilatation of the entire extrahepatic bile duct
    - IB: Fusiform dilatation of a segment of the extrahepatic bile duct
    - IC: Fusiform dilatation of the CBD portion of the extrahepatic bile duct

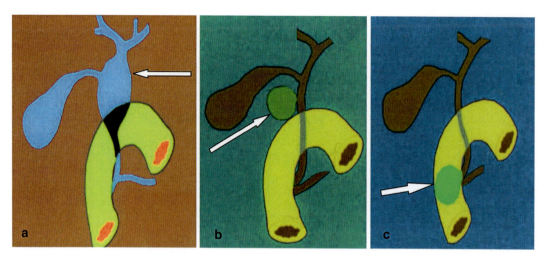

Fig. 41.1 Type I (**a**), type II (**b**) and type III (**c**) choledochal cyst

Fig. 41.2 Type IVa (**a**) and V (**b**) choledochal cyst

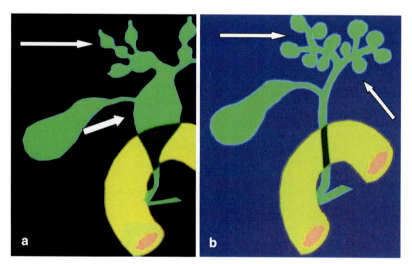

- Type II: isolated diverticulum protruding from the CBD. This comprises >5% of all types of choledochal cysts (Fig. 41.1b).
- Type III or choledochocele: cystic dilatation of the intraduodenal portion of the extrahepatic CBD (choledochocele). It comprises approximately 5% of all choledochal cysts (Fig. 41.1c).
- Type IVa: characterized by multiple dilatations of the intrahepatic and extrahepatic biliary tree (Fig. 41.2).
- Type IVb: Multiple dilatations involving only the extrahepatic bile ducts.
- Type V or Caroli's disease: cystic dilatation of intra hepatic biliary ducts (Fig. 41.3).
- The term forme fruste choledochal cyst was proposed by Lily et al. to describe one of these variants in which the cystic dilatation of the common duct is minimal or absent but there is a long pancreatobiliary union, partial obstruction of the lower common bile duct, and histopathological changes identical to choledochal cyst in the wall.

Diagnosis

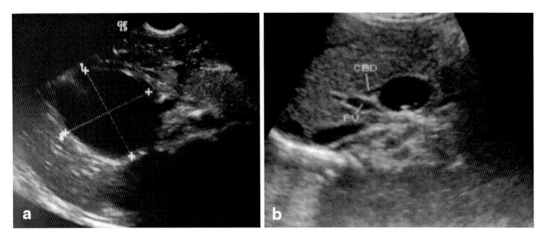

Fig. 41.3 Abdominal ultrasound showing choledochal cyst. Note also the portal vein and proximal part of the common bile duct

Clinical Features

- The classic triad for choledochal cysts is:
  - Pain
  - Jaundice
  - Abdominal mass
- This is found in only a minority (20–60%) of children at the time of presentation.
- Infants commonly present with:
  - Elevated conjugated bilirubin (80%)
  - Failure to thrive
  - An abdominal mass (30%)
- In patients older than 2 years of age:
  - Abdominal pain is the most common presenting symptom
  - This is usually associated with intermittent jaundice
  - Recurrent cholangitis and pancreatitis
- The most common complications of a choledochal cyst are:
  - Cholangitis, pancreatitis, biliary cirrhosis, liver abscess, cholelithiasis, portal hypertension, cyst rupture, malignant degeneration.
  - The risk of complications increases with age and the most important complication is malignant degeneration, with an incidence of 2.5–26%.

Diagnosis

- Diagnosis of choledochal cyst can be made by ultrasonography, which is the most useful initial investigation (Fig. 41.3).

Fig. 41.4 Abdominal CT scan showing choledochal cyst

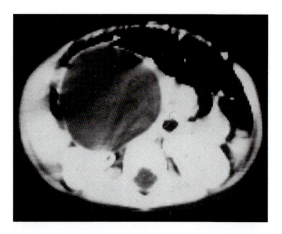

Fig. 41.5 a and **b**, ERCP and PTC showing choledochal cyst. Note also the intrahepatic biliary dilatation (type IVa choledochal cyst) and gallbladder on top of the cyst

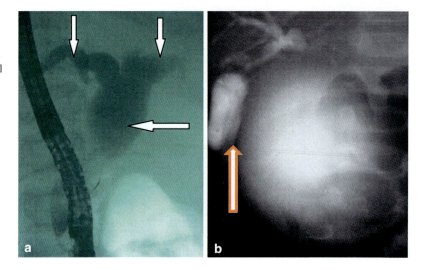

- Computed tomography (CT) scan is a valuable and accurate investigation in diagnosing choledochal cyst (Fig. 41.4).
- Endoscopic retrograde cholangiopancreatography (ERCP), Percutaneous transhepatic cholangiography (PTC), and MRCP (Magnetic resonance cholangiopancreatography) are reserved for patients in whom confusion remains after evaluation by less invasive investigation (Fig. 41.5).
- A less invasive and reliable investigation is HIDA (Hepatobiliary Iminodiacetic Acid) scan (Fig. 41.6).
- MRCP is helpful in the diagnosis and delineating the anomalous pancreaticobiliary junction.

Treatment

- An intraoperative cholangiography is mandatory to define the precise anatomy (Fig. 41.7).
- In the past, the treatment of choledochal cysts consisted of internal drainage by cystenterostomy, but because of the increased risk of carcinoma, high rate of recurrent cholangitis, and pancreatitis, drainage was abandoned in favor of cyst excision (Figs. 41.8 and 41.9).

Treatment

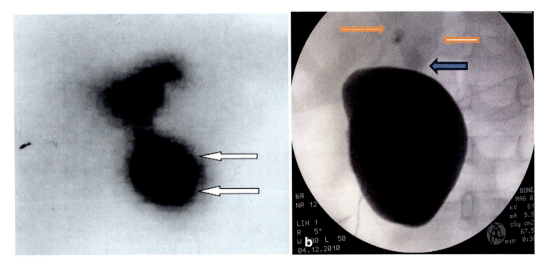

Fig. 41.6 HIDA scan showing choledochal cyst (**a**) and intraoperative cholangiogram (**b**) showing a large choledochal cyst. Note also the proximal part of the common hepatic duct and the two hepatic ducts

Fig. 41.7 An intraoperative cholangiogram through the gallbladder showing the gallbladder, cystic duct, and choledochal cyst. Note also the two hepatic bile ducts and part of common hepatic duct

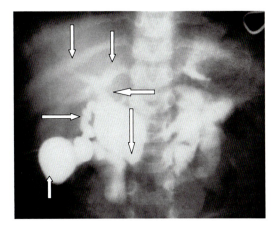

- The treatment of choice of choledochal cyst is complete excision. Surgical management varies according to the type of cyst.
- Patients who present late after development of advanced liver cirrhosis and portal hypertension are not good candidates for excisional surgery.
- Appropriate antibiotics therapy and supportive care should be given to patients presenting with cholangitis.
- Type I cyst is treated with total surgical excision with Roux-en-Y hepaticojejunostomy.
- Hepaticoduodenostomy is associated with a high rate of duodenogastric reflux (33%) when compared to hepaticojejunostomy.
- In difficult cases where the cyst wall is adherent posteriorly to the portal vein, Lilly in 1978 advocated excising the cyst from within. The cyst is opened and the cyst wall is excised from inside, leaving the fibrotic posterior wall behind.
- A lower complication rate and less hepatic fibrosis were reported in neonates who underwent excision of choledochal cyst in the first 30 days of life. This stresses the importance of antenatal diagnosis.

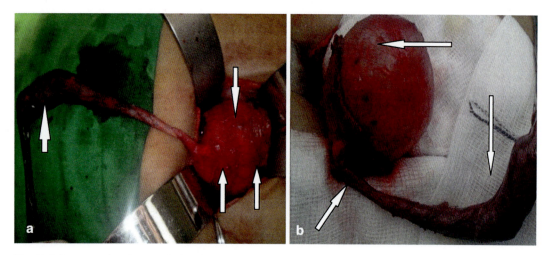

Fig. 41.8 Intraoperative photograph showing the dissected gallbladder attached to the choledochal cyst

Fig. 41.9 Intraoperative cholangiogram showing the already dissected choledochal cyst. Note its attachment to the proximal common bile duct representing type IB of choledochal cyst

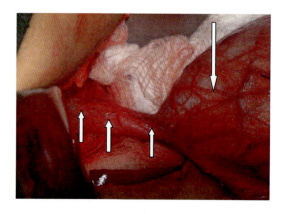

- Type II is treated with simple cyst excision. The CBD should be closed transversely over a T-tube to avoid stricture formation.
- Type III is treated with endoscopic sphincterotomy if small in size, otherwise it should be excised via a transverse duodenotomy.
- Type IV: require complete resection of the extrahepatic biliary tree when possible. Regarding intrahepatic ducts, surgery should be individualized depending on:
  - The lobes affected.
  - The presence of strictures or stones.
  - The presence of cirrhosis or malignancy.
  - If intrahepatic cysts are localized into one lobe, hepatic lobectomy is the preferred approach.
- For diffuse intrahepatic disease, liver transplantation should be considered.
- Type V (Caroli's disease):
  - If unilateral or segmental with cirrhosis: resection of the involved part of liver is the treatment of choice.
  - Ursodeoxycholic acid may improve bile flow, reducing the incidence of biliary sludge, stones, and cholangitis.

- In the absence of cirrhosis or malignancy, Roux-en-Y hepaticojejunostomy with bilateral transhepatic silastic stents may be indicated to improve biliary drainage (stents left for 6–12 months).
- Patients with Caroli's disease and liver failure may warrant liver transplantation.

- Recently and with advancement in minimal invasive surgery, laparoscopic complete cyst excision and hepaticoduodenostomy for choledochal cyst were shown to be feasible and safe. This however requires experienced laparoscopic surgeons.
- Complications after surgery for choledochal cyst have been mainly observed with types I, IV, and V.
- The overall morbidity rate is < 10%.
- Postsurgical complications include:
    - Cholangitis
    - Biliary stone formation
    - Anastomotic stricture
    - Residual debris
    - Biliary stone formation
    - Pancreatitis
    - Intrahepatic bile duct dilatation.

Recommended Reading

Chijiiwa K, Koga A. Surgical management and long-term follow-up of patients with choledochal cysts. *Am J Surg.* 1993;165(2):238–42.

Miyano T, Yamataka A. Choledochal cysts. *Curr Opin Pediatr.* 1997;9(3):283–8.

Todani T, Watanabe Y, Narusue M, Tabuchi K, Okajima K. Congenital bile duct cysts: classification, operative procedures, and review of thirty-seven cases including cancer arising from choledochal cyst. Am J Surg. 1977;134(2):263–9.

Chapter 42
Biliary Atresia

Introduction

- Biliary atresia is also known as progressive obliterative cholangiopathy.
- Biliary atresia causes a progressive damage of the extrahepatic and intrahepatic bile ducts with cholestasis as a result of obstructive cholangiopathy secondary to inflammation, leading to fibrosis, and if not recognized and treated, it leads to biliary cirrhosis and liver failure.
- It is the most common cause of surgical jaundice in infants.
- The cause of biliary atresia is not known.
- The incidence of biliary atresia is variable and ranges from 1:10,000 to 1:15,000 live births.
- Biliary atresia seems to affect girls slightly more often than boys.
- Asians and African-Americans are affected more frequently than Caucasians. Biliary atresia is known to be more common in Chinese and Japanese.
- Biliary atresia should be recognized and distinguished from neonatal jaundice. Infants with prolonged jaundice should be thoroughly investigated for biliary atresia.
- Biliary atresia should be considered in all neonates with direct hyperbilirubinemia.
- Physiologic unconjugated hyperbilirubinemia rarely persists beyond 2 weeks of age. Infants with prolonged physiologic jaundice must be evaluated for other causes.
- A high index of suspicion is important to make the diagnosis of biliary atresia because surgical treatment by age 2 months has clearly been shown to improve the outcome and establishment of bile flow and to prevent the development of biliary cirrhosis.
- In 1959, Kasai introduced his operation for what was considered non-correctable biliary atresia.
- The success of Kasai operation is most effective when performed before the patient reaches 2 months of age.

Etiology

The exact cause of biliary atresia is not known and many factors have been incriminated in its pathogenesis, including:

1. Reovirus 3 infection.
2. Congenital malformation. Early studies postulated a congenital malformation of the biliary ducts leading to their obstruction.
3. Congenital cytomegalovirus (CMV) infection.
4. Autoimmunity.

Fig. 42.1 Classification of biliary atresia

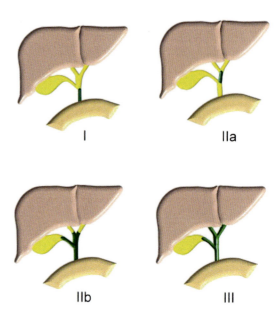

5. A possible association with the gene GPC1, which encodes a glypican 1-a heparan sulfate proteoglycan, has been reported in the pathogenesis of biliary atresia. This gene is located on the long arm of chromosome 2 (2q37).
6. Identification of active and progressive inflammation and destruction of the biliary system on histological studies suggest that extrahepatic biliary atresia represents an acquired lesion. Infectious agents seem to be the most possible cause.

Classification

There are three types of biliary atresia (Fig. 42.1):

- Type I: Atresia involving the common bile duct. The proximal bile ducts are patent.
- Type II: Atresia involving the common hepatic duct. This is usually associated with cystic structure at the porta hepatis.
  - Type IIa: The cystic and common bile ducts are patent.
  - Type IIb: The cystic, common bile duct, and hepatic ducts are all obliterated.
- Type III: Atresia involving the right and left hepatic ducts up to the porta hepatis. This is the commonest type seen in >90% of cases.

Clinically, biliary atresia occurs in two distinct forms:

- The fetal-embryonic form:
  - Appears in the first 2 weeks of life.
  - About 10–20% of affected neonates have associated congenital defects.
- The postnatal form:

Clinical Features

Fig. 42.2 An intraoperative photograph showing polysplenia in a patient with biliary atresia

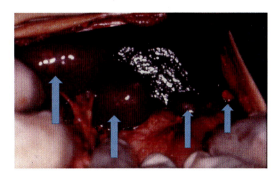

- Appears in neonates and infants aged 2–8 weeks.
- Progressive inflammation and obliteration of the extrahepatic bile ducts occur after birth.
- Not associated with congenital anomalies.
- Infants may have a short jaundice-free interval.

Associated Anomalies

- Associated anomalies are seen in about 20% of biliary atresia cases. These include:
  - Cardiac malformations
  - Polysplenia
  - Situs inversus
  - Absent vena cava
  - A preduodenal portal vein
- This complex of anomalies is also termed the polysplenia syndrome (polysplenia, absent inferior vena cava, bilobed symmetric liver, malrotation, preduodenal portal vein, bilobed lungs, and cardiac anomalies) and is seen in 10–20% of patients with biliary atresia (Fig. 42.2).

Clinical Features

- The initial symptoms of biliary atresia are indistinguishable from neonatal jaundice.
- Infants with biliary atresia are typically full term.
- The symptoms are seen usually between 1 and 6 weeks of life.
- These include:
  - Jaundice which is prolonged.
  - Clay-colored stools. The color of the stools may be slightly yellow due to the intestinal epithelial cells, which are shed in the stools. These cells are stained yellow from the generalized jaundice.
  - Dark urine.
- Hepatomegaly may be present early, and the liver is often firm or hard to palpation.
- Splenomegaly suggests progressive cirrhosis with portal hypertension.

Differential Diagnosis

The list of causes of neonatal jaundice is long and includes the following:

- Alagille syndrome
- Biliary hypoplasia
- Caroli disease and choledochal cyst
- Cystic fibrosis
- Cytomegalovirus infection
- Galactosemia
- Neonatal hemochromatosis
- Herpes simplex virus infection
- Lipid storage disorders
- Rubella
- Syphilis
- Toxoplasmosis

Investigations

- Serum bilirubin (total and direct): Conjugated hyperbilirubinemia, defined as any level exceeding either 2 mg/dL or 20% of total bilirubin, is always abnormal.
- Alkaline phosphatase.
- 5' nucleotidase, gamma-glutamyl transpeptidase (GGTP), serum aminotransferases, serum bile acids: A markedly elevated alanine aminotransferase level (>800 IU/L) is more in favor of neonatal hepatitis.
- Serum alpha1-antitrypsin.
- Sweat chloride test to exclude cystic fibrosis.
- Ultrasonography: Ultrasonography has been found unreliable in the evaluation of biliary atresia, but it may demonstrate absence of the gallbladder and no dilatation of the biliary tree. It is useful in excluding other causes, mainly choledochal cyst.
- Hepatobiliary isotope scan: This is useful in evaluating infants with biliary atresia. Intestinal excretion of the isotope confirms patency of the extrahepatic bile ducts. This test has been associated with a 10% rate of false-positive or false-negative diagnostic errors. The use of phenobarbitone (5–10 mg/kg/day) for about 5 days prior to the test reduces the number of false positives (Fig. 42.3). In those with biliary atresia, there is normal uptake by the liver and failure of secretion of the isotope, while in neonatal hepatitis there is poor liver uptake of isotope.
- Duodenal intubation and test of duodenal secretions for bile.
- Endoscopic retrograde cholangiopancreatography (ERCP) is useful in the presence of equipment and personnel experienced in this.
- Percutaneous liver biopsy is the most valuable study for evaluating neonatal cholestasis. When examined by an experienced pathologist, an adequate biopsy specimen can differentiate between obstructive and hepatocellular causes of cholestasis, with 90% sensitivity and specificity for biliary atresia.
- Intraoperative cholangiography: this procedure definitively demonstrates anatomy and patency of the extrahepatic bile ducts (Figs. 42.4, 42.5, and 42.6).
- Laparoscopy is valuable for the diagnosis of biliary atresia including liver biopsy and intraoperative cholangiogram.

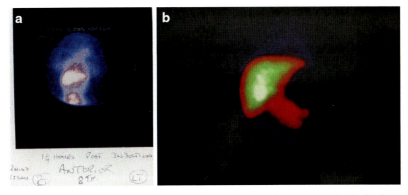

Fig. 42.3 HIDA scan in two patients with obstructive jaundice showing no isotope secretion in the first one, suggestive of biliary atresia, and normal secretion of isotope in the second one

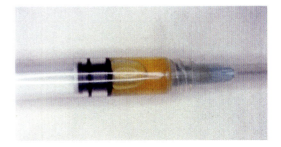

Fig. 42.4 Bile aspirated from the gallbladder at the time of cholangiography. This indicates patent bile ducts

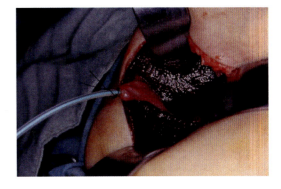

Fig. 42.5 Intraoperative photograph in a patient with biliary atresia. Note the small contracted gallbladder and slightly cirrhotic liver

Treatment

- Once biliary atresia is suspected, surgical intervention in the form of intraoperative cholangiogram and Kasai portoenterostomy is indicated.
- This procedure is not usually curative, but ideally does buy time until the child can achieve growth and undergo liver transplantation.
- A considerable number of these patients, even if Kasai portoenterostomy has been successful, eventually undergo liver transplantation.

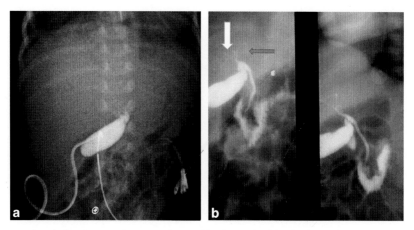

Fig. 42.6 Intraoperative cholangiograms in two patients with obstructive jaundice. In **a** there are no bile ducts seen, indicative of biliary atresia; and in **b** there is biliary hypoplasia. Note the small but patent bile ducts in **b**

- In the unusual circumstance of patent common bile duct, a modified portoenterostomy may be considered. The fact that this is a progressive disease must be kept in mind and these patients may subsequently require classic Kasai portoenterostomy.

Postoperative Care

- In the immediate postoperative period, high-dose pulse therapy with methylprednisolone or low dose has been used as both an anti-inflammatory agent and as a nonspecific stimulant of bile salt secretion.
- Ursodeoxycholic acid has also been shown to enhance bile flow.
- In order to prevent cholangitis postoperatively, prophylaxis with trimethoprim–sulfamethoxazole has been used on a long-term basis.

Postoperative Complications and Outcome

- About 60–80 % of patients drain bile following Kasai portoenterostomy.
- Age at the time of surgery remains the most important factor in determining the outcome.
- The earliest common complication is an unsuccessful anastomosis with failure to achieve bile drainage.
- The following factors have been shown to predict the long-term outcome after Kasai portoenterostomy:

  – Age younger than 2 months at operation
  – Preoperative liver histology and ductal remnant size
  – The presence of bile in hepatic lobular zone 1
  – Absence of portal hypertension and liver cirrhosis
  – Postoperative decline and disappearance of jaundice

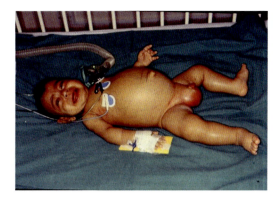

Fig. 42.7 A clinical photograph of a child with advanced biliary atresia. Note the abdominal distension secondary to ascites

- About 30% of the patients fail to have adequate bile flow following surgery. These patients develop progressive fibrosis and biliary cirrhosis. These patients are candidates for orthotopic liver transplantation.
- More than 60% of those who achieve initial response subsequently develop complications related to progressive liver disease and portal hypertension. These will require liver transplantation (Fig. 42.7).
- Cholangitis develops in 50% of patients following Kasai portoenterostomy.
- Hepatocellular carcinoma is a rare risk in those with liver cirrhosis.
- Liver transplantation is the only option for long-term survival in the majority of patients with biliary atresia.
- Children with biliary atresia have the promise of long-term survival with a combination of Kasai portoenterostomy and liver transplantation.
- Re-exploration should be considered for patients following Kasai portoenterostomy when:
  - They become jaundiced after an initial jaundice free phase postoperatively
  - They have favorable hepatic and biliary duct remnant histology but do not successfully drain bile
  - They may have had an inadequate initial surgery

Recommended Reading

Bassett MD, Murray KF. Biliary atresia: recent progress. J Clin Gastroenterol. 2008;42(6):720–9.
Okazaki T, Kobayashi H, Yamataka A, Lane GJ, Miyano T. Long-term postsurgical outcome of biliary atresia. J Pediatr Surg. 1999; 34(2):312–5.
Utterson EC, Shepherd RW, Sokol RJ, et al. Biliary atresia: clinical profiles, risk factors, and outcomes of 755 patients listed for liver transplantation. J Pediatr. 2005;147(2):180–5.
Visser BC, Suh I, Hirose S, Rosenthal P, Lee H, Roberts JP, Hirose R. The influence of portoenterostomy on transplantation for biliary atresia. Liver Transpl. 2004;10(10):1279–86.

Chapter 43
Pancreatitis and Pancreatic Pseudocyst in Children

Introduction

- Pancreatitis is uncommon in children, is associated with significant morbidity and mortality, and represents a diagnostic challenge for clinicians.
- In adults, pancreatitis is commonly caused by alcohol abuse or gallstone disease. The etiology of pancreatitis in children is however diverse.
- The causes of pancreatitis in children include:
    - Abdominal trauma (23 %)
    - Anomalies of the pancreaticobiliary system (15 %)
    - Multisystem disease (14 %)
    - Drugs and toxins (12 %)
    - Viral infections (10 %)
    - Hereditary disorders (2 %)
    - Metabolic disorders (2 %)
    - Unknown etiology (25 %)
- Pancreatitis is classified into:
    - Local or diffuse
    - Acute, chronic, familial, necrotic, or hemorrhagic
- Occasionally, pancreatitis is complicated by the formation of a pseudocyst.
- Pancreatic pseudocyst is a localized cystic swelling filled with pancreatic fluids and enzymes, and has a wall made up of fibrous and granulation tissue with no epithelial linings.
- In general, the prognosis of children with acute pancreatitis is excellent, but it can be complicated by the formation of pseudocysts in 10–23 % of patients. This is more often in chronic than acute pancreatitis patients.
- The frequency of pseudocyst formation is > 50 % when pancreatitis is associated with abdominal trauma.

Etiology

- Common causes of pancreatitis include:
    - Blunt abdominal trauma:

- Motor vehicle accident
- Child abuse
- Bicycle accident where the abdomen is compressed by the handlebars
- Systemic infection including:
  - Mumps
  - Rubella
  - Coxsackie virus B
  - Cytomegalovirus
  - Human immunodeficiency virus
- Pancreaticobiliary malunion
- Congenital anomalies of the pancreatobiliary junction.
- Pancreas divisum
- Congenital sphincter of Oddi abnormality
- Choledochal cysts
- Choledocholithiasis
- Use of hyperalimentation
- Medications including:
  - Azathioprine
  - Tetracycline
  - l-Asparagine
  - Valproic acid
  - Steroids
  - Immunosuppressive agents
- Metabolic diseases including:
  - Hypertriglyceridemia
  - Hypercalcemia
  - Cystic fibrosis
- Hereditary pancreatitis: This is characterized by an alteration in the long arm of chromosome 7, which yields an aberrant trypsinogen protein that may induce autodigestion of the pancreas

Acute Pancreatitis

Clinical Features

- In children, the clinical features of acute pancreatitis are variable.
- Most commonly, children with acute pancreatitis present with:
  - Abdominal pain (87%)
  - Vomiting (64%)
  - Abdominal tenderness (77%)
  - Abdominal distension (18%)
  - Other, less common clinical signs include:
    - Fever
    - Tachycardia
    - Hypotension
    - Jaundice
    - Abdominal guarding
    - Rebound tenderness
    - Decreased bowel sounds

- Acute hemorrhagic pancreatitis:
  - Rarely occurs in children.
  - This is a life-threatening condition with a mortality rate approaching 50% because of:
    - Shock
    - Systemic inflammatory response syndrome with multiple organ dysfunction
    - Acute respiratory distress syndrome
    - Disseminated intravascular coagulation
    - Massive gastrointestinal (GI) bleeding
    - Systemic or peritoneal infection
  - Physical examination findings associated with hemorrhagic pancreatitis may include:
    - A bluish discoloration of the flanks (Grey Turner sign)
    - Periumbilical region bluish discoloration (Cullen sign)
    - Pleural effusions
    - Hematemesis
    - Melena
    - Coma

Diagnosis

- Serum amylase and lipase levels.
- The magnitude of enzyme elevation does not correlate with the severity of acute pancreatitis.
- Serum amylase levels peak 48 h after onset and are typically elevated for as long as 4 days.
- Serum or urinary amylase levels and their ratio aid in the diagnosis of acute pancreatitis.
- Amylase levels can be within normal limits in 10–15% of patients with acute pancreatitis.
- Serum lipase is more specific than amylase for acute pancreatitis, and typically, lipase levels remain elevated 8–14 days longer than amylase levels.
- Other laboratory abnormalities found in patients with pancreatitis may include:
  - Coagulopathies
  - Leukocytosis
  - Hyperglycemia
  - Glucosuria
  - Hypocalcemia
  - Hyperbilirubinemia
  - Elevated gamma glutamyl transpeptidase
- Urinary levels of trypsin activator peptide (TAP) may help determine the severity of the pancreatitis.
- Abdominal X-ray may demonstrate nonspecific findings:
  - A distended loop of small intestine (sentinel loop)
  - Calcifications
  - Radiopaque gallstones
  - Dilation of the transverse colon (cutoff sign)
  - Ascites
  - Peripancreatic extraluminal gas bubbles
  - Ileus
  - Left-sided basal pleural effusion
  - Blurring of the left psoas margin

Fig. 43.1 Abdominal CT scan showing posttraumatic pancreatic pseudocyst in a child. Note its relation to the pancreas and stomach

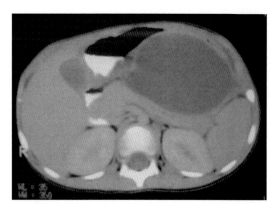

- Pancreatic calcifications from chronic or recurrent pancreatitis
- Imaging studies are normal in 20% of children with acute pancreatitis

- Ultrasonography and computed tomography (CT) scanning are the preferred imaging modalities used to diagnose and follow the course of pancreatitis and pancreatic pseudocysts (Fig. 43.1).
- Abdominal magnetic resonance imaging (MRI).
- Endoscopic retrograde cholangiopancreatography (ERCP) is useful for the diagnosis of various ductal abnormalities or obstructions and may serve as a therapeutic intervention (i.e., sphincterotomy, stone extraction, stent placement).
- Magnetic resonance cholangiopancreatography (MRCP) is a noninvasive alternative to ERCP but lacks therapeutic capabilities.

Medical Management

- Adequate rehydration.
- Analgesia.
- Pancreatic rest.
- Antacids or H2-histamine blockers are useful to prevent gastritis and reduce duodenal acid exposure.
- In severe pancreatitis, oral intake is restricted and parental nutrition is started within 3 days to prevent catabolism.
- In cases of intractable vomiting or ileus, nasogastric suction is beneficial to prevent vomiting, manage ileus, and provide pancreatic rest.
- Antibiotic therapy is indicated for systemic infections or sepsis.

Surgical Management

- Surgical intervention is indicated for:
  - The management of congenital anatomic defects (e.g., pancreatic divisum).
  - The management of complications associated with acute pancreatitis:
    - Pancreatic ascites
    - Intra-abdominal abscess
    - Pancreatic pseudocyst

- Acute pancreatic pseudocysts are managed with observation for 4–6 weeks because most resolve spontaneously.
- Chronic pancreatic pseudocysts (>3 mo) are best treated by surgical interventions such as:
  - Ultrasonography-guided or CT-guided percutaneous drainage
  - Endoscopic drainage
  - Internal drainage via cyst gastrostomy or enterostomy
- Surgery for pancreatic ductal disruption or compromise (i.e., acute traumatic pancreatitis with ductal injury) is indicated after medical failure.
- ERCP or intraoperative pancreatic ductography is valuable in determining the site of ductal disruption and directs surgical decision making to the most appropriate operative procedure.
- Operative management of chronic pancreatitis in children is controversial.
- Indications for operative intervention include:
  - Unsuccessful conservative medical therapy
  - Intractable pain
  - Impaired nutrition
- Surgical options include:
  - Distal pancreatectomy with Roux-en-Y pancreaticojejunostomy (Duval procedure)
  - Lateral pancreaticojejunostomy (Puestow procedure)
  - ERCP sphincteroplasty
  - Total pancreatectomy and islet cell transplantation

Pancreatic Pseudocyst

- Pancreatic pseudocysts are often caused by:
  - Acute or chronic pancreatitis
  - Abdominal trauma
  - Alcohol-induced pancreatitis
- Pseudocysts are more often present in chronic pancreatitis patients than in acute pancreatitis patients.

Clinical Features

- Pancreatic pseudocyst is commonly asymptomatic.
- Children with pancreatic pseudocysts may present with:
  - Abdominal pain
  - Nausea and vomiting
  - A palpable tender epigastric mass
  - Abdominal distension and fullness
  - Jaundice
  - Chest pain
  - Anorexia
  - Weight loss
  - Fever

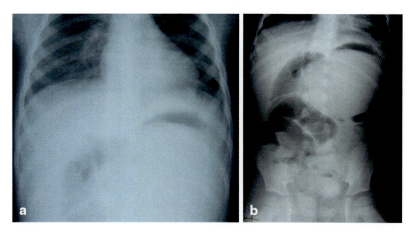

Fig. 43.2 Chest (**a**) and abdominal (**b**) X-ray in a child with pancreatic pseudocyst. Note the soft tissue density in the upper abdomen and the dilated pushed small bowel loops

- Ascites
- GI hemorrhage

- Pancreatic pseudocysts may:
  - Become infected
  - Rupture
  - Cause intestinal obstruction
  - Cause jaundice or sepsis
  - Although pseudocyst formation is an uncommon sequela of acute or chronic pancreatitis in children, complications of pancreatic pseudocysts include:
    - Spontaneous rupture
    - Hemorrhage
    - Infection

- Mediastinal pseudocysts are a rare form of pancreatic pseudocysts in the abdomen which may cause:
  - Dysphagia
  - Dyspnea
  - Airway obstruction
  - Cardiac tamponade

Diagnosis

- Chest and abdominal X-ray (Fig. 43.2).
- The most common and effective method of diagnosing a pancreatic pseudocyst is with abdominal ultrasound and CT scan (Figs. 43.3 and 43.4).
- A pseudocyst generally appears as a fluid-filled mass.
- Transabdominal ultrasound can be used to identify pseudocysts.

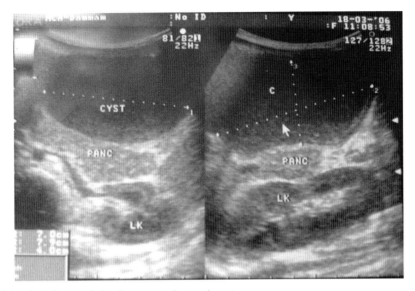

Fig. 43.3 Abdominal ultrasound showing pancreatic pseudocyst

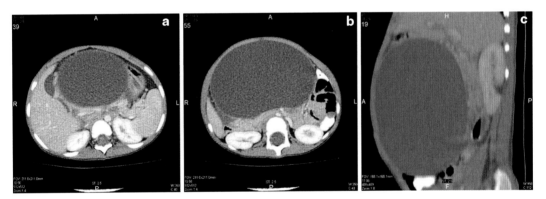

Fig. 43.4 a–c, Abdominal CT scan showing a large pancreatic pseudocyst in a child

Treatment

- Not all pseudocysts require surgical treatment.
- Many pancreatic pseudocysts improve and disappear by themselves.
- If the cysts are small and are not causing symptoms, careful observation with periodic CT scans is recommended.
- Pseudocysts that persist over many months or that cause symptoms or complications require treatment.
- Approximately 60% of pancreatic pseudocysts that are caused by blunt trauma require surgical intervention.

- There are three main methods for draining a pancreatic pseudocyst:
  - Endoscopic drainage
  - Percutaneous catheter drainage
  - Open surgery
- Percutaneous drainage:
  - This is done under the guidance of a CT scan or ultrasound.
  - A drainage catheter is placed into the fluid cavity to drain the fluid, which is then collected over several weeks into an external collection system.
  - The catheter is removed when the drainage becomes minimal.
  - Once the catheter is to be removed, contrast is injected into the cyst cavity to determine the remaining size and to monitor its progress.
  - The success rate of percutaneous drainage is around 50%.
  - Unsuccessful drainages are mostly caused by large ductal leaks or blockage of the main pancreatic duct.
- Acute pancreatic pseudocysts <5 cm in diameter are managed with observation for 4–6 weeks because most resolve spontaneously.
- Pancreatic pseudocysts >5 cm in diameter may require surgical intervention; however, conservative therapy is required for approximately 4–6 weeks to allow the cyst wall to mature.
- Chronic pancreatic pseudocysts (>3 months duration) are best treated by surgical interventions.
- Surgical approaches for internal drainage are largely determined by the anatomic location of the pseudocyst.
  - If the pseudocyst is adherent to the posterior wall of the stomach, cystogastrostomy is performed.
  - If the cyst is present in the head of the pancreas, cystoduodenostomy is performed.
  - For other cysts not adherent to the stomach or duodenum, cystojejunostomy is preferred.
  - Distal pancreatectomy is considered when the pseudocyst is in the tail of the pancreas.
- Endoscopic drainage is becoming the preferred method of draining pseudocysts because:
  - It is less invasive.
  - It does not require external drain.
  - It has a large long-term success rate.
  - Drainage is usually achieved with a transpapillary approach with ERCP.
  - Sometimes a direct drainage across the stomach or duodenal wall is used instead.
  - The transpapillary approach is used when the pseudocyst is in communication with the main pancreatic duct, and is also successful in patients with pancreatic duct disruption.
  - Transgastric or transduodenal approaches are used when the pseudocyst is next to the gastroduodenal wall.
  - Endoscopic ultrasound is a valuable investigation prior to endoscopic drainage.
  - The endoscopic method depends on the presence of a bulge into the stomach or duodenum to determine the site for catheterization.
  - In patients with chronic pseudocysts, this approach has a 90% success rate.
  - Recurrence after drainage is around 4%, and the complication rate is below 16%.
  - Inherent risks include:
    - Missing the pseudocyst
    - Injuring nearby vessels
    - Inefficient placement of the catheter

Recommended Reading

Benifla M, Weizman Z. Acute pancreatitis in childhood: analysis of literature data. J Clin Gastroenterol. 2003;37(2):169–72.
Ford EG, Hardin F, Mahour GH, Woolley MM. Pseudocysts of the pancreas in children. Am Surg. 1990;56(6):384–7.
Lerner A, Branski D, Lebenthal E. Pancreatic diseases in children. Pediatr Clin North Am. 1996;43(1):125–56.
Werlin SL. Pancreatitis in children. J Pediatr Gastroenterol Nutr. 2003;37:591–5.

Chapter 44
Congenital Pancreatic Cysts

Introduction

- Pancreatic cysts are relatively rare and commonly seen in adults.
- In the pediatric age group, pancreatic cysts are very rare.
- Pancreatic cysts are classified into six types:
  - Congenital
  - Retention
  - Duplication
  - Pseudocysts
  - Neoplastic
  - Parasitic cysts
- Clinically and radiologically, it is difficult to differentiate between these types.
- This may be also difficult pathologically for the first three types, which are also called true cysts.
- Congenital, retention, and duplication cysts are true developmental cysts and are lined by true epithelium.
- This is in contrast to the pseudopancreatic cyst, which does not have an epithelial lining.
- Among these, pancreatic pseudocysts whether post traumatic or post inflammatory following acute pancreatitis are the commonest.
- The majority of pancreatic cysts in children are also pseudocysts resulting from trauma, acute pancreatitis, or infection.
- True congenital pancreatic cysts on the other hand are extremely rare and pose unique surgical challenges.
- The site of origin of congenital pancreatic cysts is variable
  - The majorities are localized in the tail or neck of the pancreas (62%).
  - Localization in the head of the pancreas was reported in 32% of cases.
- Congenital pancreatic cysts originating in the neck and tail of the pancreas are often confused with duplication cyst of the stomach and pancreatic pseudocysts, while those originating in the head of the pancreas are often confused with choledochal cyst or duplication cyst of the duodenum.
- They are generally asymptomatic discovered as an incidental abdominal swelling but may cause abdominal distention and may become symptomatic as a result of pressure on adjacent viscera.
- They can attain a large size and are difficult to diagnose preoperatively as they may be confused with pancreatic pseudocysts or duplication cyst of the pancreas, stomach, or duodenum.
- Because preoperative diagnosis of congenital pancreatic cyst is difficult, this condition should be considered in the differential diagnosis of cystic lesions of the pancreas in infants and children.

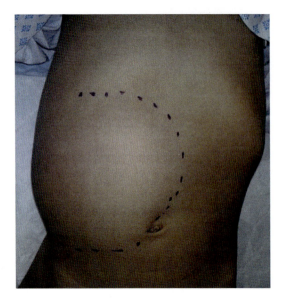

Fig. 44.1 A clinical photograph showing a large congenital pancreatic cyst

- Complete excision is the treatment of choice for congenital pancreatic cysts, but if this is not feasible, a form of internal drainage, a cystoduodenostomy, or a Roux-in-Y cystojejunostomy should be done.

Embryology

- The exact embryological origin of congenital pancreatic cyst is not known.
- It is believed to arise from a developmental anomaly of the pancreatic ductal system.
- Embryologically, the pancreatic ducts are replaced by permanent ones as they grow, and persistence or failure of these embryonic ducts to regress may lead to their obstruction forming cysts that fill with fluid.
- There are also reports of congenital pancreatic cysts arising from occlusion of the pancreatic duct.

Clinical Features

- Congenital pancreatic cysts are extremely rare and generally asymptomatic, but they can attain a large size (Fig. 44.1).
- They may however be symptomatic as a result of pressure on adjacent structures leading to:
    - Abdominal distention
    - Vomiting
    - Jaundice
    - Pancreatitis
- The majority of patients present before the age of 2 years, and associated anomalies were found in 30% of cases. These include:
    - Asphyxiating thoracic dysplasia (Jeune syndrome)
    - Short-limb dwarfism

Diagnosis 311

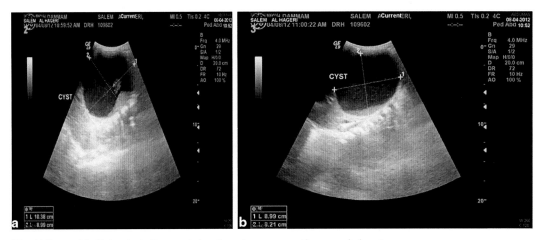

Fig. 44.2 a and b Abdominal ultrasound showing a large pancreatic congenital cyst

Fig. 44.3 Abdominal CT scan showing a very large congenital pancreatic cyst. Note the thick wall of the cyst

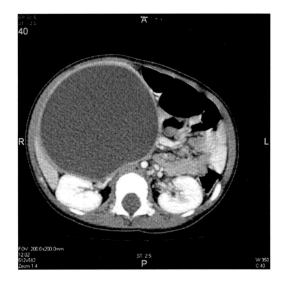

- Polydactyly
- von Hippel–Lindau disease
- Beckwith–Wiedemann syndrome
- Hemihypertrophy
- Renal tubular ectasia
- Anorectal malformation
- Polycystic kidneys

Diagnosis

- Modern imaging techniques usually show a well-defined unilocular cyst; however, even with the combined use of laboratory data, clinical features, and diagnostic imaging, it may be difficult to accurately differentiate congenital pancreatic cyst from other nearby cystic lesions of the abdomen. This is specially so if they are large in size (Figs. 44.2, 44.3, 44.4 and 44.5).

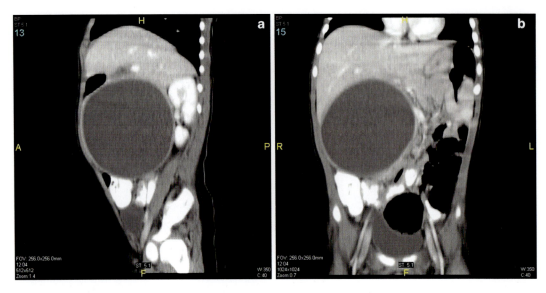

Fig. 44.4 a and **b** Abdominal CT scan showing a very large congenital pancreatic cyst

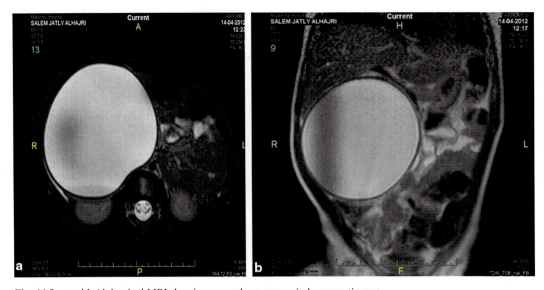

Fig. 44.5 a and **b** Abdominal MRI showing a very large congenital pancreatic cyst

- Pathologically, the cysts are lined by cuboidal epithelium and pancreatic tissue may be seen in the wall of the cyst.
- These cysts also show a high amylase level in the fluid content.

Treatment

- Once diagnosed, the treatment is surgery. A variety of procedures were described to treat congenital pancreatic cyst depending on its location and feasibility. These include cystoduodenostomy, a Roux-en-Y cystojejunostomy, total cystectomy, and total cystectomy with distal pancreatectomy.
- The treatment of congenital pancreatic cyst is surgical.

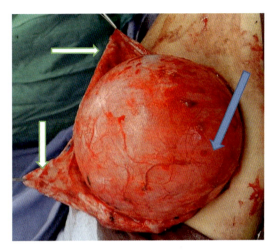

Fig. 44.6 Intraoperative photograph showing a very large congenital pancreatic cyst. Note the stretched pancreatic tissue

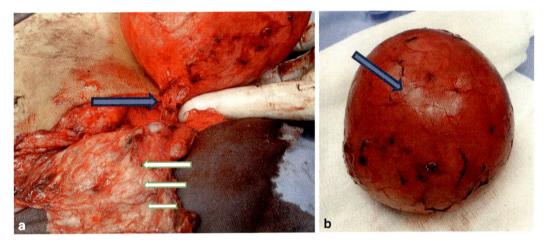

Fig. 44.7 Intraoperative photograph showing a very large congenital pancreatic cyst. Note its attachment to the pancreas (*blue arrow*) and the stretched pancreatic tissue (*white arrows*; **a**) and the already removed cyst (**b**)

- The type of surgical treatment depends on the site and size of the cyst.
- Total excision is the treatment of choice. This is usually feasible for those cysts located in the body and tail, which may necessitate distal pancreatectomy (Figs. 44.6 and 44.7).
- Cysts located in the head of the pancreas are difficult to excise totally and are better managed via internal drainage by either cystoduodenostomy or Roux-en-Y cystojejunostomy.

Recommended Reading

Agarwala S, Lal A, Bhatnagar V, Dinda AK, Mitra DK. Congenital true pancreatic cyst: presentation and management. Trop Gastroenterol. 1999;20:87–8.

Basturk O, Coban I, Adsay NV. Pancreatic cysts: pathologic classification, differential diagnosis, and clinical implications. Arch Pathol Lab Med. 2009;133(3):423–38.

Boulanger SC, Borowitz DS, Fisher JF, Brisseau GF. Congenital pancreatic cysts in children. J Pediatr Surg. 2003;38(7):1080–2.

Castellani C, Zeder SL, Spuller E, Höllwarth ME. Neonatal congenital pancreatic cyst: diagnosis and management. J Pediatr Surg. 2009;44(2):e1–4.

Chapter 45
Intestinal Polyps and Polyposis Syndromes

Introduction

- Intestinal polyps are abnormal mucosal or submucosal growths that bulge into the lumen of the intestine.
- Gastrointestinal polyps in children commonly occur in the rectum or colon.
- Most colon polyps in children are benign.
- Intestinal polyps occur in children between 1 and 6 years of age, but polyps can occur at any age.
- Intestinal polyps may occur anywhere in the gastrointestinal tract (GI), but juvenile polyps are most common in the colon and rectum.
- Intestinal polyps may also occur as part of a polyposis syndrome or may run in families.
- Intestinal polyposis syndromes require frequent monitoring by a pediatric gastroenterologist.
- Polyps may be pedunculated or sessile.
- Although intestinal polyposis syndromes are relatively rare, awareness of the health risks is important for patients and their families.
- Intestinal polyposis syndromes can be divided, based on histology into
  - Familial adenomatous polyposis (FAP)
  - Hamartomatous polyposis syndromes
  - Hereditary-mixed polyposis syndrome (HMPS)
- Polyps in the pediatric population occur less frequently than in adults, with the most common lesions being the juvenile "inflammatory" polyp and the hamartomatous Peutz–Jeghers polyps.
- Intestinal polyps with malignant potential include adenomatous polyps that are associated with polyposis syndromes such as:
  - FAP
  - Gardener's syndrome
  - Turcot's syndrome
- The etiology, diagnosis, clinical presentation, and management of these intestinal polyps depend on the type of polyp or polyposis syndrome.
- The presentation of intestinal polyps include:
  - A change in bowel habits
  - Abdominal pain
  - Rectal bleeding
  - Rectal prolapse
  - Intussusception

- The intussusceptions due to polyps are almost always small bowel—small bowel and therefore not amenable to hydrostatic or air reduction.
- Hydrostatic reduction of an intussusception due to polypoid disease is rarely successful and would not be a definitive treatment.
- Surgical treatment with enterotomy and polypectomy, or segmental bowel resection to remove the lead point, is required.
- A few children present with more life-threatening symptoms from polyps such as intestinal obstruction or perforation

Classification

Intestinal polyps are classified into:

1. Juvenile polyps
2. Inherited hamartomatous polyposis syndromes

   - Peutz–Jeghers syndrome
   - Juvenile polyposis syndrome
   - Cowden's syndrome
   - Ruvalcaba–Myhre–Smith syndrome

3. Inherited adenamatous polyposis syndromes

   - Familial polyposis coli
   - Gardner's syndrome
   - Turcot's syndrome

4. Noninherited polyposis

   - Lymphoid polyposis
   - Cronkhite–Canada syndrome

Juvenile Polyps

- Juvenile polyps are the most common intestinal polyps in children.
- The juvenile polyp is usually 1–3 cm in size, is smooth and pink, and bleeds easily.
- Juvenile polyps are one of the most common causes of rectal bleeding in children.
- They are hamartomatous polyps limited to the colon.
- They are also referred to as inflammatory polyps or retention polyps.
- Juvenile polyps make up more than 90% of all colon polyps in children.
- They typically present with lower intestinal bleeding. The bleeding can be significant, but is typically self-limited.
- Juvenile polyps typically present between 3 and 10 years of age. Sporadic juvenile polyps are uncommon before 2 years of age and are rare in the first year of life.
- Low-rectal polyps can prolapse (Fig. 45.1).
- Colo-colonic intussusception is unusual and rarely leads to prolapse of the intussusceptum.
- Juvenile polyps are variable in size, with clinical symptoms developing from polyps that range in size from <0.5 cm up to ≥3 cm.
- Most juvenile polyps are pedunculated and bleed easily (Fig. 45.2).

Classification

Fig. 45.1 a and **b** Intraoperative photographs showing prolapsed rectal polyps

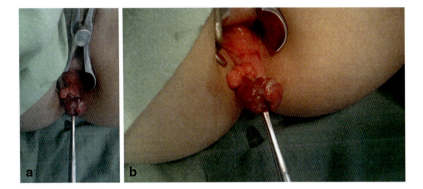

Fig. 45.2 Intraoperative colonoscopic photograph showing a *large* colonic polyp diagnosed and removed via colonoscopy

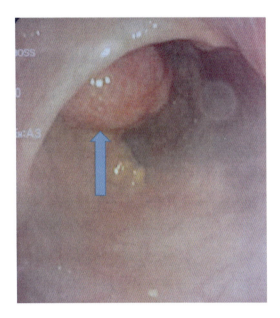

- They are mucosal lesions that contain dilated, mucous-filled glands with inflammation in the lamina propria; on cut surface, they often appear cystic. This combination of findings leads to the common reference to these as inflammatory or retention polyps.
- Juvenile polyps are hamartomas.
- In contrast to juvenile polyposis syndrome, juvenile polyps are not neoplastic and are not associated with malignant transformation. There have been reports of adenomatous changes in juvenile polyps and though rare, dysplasia may confer an increased risk of carcinoma.
- Many of these polyps simply outgrow their blood supply, become ischemic, and autoamputate.
- Juvenile polyps are usually confined to the rectosigmoid colon. However, between 50 and 60 % of patients have more than one polyp.
- About 25 % of patients have polyps in the cecum or ascending colon.
- Patients with an isolated episode of bleeding that is self-limited and who pass tissue in the stool should be observed.
- Patients with persistent or recurrent bleeding, or who are having pain or other symptoms should have a colonoscopy (Fig. 45.3).
- When the diagnosis is made with colonoscopy, a polypectomy can safely be performed.

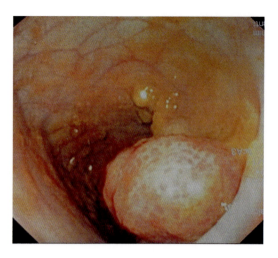

Fig. 45.3 Intraoperative colonoscopic photograph showing a *large* juvenile polyp which bleeds easily. This was removed endoscopically

- The recent evidence that patients can have more than one polyp and that polyps may be found in the cecum and ascending colon makes colonoscopy more preferable to the traditional recommendation of proctoscopy or flexible sigmoidoscopy.

Familial Juvenile Polyposis Syndrome

- Juvenile polyposis syndrome is a rare polyposis syndrome that runs in families.
- Compared to children having a single juvenile polyp, those with Juvenile polyposis syndrome have multiple polyps.
- The exact number of juvenile polyps necessary to diagnose a polyposis syndrome is controversial.
- Patients with familial juvenile polyposis are diagnosed when the following criteria are met:
  - More than five (some say ten) juvenile polyps in the colon
  - Multiple juvenile polyps throughout the GI tract
  - Any number of juvenile polyps with a family history of juvenile polyposis
- Although most polyps develop in the colon and small bowel, they can also occur in the stomach.
- These polyps are hamartomas and the term "juvenile" refers to the type of polyps seen in these patients, not the age of onset.
- Familial juvenile polyposis is an autosomal dominant disorder with varied presentation. About 75% of patients will have a parent with the syndrome, but 25% do not have a family history suggesting a new mutation.
- Mutations in the *BMPR1A* or *SMAD4* gene have been identified, but together these account for only 40% of patients.
- Children with first-degree relatives who have juvenile polyposis syndrome should undergo screening colonoscopy starting at age 12 years.
- Associated congenital extra colonic anomalies are found in as many as 20% of these patients including:
  - Macrocephaly, hydrocephalus, and spina bifida
  - Congenital heart disease
  - Urogenital anomalies including undescended testes, bifid uterus and vagina, abnormal pelvi-ureteric junction insertion, unilateral renal agenesis

- Osteoma
- Malrotation, Meckel diverticulum
- Familial juvenile polyposes affect 1:100,000 live births.
- Familial juvenile polyposes have a cumulative risk of malignancy >50%.
- Surgical treatment options:
  - Endoscopic removal of the colon polyps followed by yearly endoscopy with surveillance biopsies.
  - Laparotomy, enterotomies, and polypectomies.
  - If there are clusters of polyps in isolated areas, limited segmental resection may be appropriate.
  - Patients with numerous polyps in the colon will require proctocolectomy with ileoanal anastomosis.
- Prophylactic colectomy with ileorectal anastomosis is recommended for children with familial juvenile polyposis who have:
  - Severe or repeated bleeding
  - Hypoprotinemia
  - Failure to thrive

Peutz–Jeghers Syndrome

- The broad category of hamartomatous polyposis syndromes encompasses several syndromes, mainly:
  - Peutz–Jeghers syndrome (PJS)
  - Phosphatase and tensin homolog (*PTEN*)-associated hamartomatous syndromes including:
    - Cowden syndrome
    - Bannayan–Riley–Ruvalcaba syndrome (BRR)
  - Familial juvenile polyposis syndrome
  - Cronkhite–Canada syndrome
- The association of intestinal polyposis with mucocutaneous pigmentation was first reported in three generations of a Dutch family by Peutz in 1921. In 1949, Jeghers reported ten similar patients establishing the now well-known syndrome.
- In PJS:
  - There are hamartomatous polyps which can occur anywhere within the GI, most commonly in the jejunum.
  - There are characteristic melanin spots on the lips, around the mouth, on the inside of cheeks and digits.
- Patients with Peutz–Jeghers syndrome have multiple pedunculated hamartomatous polyps distributed as follows:
  - The small intestine (78%)
  - Colon (42%)
  - Stomach (38%)
  - Rectum (28%)
- PJS has an estimated prevalence of between 1:120,000 and 1:200,000 live births.
- These polyps are often large and may cause intussusception with intestinal obstruction.

- Polyps within ureter, bladder, and renal pelvis have also been reported in patients with PJS as well as nasal and bronchial polyps.
- PJS often runs in families but may occur without any known family member affected.
- These children often require multiple surgeries due to recurrent intussusception.
- PJS has been localized via gene linkage and logarithm of odds (LOD) score to mutations in band 19p13.3–13.4, which is now known to encode a serine-threonine kinase (STK11/LKB1) within this region.
- Approximately 80% of patients with PJS have this gene mutation.
- PJS is inherited as an autosomal dominant.
- Surgical management:
  - Most episodes of abdominal pain in patients with the Peutz–Jeghers syndrome which are usually due to intussusceptions are self-limited and resolve without surgical intervention.
  - The main indication for operative treatment is the presence of intestinal obstruction.
  - If an operation is not delayed too long, the intussusception can be reduced followed by an enterotomy and polypectomy without segmental small bowel resection.
  - The entire GI should be palpated and any other polyps removed.
  - If the patient presents late and the intussusception cannot be reduced, resection with primary anastomosis should be performed.
- Patients with Peutz–Jeghers syndrome are at increased risk of:
  - Gastrointestinal malignancies of:
    - Small intestines
    - Colon
    - Pancreatico-biliary
  - Extraintestinal malignancy of the:
    - Breast
    - Ovary
    - Cervix
    - Germ cell tumors
  - Development of gynecomastia commonly precedes the development of gynecologic or testicular malignancy.
  - It is estimated that the risk of cancer is increased 18-fold over the general population.
- None of these cancers occurs at a frequency that justifies prophylactic removal of the organs, but awareness of the risk should guide surveillance.

Familial Adenomatous Polyposis

- FAP is the most common intestinal polyposis syndrome with an estimated frequency of 1:13,000 births.
- It is inherited as an autosomal dominant disorder.
- FAP runs in families but may occur sporadically.
- Polyps begin to occur in childhood and sometimes more than 1000 polyps can be present.
- Colon cancer occurs in almost every patient with FAP by the age of 50 years.
- Children with FAP are at a high risk for developing cancers at various sites including:
  - Large intestines
  - Small intestines
  - Thyroid

- Pancreas
- Liver

- Hepatoblastoma is the most common cancer found in children less than 5 years old with FAP.
- FAP arises from germ-line mutations in the adenomatous polyposis coli (*APC*) gene on band 5q21–22.
- The presentation and severity is related to the site of the *APC* gene mutation. Proximal *APC* mutations (proximal to codon 1249) produce a milder attenuated phenotype with sparse polyposis. *APC* mutations between codons 1250 and 1330 present with tremendous degrees of polyposis.
- There are other variants of FAP including:
  - Gardner syndrome
  - Turcot syndrome
  - MYH-variant
- FAP presents with multiple adenomatous polyps throughout the colon. Eighty percent of these polyps present in the left colon.
- Diagnosis of FAP is based upon the finding of f100 adenomas in the colon.
- Patients with FAP and their first-degree relatives are recommended to undergo genetic counseling and genetic testing for detection of the truncated protein product of the mutated *APC* gene.
- Current therapies with nonsteroidal anti-inflammatory drugs have been shown to cause regression of adenomatous polyps; however, progression to adenocarcinoma in patients with FAP is inevitable without definitive surgery involving removal of the colon and rectum.
- The optimal operative treatment is a proctocolectomy with restorative ileoanal reconstruction with an ileal pouch.
- Most advocate surgical intervention when the patient is about 15 years old and is able to understand and participate in treatment decisions.
- Screening for extracolonic lesions such as duodenal polyps and hepatoblastoma is advocated.
- Mortality from duodenal cancer ranks second to colon cancer in patients with FAP.

Gardner Syndrome

- Eldon J. Gardner, a teacher of genetics, described this variant of FAP.
- In 1951, he described colonic polyposis in a Utah family whose nine members died due to colon cancer within three generations.
- Gardner syndrome is characterized by:
  - Colonic adenomatous polyps
  - Multiple osteomas
  - Mesenchymal tumors of the skin and soft tissues
  - Congenital hypertrophy of the retinal pigment epithelium
  - Carcinoma of the ampulla of Vater, adrenal, and thyroid glands
- Gardner syndrome is inherited as an autosomal dominant, with nearly 100% penetrance of the *APC* mutation by age 40 years.
- Women with Gardner syndrome have an increased risk for the development of thyroid cancer and desmoid tumors.
- Physical features commonly associated with Gardner syndrome, in addition to those listed above for FAP, include the following:

- Skin: epidermal cysts and sebaceous cysts (commonly on the back)
- Craniofacial: osteomas (including the mandible), skin fibromas, and dental anomalies (supernumerary teeth, impacted teeth, missing teeth, root anomalies)
- Endocrine: Cushing's syndrome (adrenal carcinoma), multiple endocrine neoplasia 2B

- Symptoms may present anywhere from 2 months of age to 20 years of age.
- Usually, the extracolonic manifestation of skin tumors and osteomas present before the adenomatous polyps.
- Osteomas of the skull and long bones present in about 50% of patients with this syndrome.
- Skin manifestations throughout the body include:
  - Sebaceous cysts (66%)
  - Lipomas
  - Fibromas
  - Pigmented lesions
  - Mesenchymal tumors
  - Desmoid tumors (3.5–12.4% of patients)
  - Intraabdominal desmoid tumors
- Extracolonic manifestations including:
  - Periampullary adenomas
  - Papillary carcinoma of the thyroid gland
  - Hepatoblastoma
  - Osteomas of the mandible and skull
  - Epidermal cysts
  - Desmoid tumors.

Turcot Syndrome

- The Turcot syndrome is a rare autosomal recessive disorder.
- It is characterized by:
  - Colonic adenomatous polyps.
  - Brain tumors (glioblastoma multiforme, medulloblastoma).
  - The colonic adenomatous polyps frequently become malignant in those younger than 30 years old.
- It was initially described in 1959 by a Canadian surgeon, Jacques Turcot.
- Turcot syndrome is associated with mutations in the following genes: bands 7p22, 5q21–22, and 3p21.3.
- Several patients with manifestations of Turcot syndrome have documented *APC* mutations in addition to ocular fundus lesions and jaw lesions consistent with Gardner syndrome; however, patients with Turcot syndrome have a lower degree of colonic polyposis (20–100 total).
- The inheritance of Turcot syndrome is autosomal recessive.
- The incidence of brain tumors in patients with this variant of FAP is most significant in patients before the age of 20.

MYH-associated Polyposis

- MYH-associated polyposis, or *MutYH*-associated polyposis (MAP), occurs in a small number of patients with FAP.
- The syndrome results not from a mutation in the *APC* gene but in the human *MutY* homolog gene.
- Unlike FAP, MAP is autosomal recessive, with complete penetrance by age 60 years.

Cowden Syndrome

- In 1963, Lloyd and Dennis initially described the features associated with Cowden disease.
- In 1972, Weary et al. described the manifestations of Cowden disease and classified it as a multiple hamartomatous syndrome with autosomal dominant inheritance.
- Cowden syndrome is relatively uncommon, estimated to affect 1:200,000 live births.
- It is an autosomal dominant disorder and 85% of patients have a mutation in the tumor suppressor gene PTEN on chromosome 10q.
- Individuals with Cowden disease usually present at age 10–30 years with:
  - Hyperplastic hamartomatous polyps throughout the GI tract including the esophagus.
  - Most of these polyps occur in the colon followed by the stomach.
  - Gastrointestinal cancer is not increased in these patients.
  - Glycogenic acanthosis of the esophagus.
  - Orocutaneous hamartomas of the face.
  - Pulmonary hamartomas.
  - Malignancies at various sites including:
    - Breast (75%).
    - Thyroid.
    - Adenocarcinoma of the colon which is rare.
    - Female patients with Cowden syndrome are at increased risk of breast neoplasia and neoplasia of the urogenital system mainly ovarian tumors.
    - Dysplastic gangliocytomas of the cerebellum.
    - Renal cell adenocarcinoma.
    - Merkel cell carcinomas.
- Cowden disease is typically associated with the following features:
  - Developmental delay
  - Macrocephaly (38%)
  - Cerebellar dysfunction
  - Scoliosis
  - Cutaneous hamartomas
  - Thyroid disease (>50%)
  - Chronic diarrhea
  - Visceral arteriovenous malformations
- Manifestations of Cowden disease include the following:
  - Skin:
    - Multiple hamartomas of skin and mucus membranes
    - Verrucous lesions
    - Papules of gingival and buccal mucosa

- Facial trichilemmomas (benign tumors of the lower outer root sheath epithelium of a hair follicle)
- Head and central nervous system (CNS):
  - Craniomegaly
  - Adenoid facies
  - Ataxia
  - Increased intracranial pressure
  - Cerebellar degeneration
  - Mental retardation
  - Tremors
  - Tonsillar herniation
  - Seizures
- Endocrine:
  - Thyroid hamartomas and carcinoma
- Chest:
  - Breast hamartomas and carcinomas
  - Pectus excavatum
- Gastrointestinal:
  - Intestinal hamartomatous polyps
- Tumors:
  - Dysplastic cerebellar gangliocytoma
  - Breast carcinoma
  - Ovarian carcinomas
  - Merkel cell skin carcinomas
  - Renal cell adenocarcinomas
  - Thyroid carcinomas
- Spine:
  - Scoliosis

Bannayan–Zonana Syndrome

- BRR syndrome, also termed Bannayan–Zonana syndrome, was first described by Riley and Smith in 1961, was next described by Bannayan in 1971, and was further characterized by Zonana et al. in 1975.
- BRR syndrome is characterized by:
  - Hamartomatous polyps of the colon and tongue
  - Macrocephaly
  - Lipomas
  - Hemangiomas

- BRR syndrome is rare with probable autosomal dominant inheritance.
- BRR syndrome and Cowden disease have both been mapped to chromosome 10q23.3, which encodes the *PTEN* gene, a phosphatase that functions within the phosphatidylinositol 3-kinase pathway.
- Common findings associated with BRR include the following:
    - General:
        - Increased weight and length at birth
        - Macrocephaly
        - Scaphocephaly
        - Broad thumb and hallux
    - Central nervous system:
        - Hypotonia
        - Myopathy
        - Developmental delay
        - Mild mental retardation
    - Cardiovascular:
        - Arteriovenous malformation
        - Congenital heart disease
    - Pulmonary:
        - Pectus excavatum
    - Gastrointestinal tract:
        - High palate
        - Hamartomatous intestinal polyps (colon, tongue)
    - Genitourinary:
        - Enlarged penis
        - Spotted pigment of glans penis
        - Testicular enlargement
    - Ocular:
        - Pseudo papilledema, exotropia

Cronkhite–Canada Syndrome

- Cronkhite–Canada syndrome is characterized by:
    - Multiple intestinal polyps, sparing the esophagus
    - Hyperpigmentation of the skin
    - Alopecia
    - Atrophy of nail beds
    - Severe protein-losing enteropathy with electrolyte disturbances
- Cronkhite–Canada syndrome is considered to be rare, sporadic, and acquired rather than inherited and is associated with a high mortality rate.
- Usually presents at an average age of 62 years.
- Cronkhite–Canada syndrome has a 5-year mortality rate of 55%, secondary to:
    - Life-threatening GI bleeding
    - Intussusception
    - Protein-losing enteropathy
- Cronkhite–Canada syndrome has an association with colorectal cancer.

Hereditary-mixed Polyposis Syndrome

- This is extremely rare.
- It is characterized by familial presentation of colorectal polyps that have mixed histologic elements with both adenomatous and hyperplastic features.

Gorlin Syndrome

- Gorlin and Goltz initially described this syndrome (GS) in 1960, also termed nevoid basal cell carcinoma syndrome.
- Herzberg and Wiskemann further associated GS with medulloblastoma in 1963.
- GS has an increased risk for the following malignant tumors:
    - Basal cell carcinoma
    - Ovarian carcinoma
    - Medulloblastoma
- GS is caused by an autosomal dominant mutation localized to band 9q22.3–31, which encodes a human analogue to the Drosophila *PTCH* gene, a tumor suppressor gene.
- The prevalence of GS is about 1:57,000 births.
- Patients with Gorlin syndrome may present with:
    - Hamartomatous gastric polyps.
    - Congenital hydrocephalus.
    - Cleft lip and palate.
    - Lung cysts.
    - Rib and vertebral anomalies.
    - Cardiac anomalies.
    - Palmar pits.
    - Lymphomesenteric cysts.
    - Ovarian fibromas and carcinomas.
    - Scoliosis, kyphoscoliosis, cervical anomalies, rib anomalies, brachydactyly, short fourth metacarpal, and thumb.
    - Enamel hypoplasia.
    - Medulloblastoma when younger than 5 years.
    - Dental anomalies and basal cell carcinoma can appear in adolescents.
    - Calcification of the falx cerebri (65%).
    - Bridged sella (68%).
    - Flame-shaped lucencies in the phalanges, carpals, and metacarpals (30%).
    - Bifid ribs (26%).
    - Calcification of the tentorium cerebri (20%).
    - Hemivertebrae (15%).
    - Fused vertebral bodies (10%).

Lymphoid Polyposis

- Lymphoid polyps are focal hyperplasia of lymphoid follicles in the colon.
- Though recognized in children, these are rare polyps that are considered benign and have an overlying normal colonic mucosa.

Classification

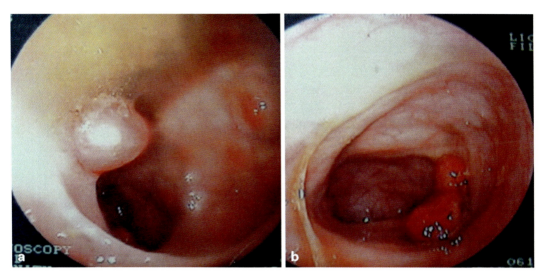

Fig. 45.4 a and **b** Colonoscopic photographs showing multiple colonic polyps in a child who presented with bleeding per rectum. Histology showed these polyps to be lymphoid polyps

- Treatment for these polyps is local excision to differentiate this benign polyposis from malignant lymphoma of the colon (Fig. 45.4).

Ruvalcaba–Myhre–Smith Syndrome

- Described in 1980, it is an autosomal dominant inherited disorder.
- It is characterized by:
    - Juvenile polyps
    - Macrocephaly
    - Pigmented macules of the genitals
    - Macrocephaly
    - Additional features include:
        - Mental retardation
        - Abnormal lipid storage
        - Delayed motor skills
        - Ocular abnormalities
- There has been no evidence of increased risk of colorectal cancer in patients with this disorder.

Recommended Reading

Calva D, Howe JR. Hamartomatous polyposis syndromes. Surg Clin North Am. 2008;88(4):779–817.
Erdman SH, Barnard J. Gastrointestinal polyps and polyposis syndromes in children. Curr Opin Pediatr. 2002;14:576–82.
Sidhu R, Sanders DS, McAlindon ME, Thomson M. Capsule endoscopy and enteroscopy: modern modalities to investigate the small bowel in paediatrics. Arch Dis Child. 2008;93(2):154–9.

Chapter 46
Congenital Diaphragmatic Hernia

Introduction

- The diaphragm is a musculotendinous structure that separates the organs in the abdominal cavity from those in the chest. It is composed of a central tendon surrounded by a muscular rim in addition to the right and left diaphragmatic cura.
- There are several different types of diaphragmatic hernia (Fig. 46.1):
  - Bochdalek hernia: The most common type of congenital diaphragmatic hernia is a posterolateral (Bochdalek hernia) hernia (Fig. 46.2).
  - Morgagni's hernia: The Morgagni defect occurs posterior to the sternum and results from failure of sternal and costal fibers to fuse (Fig. 46.3).
  - Hiatal hernia: The hiatus hernia occurs through the esophageal hiatus and is divided into three types (Figs. 46.4, 46.5, 46.6, and 46.7):
    - Sliding
    - Rolling
    - Mixed sliding and rolling
  - Central tendon hernia: This hernia is a rare diaphragm defect involving the central tendinous portion of the diaphragm.
  - Anterolateral hernia: Occurs anterolaterally through a defect in the muscular part of the diaphragm.
  - Eventration of diaphragm: There is incomplete mascularization of the diaphragm. This leads to elevation of a portion or all of the intact diaphragm that is thinned as a result of incomplete muscularization (Fig. 46.8).
  - Latrogenic diaphragmatic hernia: Occurs as a result of diaphragmatic injury during surgery.
  - Traumatic diaphragmatic hernia: Occurs following penetrating and blunt abdominal and thoracic trauma (Fig. 46.9).
  - Congenital diaphragmatic hernia is the commonest of all types of diaphragmatic hernias occurring through a posterolateral defect in the diaphragm and ranging in size from a small defect in the diaphragm to its complete absence (agenesis of diaphragm).
- Lazarus Riverius (1589–1655) in 1679 reported the first case of a congenital diaphragmatic hernia in a 24-year-old male following postmortem examination.
- In 1946, Gross reported the first successful repair of a neonatal diaphragmatic hernia in the first 24 h of life.

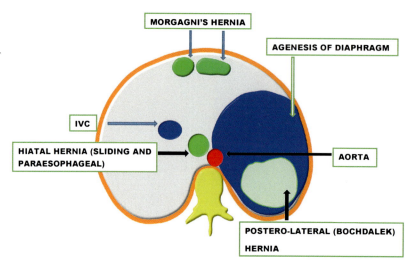

Fig. 46.1 Diagrammatic representation of the diaphragm showing the different types and sites of hernias

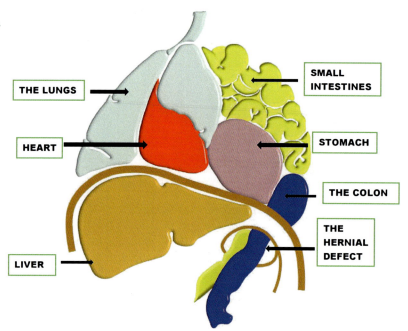

Fig. 46.2 Diagrammatic representation of left Bochdalek hernia

- Congenital diaphragmatic hernia occurs in 1 of every 2500–5000 live births.
- Congenital diaphragmatic hernia occurs equally in males and females.
- Most congenital diaphragmatic hernias occur posterolaterally through the foramen of Bochdaleck.
- Approximately 85% occur on the left side and 15% occur on the right side.
- Bilateral hernias are uncommon and are usually fatal.
- The term "posterolateral" diaphragmatic hernia may be a misnomer because, frequently, much larger areas of the diaphragm defects are found and only a posterior rim of muscle can be found (Fig. 46.10).
- A hernia sac is present in 10–20% of congenital diaphragmatic hernias (Fig. 46.11).
- Over the past 20 years, pulmonary hypertension and pulmonary hypoplasia have been recognized as the two cornerstones of the pathophysiology of congenital diaphragmatic hernia.

Introduction

Fig. 46.3 a and **b** Intraoperative photograph showing bilateral Morgagni's hernia. Note that the left one is larger than the right

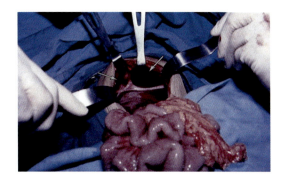

Fig. 46.4 Barium enema showing the colon herniating through a Morgagni's hernia. Note the anterior retrosternal position of the hernia

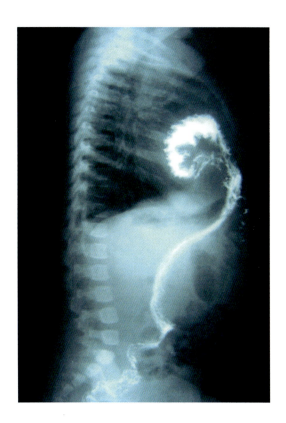

Fig. 46.5 Diagrammatic representation of a paraesophageal and sliding hernia

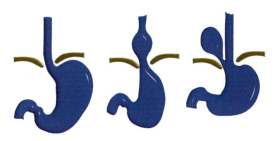

Fig. 46.6 a and **b** Barium meal showing paraesophageal hernia

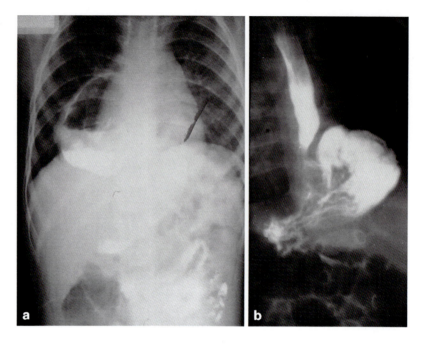

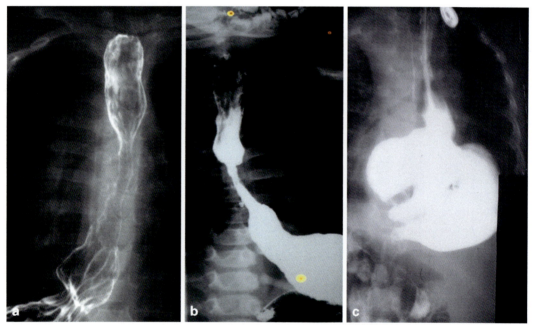

Fig. 46.7 Barium meal showing sliding hiatal hernia in the first tow and combined paraesophageal and sliding hiatal hernia in the third

Fig. 46.8 Anteroposterior (**a**) and lateral (**b**) chest x-rays showing eventration of right diaphragm

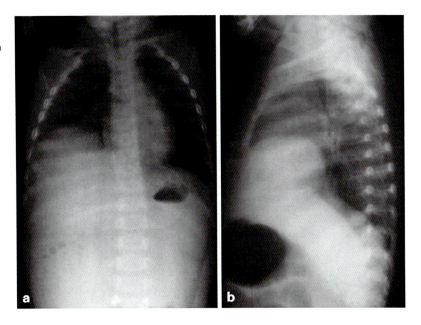

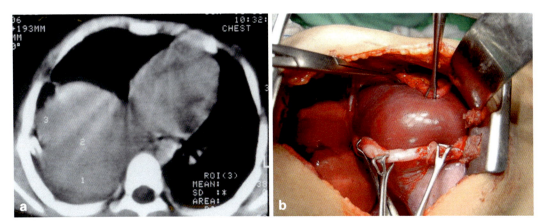

Fig. 46.9 CT-scan of the chest showing traumatic diaphragmatic hernia on the right side with herniation of the liver into the chest and intraoperative photograph showing traumatic rupture of the right diaphragm with herniation of the liver into the chest. Note the extent of the tear in the diaphragm

- Although congenital diaphragmatic hernia is usually a disorder of the newborn period, about 10% of patients may present after the newborn period and even during adulthood.
- Familial congenital diaphragmatic hernia is rare (<2% of all cases), and both autosomal recessive and autosomal dominant patterns of inheritance have been reported.

Embryology

- The diaphragm is derived from four embryonic structures:
    - The septum transversum

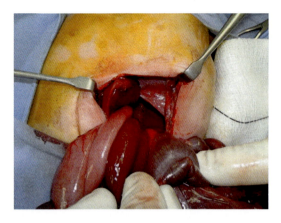

Fig. 46.10 Intraoperative photograph showing a left diaphragmatic hernia. Note the size of the defect which does not correspond to a real posterolateral defect

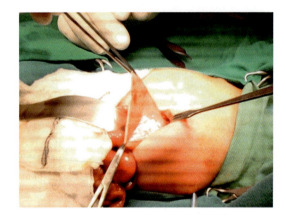

Fig. 46.11 Intraoperative photograph showing a hernia sac in a left congenital diaphragmatic hernia

- The pleuroperitoneal membranes
- The mesoderm of the body wall
- The esophageal mesenchyme

- At around 4–5 weeks' gestation, the septum transversum forms like a semicircular shelf, which separates the heart from the liver.
- As the septum transversum develops, it separates the thoracic cavity from the peritoneal cavity but allows pericardioperitoneal canals on either side of the esophagus.
- At around the fifth week of gestation, the pleuroperitoneal membranes develop along a line connecting the root of the 12th rib with the tips of the 7th to 12th ribs.
- The pleuroperitoneal membranes then grow ventrally and fuse with the septum transversum and the dorsal mesentery of the esophagus.
- At 6–7 weeks' gestation, the pleuroperitoneal canals close; the left side closes after the right.
- The left and right crura of the diaphragm develop from the mesentery of the esophagus.
- The mesoderm of the body wall forms the outer rim of diaphragmatic muscle.
- The posterolateral diaphragmatic hernia results from failure of closure of the pleuroperitoneal canals.
- Some intestines and other viscera enter the thorax through this defect and lead to compression of the developing lung at the pseudoglandular stage of lung development. This occurs around the tenth week of gestation.
- This will also lead to shift of the mediastinum to the contralateral side. This causes compression of the heart and the contralateral lung as well.

- Lung compression results in pulmonary hypoplasia that is most severe on the side of the hernia but both lungs may be affected.
- The timing of herniation of bowel into the chest is crucial. The earlier the herniation, the more severe is the pulmonary hypoplasia.

Pathophysiology

- As a result of bowel herniation and compression on the developing lungs, both lungs develop abnormally. This is more severe on the affected side and the degree of pulmonary hypoplasia is variable.
- The bronchi are less numerous, and the number of alveoli is reduced.
- This will lead to a decreased alveolar capillary membrane for gas exchange.
- The pulmonary vessels are also affected. The cross-sectional area of the pulmonary vessels is reduced and there is an increase in muscle layer (muscularization) of the pulmonary arteries and arterioles.
- This will result in pulmonary hypertension which leads to right-to-left shunts at atrial and ductal levels. This persistent fetal circulation leads to right-sided heart failure. A vicious cycle of progressive hypoxemia, hypercarbia, acidosis, and pulmonary hypertension results.
- Infants with congenital diaphragmatic hernias also have impairment of the pulmonary antioxidant enzyme system.
- There is also defective development of the surfactant system of the lung.
- In very severe cases, left ventricular hypoplasia may develop.
- So the pathophysiology of congenital diaphragmatic hernia involves:
  - Pulmonary hypoplasia
  - Pulmonary hypertension
  - Pulmonary immaturity
  - Pulmonary surfactant deficiencies
- The severity of hypoxemia, hypercarbia, and respiratory or metabolic acidosis depend on the degree of:
  - Pulmonary hypoplasia
  - Persistent pulmonary hypertension of newborn
  - Right-to-left shunts
  - Ventricular function.

Clinical Features

- Currently, the diagnosis of congenital diaphragmatic hernia is made prenatally on antenatal ultrasound in 46–97%.
- Antenatal ultrasonography reveals:
  - Polyhydramnios
  - An absent intra-abdominal gastric air bubble
  - Mediastinal shift
  - Hydrops fetalis

Fig. 46.12 A clinical photograph showing a newborn with left congenital diaphragmatic hernia. Note the scaphoid abdomen and barrel-shaped chest

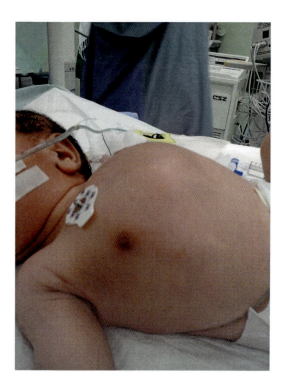

- The presentation is commonly with respiratory distress and cyanosis in the first minutes or hours of life, although a later presentation is possible.
- Clinically, infants with congenital diaphragmatic hernia have:
  - A scaphoid abdomen
  - A barrel-shaped chest (Fig. 46.12)
  - Signs of respiratory distress (retractions, cyanosis, grunting respirations)
  - Poor air entry on the affected side, with a shift of cardiac sounds
- Patients may present outside of the neonatal period with:
  - Respiratory symptoms
  - Intestinal obstruction
  - Bowel ischemia and necrosis following volvulus

Associated Anomalies

- Associated anomalies are common in infants with congenital diaphragmatic hernia (10–50 %).
- The incidence of associated cardiac anomalies is high (approximately 25 %).
- Genitourinary anomalies occur in 6–8 % of infants with congenital diaphragmatic hernia.
- Chromosome abnormalities occur in as many as 30 % of infants with congenital diaphragmatic hernia including:
  - Trisomy 13, Trisomy 18, Trisomy 21, and Turner syndrome
  - Chromosome deletions on chromosomes 1q, 8p, and 15q

- Congenital diaphragmatic hernia may occur as:
  - Nonsyndromic: as an isolated defect
  - Syndromic:
    - More than 10% of infants with congenital diaphragmatic hernia have an underlying syndromic diagnosis.
    - Dysmorphisms such as craniofacial, extremity abnormalities, or spinal dysraphism may suggest syndromic congenital diaphragmatic hernia.
- Cornelia de Lange syndrome is an autosomal dominant syndrome with characteristic facial features, hirsutism, developmental delay, and congenital diaphragmatic hernia.
- Fryns syndrome is an autosomal recessive condition that includes congenital diaphragmatic hernia, along with hypoplasia of the distal digits and other variable abnormalities of the brain, heart, and genitourinary development.
- Pallister–Killian syndrome (tetrasomy 12p mosaicism) includes coarse facial features, aortic stenosis, cardiac septal defects, abnormal genitalia, and congenital diaphragmatic hernia.

Diagnosis and Management

If the diagnosis of congenital diaphragmatic hernia is made antenatally, these patients should be referred to a tertiary care center where they can be managed appropriately.

- If the diagnosis is known at the time of delivery, bag-and-mask ventilation in the delivery room should be avoided. This is to prevent the stomach and intestines to become distended with air which further compromise pulmonary function.
- All infants with severe congenital diaphragmatic hernia who present in the first few hours of life should be intubated and ventilated.
- A nasogastric or an orogastric tube should be placed as soon as possible to help decompress the stomach and determine whether the tube is positioned above or below the diaphragm (Fig. 46.13).
- Secure an arterial line in the umbilical artery or in a peripheral artery (radial, posterior tibial) for continuous blood pressure measurement and to frequently assess pH, $PaCO_2$, and PaO_2. Note that the PaO_2 is often higher from a preductal (right-hand) sampling site because of right-to-left shunt (Fig. 46.14).
- Urinary catheterization to monitor urine output and fluid resuscitation.
- Place an umbilical vein catheter to allow for administration of inotropic agents and hypertonic solutions such as calcium gluconate.
- Chromosomal studies.
- A chest radiograph (Figs. 46.15 and 46.16).
- An echocardiography should always be performed prior to surgical repair.
- The treatment of infants with congenital diaphragmatic hernia is medical to start with and it is directed towards management of pulmonary hypoplasia and persistent pulmonary hypertension.
- High-frequency ventilation:
  - The use of high-frequency ventilation in congenital diaphragmatic hernia remains controversial.
  - High-frequency ventilation is recommended for infants with hypercarbia and hypoxemia resistant to conventional ventilation or requiring high PIP (>30 cm H_2O).
  - Patients with congenital diaphragmatic hernia often have hypercarbia because of pulmonary hypoplasia.

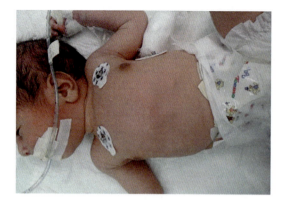

Fig. 46.13 A clinical photograph of a newborn with congenital diaphragmatic hernia. Note the endotracheal tube and orogastric tube

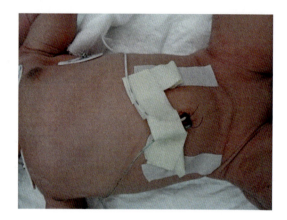

Fig. 46.14 A clinical photograph showing a newborn with congenital diaphragmatic hernia. Note the umbilical arterial and venous lines

- High-frequency ventilation avoids the use of high peak inspiratory pressures and may help lower and normalize $PaCO_2$.
- A low $PaCO_2$ is beneficial as it causes pulmonary vasodilation.

- Exogenous surfactant:
  - Administer exogenous surfactant to newborns with congenital diaphragmatic hernia.
  - Surfactant therapy is associated with an improvement in oxygenation in some neonates with congenital diaphragmatic hernia.
  - Surfactant is administered within 24 h of birth in neonates with congenital diaphragmatic hernia and a poor prognosis.

- Continuous monitoring of oxygenation, blood pressure, and perfusion. This may require the use of volume expanders (crystalloids and colloids) and inotropic agents (dopamine and dobutamine; Fig. 46.17).
- Maintain glucose and ionized calcium concentrations.
- Inhaled nitric oxide:
  - Is beneficial for the treatment of persistent pulmonary hypertension.
  - It is a highly selective pulmonary vasodilator and has been used to treat infants with persistent pulmonary hypertension of newborn.
  - It produces pulmonary vasodilatation.
  - It decreases the ventilation–perfusion mismatch.

Diagnosis and Management

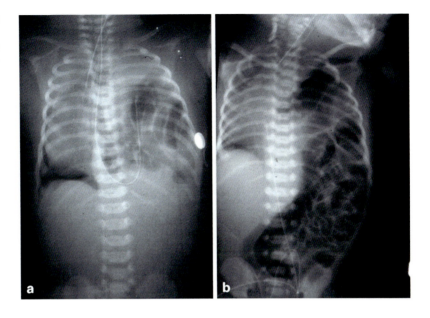

Fig. 46.15 a and b Chest x-rays showing left congenital diaphragmatic hernia. Note the nasogastric tube curving into the chest in the right x-ray

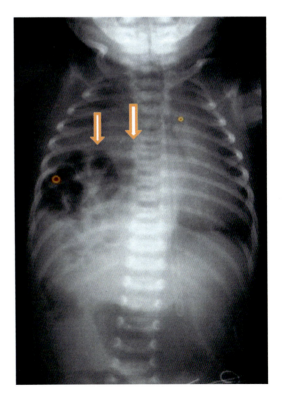

Fig. 46.16 Chest x-ray showing right congenital diaphragmatic hernia

- It reverses the ductal shunting observed in persistent pulmonary hypertension of newborn.
- The efficacy of nitric oxide improves if given after surfactant therapy.
- The appropriate targets for partial pressure of oxygen in the blood (PaO_2) and partial pressure of carbon dioxide in the blood ($PaCO_2$) are controversial. A PaO_2 concentration >50 mm Hg is sufficient for adequate oxygen delivery at the tissue level.

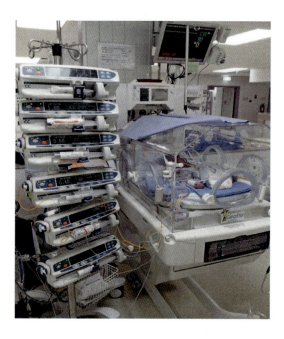

Fig. 46.17 A clinical photograph of a newborn with congenital diaphragmatic hernia. Note the extent of monitoring and supportive measures

- Venoarterial or venovenous extracorporeal membrane oxygenation (ECMO) is available at few centers and commonly used for severely affected infants.
- ECMO criteria:
  - Older than weeks' gestation
  - Have a weight >2000 g
  - No major intracranial hemorrhage on cranial sonography
  - Have been on mechanical ventilator support for <10–14 days
  - No lethal congenital anomalies or inoperable cardiac anomalies
  - A pH <7.15, oxygenation index >40, and failure to respond to maximal medical treatmen.
- Fetal surgery:
  - Has been attempted for severely affected infants.
  - Harrison et al. reported the first human fetal surgery for congenital diaphragmatic hernia in 1990.
  - In 1998, a report showed that in utero repair of congenital diaphragmatic hernia did not improve survival when compared with standard treatment.
  - Currently, fetal surgery is focused on endoscopic occlusion of the fetal trachea (minimal access surgery).
  - The fetal lung secretes fluid and this fluid provides a template for lung growth. Occlusion of the fetal trachea traps this fluid and stimulates lung growth, either by retention of growth factors within the lung or stimulation of local growth factors by the gentle distension provided by the fluid.
  - So endoscopically occluding the fetal trachea promotes lung growth in those with congenital diaphragmatic hernia and decreases the chance of pulmonary hypoplasia.
- Congenital diaphragmatic hernia is no longer a surgical emergency.
- The herniated viscera in the chest does not appear to exacerbate the pathophysiology of congenital diaphragmatic hernia as long as bowel decompression with a nasogastric tube is adequate and preoperative stabilization with delayed surgical repair is the current practice.

Fig. 46.18 Chest x-ray showing left congenital diaphragmatic hernia and pneumothorax on the other side

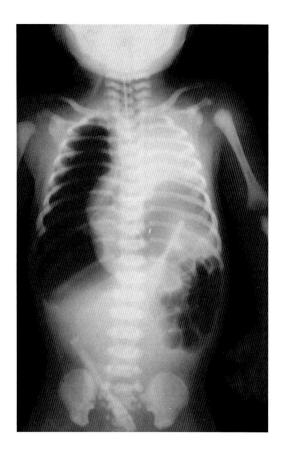

- The ideal time to repair a congenital diaphragmatic hernia is not well established but repair 24 h after stabilization is ideal.
- Chest tube drainage is necessary when a tension pneumothorax is present; however, whether routine chest drainage following surgical repair has a role is controversial (Fig. 46.18).
- A balanced intrathoracic drainage, in which a closed gated pressure system is used to maintain intrathoracic pressure within the normal physiologic range, may help minimize the risk of pulmonary injury and improve respiratory mechanics.
- Antenatal administration of corticosteroids 24 and 48 h prior to delivery was associated with significant increases in lung compliance.

Surgical Repair

- A subcostal incision is used.
- The hernial contents are reduced.
- A hernia sac if present is excised.
- The leaves of the diaphragm are dissected.
- Primary repair is done in a single layer using nonabsorbable sutures.
- If the diaphragmatic defect is large to preclude primary closure, a prosthetic patch, or rotational muscle flaps can be used.
- Malrotation is corrected and Ladd bands are lysed.

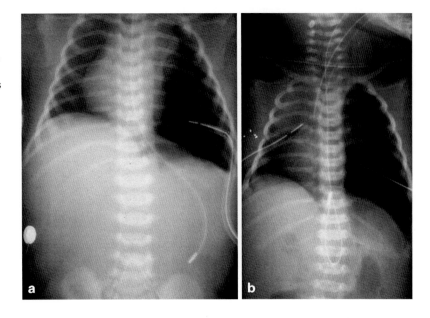

Fig. 46.19 Chest x-rays showing one chest tube following repair of left congenital diaphragmatic hernia (**a**) and in the second x-ray two chest tubes to drain a contralateral pneumothorax (**b**)

- If abdominal closure will interfere with diaphragmatic compliance or lead to abdominal compartment syndrome, then a temporary silo with delayed primary closure of the fascia or skin can be safely accomplished.
- The use of chest tubes is controversial (Fig. 46.19).
- Currently, thoracoscopic or laparoscopic repair of congenital diaphragmatic hernia is offered for late presenters and neonates requiring minimal ventilator support.
- Thoracoscopic repair provides improved visibility, less need for postoperative opioids, and decreased duration of ventilation (which may related to the patient group selected).
- The recurrence rate as high as 23 % among infants undergoing thoracoscopic repair in the newborn period.

Complications in the early postoperative period include:

- Recurrent pulmonary hypertension and deterioration in respiratory mechanics and gaseous exchange.
- Recurrent congenital diaphragmatic hernia. This is more common if a patch is used to repair the hernia (Fig. 46.20).
- Leakage of peritoneal fluid and blood into the thorax.
- Development of an ipsilateral hydrothorax or chylothorax.
- Small-bowel obstruction may occur secondary to adhesions or volvulus.

Long-Term Outcomes and Prognosis

- The exact mortality of congenital diaphragmatic hernia is difficult to determine.
- This is partially because of the "hidden mortality," which refers to infants with congenital diaphragmatic hernia who die in utero or shortly after birth, prior to transfer to a pediatric surgery center.

Fig. 46.20 Chest x-ray and barium enema showing recurrent left congenital diaphragmatic hernia with bowel loops herniating into the chest

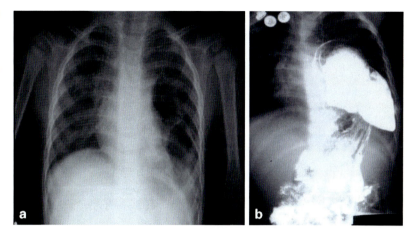

The overall reported survival rates of congenital diaphragmatic hernia range from 40 to 90 % with an average of 52 %.

- The Congenital Diaphragmatic Hernia Study Group recorded a 63 % survival rate in 1995–1996 based on data from 62 centers in North America, Europe, and Australia.
- Long-term complications in survivors of congenital diaphragmatic hernia include:
  - Long-term pulmonary disease:
    - This depends on the degree of pulmonary hypoplasia and barotrauma sustained in the neonatal period.
    - They may develop bronchopulmonary dysplasia.
    - Restrictive and/or obstructive lung disease may be observed.
  - Failure to thrive
  - Functional and anatomic esophageal abnormalities (45–85 %):
    - These are associated with significant gastroesophageal reflux in 40 % of survivors.
    - Prophylactic fundoplication at the time of primary repair for infants requiring a patch repair is advocated by some surgeons.
    - Other patients who may require fundoplication include the neurologically impaired and those with chronic lung disease.
    - Most other infants outgrow gastroesophageal reflux.
- Sensorineural hearing loss (40 %) as well as neurodevelopmental abnormalities (cognitive and developmental delay, cerebral palsy, seizure disorders, impaired vision):
  - These are seen more in those who require ECMO, hyperventilation treatment, and ototoxic medication.
- Altered musculoskeletal development results in:
  - Thoracic scoliosis
  - Pectus deformities
  - A decreased thoracic cavity
- Learning disability
- Developmental disability
- Cognitive and attention deficit
- Hyperactivity disorder
- Behavioral problems.

Recommended Reading

Bagolan P, Casaccia G, Crescenzi F, Nahom A, Trucchi A, Giorlandino C. Impact of a current treatment protocol on outcome of high-risk congenital diaphragmatic hernia. J Pediatr Surg. 2004;39(3):313–8.

Clark RH, Hardin WD Jr, Hirschl RB, et al. Current surgical management of congenital diaphragmatic hernia: a report from the Congenital Diaphragmatic Hernia Study Group. J Pediatr Surg. 1998;33(7):1004–9.

Gander JW, Fisher JC, Gross ER, Reichstein AR, Cowles RA, Aspelund G. Early recurrence of congenital diaphragmatic hernia is higher after thoracoscopic than open repair: a single institutional study. J Pediatr Surg. 2011;46(7):1303–8.

Karamanoukian HL, O'Toole SJ, Glick PL. "State-of-the-art" management strategies for the fetus and neonate with congenital diaphragmatic hernia. J Perinatol. 1996;16(2 Pt 2 Su):S40–7.

Okazaki T, Nishimura K, Takahashi T, Shoji H, Shimizu T, Tanaka T. Indications for thoracoscopic repair of congenital diaphragmatic hernia in neonates. Pediatr Surg Int. 2011;27(1):35–8.

Wung JT, Sahni R, Moffitt ST, Lipsitz E, Stolar CJ. Congenital diaphragmatic hernia: survival treated with very delayed surgery, spontaneous respiration, and no chest tube. J Pediatr Surg. 1995;30(3):406–9.

Chapter 47
Eventration of the Diaphragm

Introduction

- There are different types of congenital diaphragmatic hernia. These include:
  - Bochdalek hernia: The most common type of congenital diaphragmatic hernia
  - Morgagni hernia
  - Hiatal hernia
  - Eventration of diaphragm
  - Central tendon defects of the diaphragm
- Eventration of the diaphragm is a disorder in which all or part of the diaphragmatic muscle is replaced by fibroelastic tissue.
- Eventration of the diaphragm leads to an abnormal elevation of one leaf of an intact diaphragm as a result of:
  - Congenital aplasia or maldevelopment of the diaphragm
  - Paralysis of the phrenic nerve
- Eventration of the diaphragm is a rare anomaly.
- The exact incidence of eventration is unknown. An incidence of 1 per 1400 to 1 in 10,000 live births was reported.
- It is more common in males than in females.
- It is more likely to affect the left hemidiaphragm (Fig. 47.1).
- It is postulated that they occur embryologically because of abnormal migration of myoblasts from the upper cervical somites into two of the four embryological structures that contribute to diaphragm development: the septum transversum (beginning at 4 weeks of gestation) and the pleuroperitoneal membrane (at 8–12 weeks of gestation).
- The loss of contractility leads to muscle atrophy with elevation of the hemidiaphragm.
- It is usually congenital but may be acquired.
- Complete eventration almost invariably occurs on the left side and is rare on the right.
- It is more common in males than in females.
- Congenital eventration of the diaphragm is commonly an isolated condition.
- Sometimes it is associated with other developmental defects such as:
  - Cleft palate
  - Congenital heart disease
  - Situs inversus
  - Undescended testicle

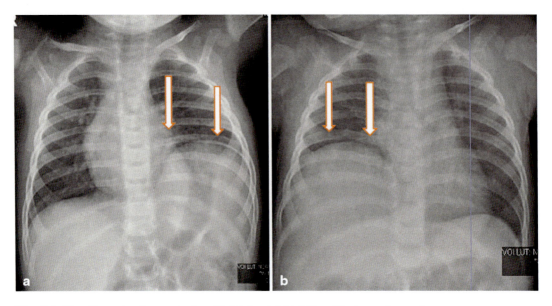

Fig. 47.1 Chest X-ray showing eventration of left (**a**) and right (**b**) hemidiaphragm (*arrows*)

Classification

- Eventration of the diaphragm is divided into two types:
    - Congenital
    - Acquired
- Congenital eventration results from:
    - Inadequate development of the muscle of diaphragm
    - Absence of the phrenic nerves
- The most common cause of acquired eventration is injury to the phrenic nerve, resulting from:
    - Traumatic birth leading to injury of phrenic nerve
    - Thoracic surgery for congenital heart disease
    - Rarely, tumors of the chest
    - Obstetric injury may be combined with lesion of brachial plexus leading to a paralysis of the Erb–Duchenne type.
- In the acquired form, the central tendon of diaphragm is normal and the diaphragm consists of normally developed muscle that is atrophic. Both sides of diaphragm are affected equally.
- The defect in congenital eventration can be:
    - Partial
    - Diffuse
- In the partial type, the defect is localized.
- In the diffuse type, the diaphragm consists of a thin membrane that is attached peripherally to normal muscles.
- Partial defects mostly affect the right hemidiaphragm (65%) of children.
- Diffuse eventration is more frequent on the left side.

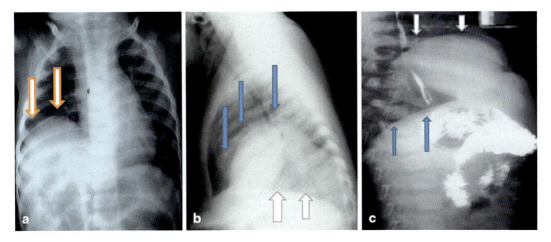

Fig. 47.2 a–c Anteroposterior and lateral chest X-rays showing eventration of right diaphragm. Note that there was no herniation of abdominal contents into the thoracic cavity

Pathophysiology

- Eventration of the diaphragm is usually asymptomatic but can cause problems as a result of:
  - Inability to properly ventilate the ipsilateral lung
  - Direct compression of the ipsilateral lung
  - Pneumonia due to chronic atelectasis
  - Paradoxical motion of the diaphragm making ventilation of the contralateral lung inefficient
- The mediastinum is very mobile and paradoxical movement of the affected diaphragm causes a shift of the heart and mediastinum toward the contralateral side. This limits effective ventilation of the opposite lung and also impedes venous return to the heart.

Clinical Features

- The clinical manifestations of eventration of diaphragm are variable, ranging from asymptomatic to life-threatening respiratory distress requiring mechanical ventilatory support.
- Eventration of diaphragm usually remains asymptomatic in early life and presents later with respiratory and occasionally gastrointestinal complications.
- The respiratory complications are more in children compared to adults.
- Recurrent chest infections are the commonest presenting complaint in patients with eventration of diaphragm.

Diagnosis

- The diagnosis of diaphragmatic eventration can usually be made on standard posteroanterior and lateral chest films (Fig. 47.2).
- In eventration, the diaphragm retains its continuity and attachments to the costal margin.

Fig. 47.3 Intraoperative photograph showing thoracotomy to repair eventration of diaphragm. Note the elevated diaphragm and the compressed lung

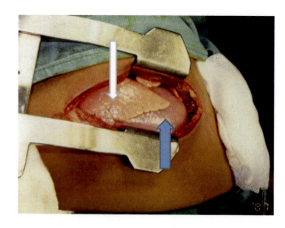

- The affected hemidiaphragm should be at least two intercostal spaces higher than the other side.
- Fluoroscopy is considered the most reliable way to document diaphragmatic paralysis. Paradoxical movement of the affected diaphragm is seen during screening.
- Ultrasonography can help in establishing the diagnosis of partial eventration and in distinguishing it from diaphragmatic nerve interruption.
- It is sometimes difficult to distinguish the radiological picture of eventration of the diaphragm from that of congenital diaphragmatic hernia (CDH). This is especially so in those who present late and have a hernia sac.

Treatment

- Patients with eventration who are asymptomatic or patients who improve without intervention may be treated conservatively.
- Conservative treatment for asymptomatic patients whose eventration is due to phrenic nerve injury is also to be advocated, with hope for recovery if possible.
- Eventration of diaphragm in children may require surgical treatment to restore normal pulmonary parenchymal volume.
- Indications for surgery:
  - Two or more recurrent ipsilateral pneumonias
  - One life-threatening pneumonia
  - Inability to wean the patient from mechanical ventilation
  - Respiratory distress related to paradoxical motion of the diaphragm
- The most commonly used treatment for this condition is diaphragmatic plication. This makes the lax diaphragm taut and moves it to a lower position. The lung is able to expand and function better than before (Figs. 47.3 and 47.4).
- Surgical approaches:
  - Thoracotomy
  - Thoracoscopic assisted
  - Laparotomy
  - Laparoscopic

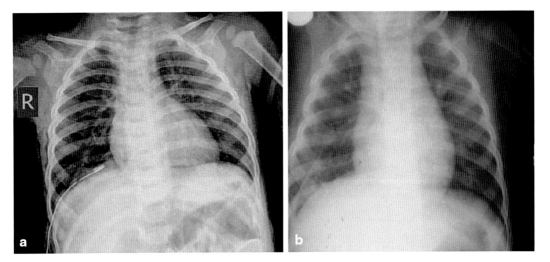

Fig. 47.4 Immediate postoperative anteroposterior chest X-ray showing a normal diaphragm following thoracoscopic plication (**a**) and a follow-up X-ray after open plication (**b**)

- Thoracoscopic surgery avoids the problems of open surgery, and its safety is well documented in children.
- For left-sided eventration, the approach can be either abdominal or thoracic.
- For eventration on the right side, a thoracic approach is preferred.
- Bilateral cases can be approached through a transverse upper abdominal incision.
- Laparoscopy can be used to repair left eventration.

Recommended Reading

Mouroux J, Venissac N, Leo F, Alifano M, Guillot F. Surgical treatment of diaphragmatic eventration using video-assisted thoracic surgery: a prospective study. Ann Thorac Surg. 2005;79:308–12.

Shah SR, Wishnew J, Barsness K, Gaines BA, Potoka DA, Gittes GK, Kane TD. Minimally invasive congenital diaphragmatic hernia repair: a 7-year review of one institution's experience. Surg Endosc. 2009;23:1265.

Chapter 48
Morgagni's Hernia

Introduction

- Congenital diaphragmatic hernia is a life-threatening malformation in infants, and a major cause of death usually secondary to pulmonary hypoplasia and pulmonary hypertension.
- The incidence of congenital diaphragmatic hernia is approximately 1 per 2000–4000 pregnancies.
- Most congenital diaphragmatic hernias in infants are diagnosed in utero and are of the Bochdalek type, resulting from a posterolateral defect in the diaphragm. This is commonly seen on the left side.
- Other types of congenital diaphragmatic hernia include:
  - Morgagni's hernia
  - Eventration of diaphragm
  - Paraesophageal hernia
  - Hernia through a defect in the central tendon of the diaphragm
- Morgagni's hernia was first described in 1769 by the Italian anatomist Morgagni. He described substernal herniation of abdominal contents into the thoracic cavity based on observations made during autopsy examinations.
- This rare anterior defect of the diaphragm is variably referred to as Morgagni's, retrosternal, or parasternal hernia.
- Morgagni's hernias result from an anterior defect in the diaphragm as a result of failure of complete fusion between the pars sternalis and the pars costalis of the hemidiaphragms.
- The foramen of Morgagni (space of Larrey) extends from the sternum medially to the eighth rib laterally. The diaphragmatic defect described by both Morgagni and Larrey is a triangular space between the muscle fibers of the diaphragm that originate from the xiphisternum and the costal margin and insert on the central tendon of the diaphragm. This potential space is referred to as the foramen of Morgagni or the space of Larrey.
- Morgagni's hernia is a rare congenital diaphragmatic hernia comprising about 4–5 % of all diaphragmatic hernias.
- The majority of Morgagni's hernias occur on the right side because the left side is protected by the heart and pericardium (Fig. 48.1).
- Morgagni's hernia can be bilateral (Fig. 48.2).
- Morgagni's hernia is slightly more common in females.

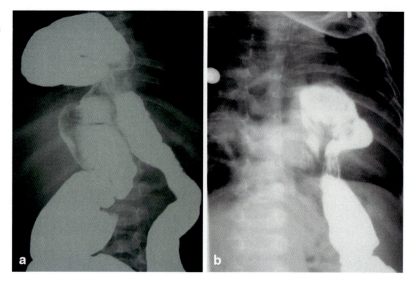

Fig. 48.1 Barium enema showing colonic herniation into a right Morgagni's hernia (**a**) and colonic herniation into a left Morgagni's hernia (**b**)

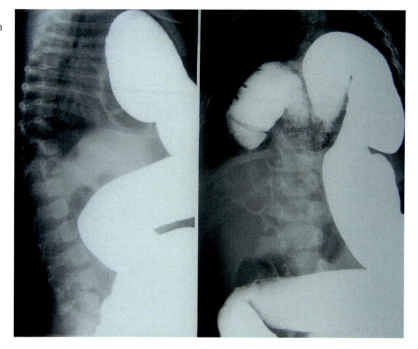

Fig. 48.2 Barium enema showing colonic herniation into bilateral Morgagni's hernia

Presentation

- Most Morgagni's hernias present later in life and are generally asymptomatic discovered accidentally or during the evaluation of other nonrelated conditions.
- Rarely Morgagni's hernia present in the newborn period with respiratory distress at birth similar to Bochdalek hernia.
- Morgagni's hernias may also be the cause of recurrent chest infections and nonspecific gastrointestinal symptoms.

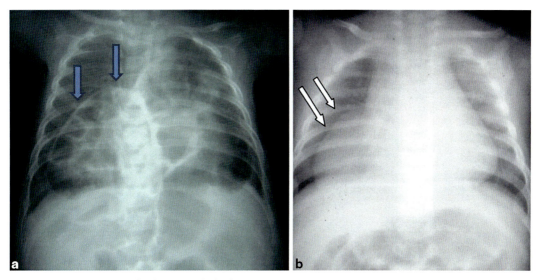

Fig. 48.3 Chest x-rays showing bowel herniation into a right Morgagni's hernia (**a**) and part of the liver herniating into a right Morgagni's hernia (**b**)

- Morgagni's hernia may also present with cough, dyspnea, and upper abdominal discomfort, fullness, bloating and vomiting.
- Morgagni's hernia may be discovered as a result of an increase in intra-abdominal pressure secondary to:
  - Trauma
  - Pregnancy
  - Obesity
  - Vetriculo-peritoneal shunt

Associated Anomalies

- Morgagnis's hernia is well known to be associated with other congenital anomalies. These include:
  - Congenital heart disease which is reported in up to 80% of patients.
  - Down's syndrome (14–35%). It is well known that children with Down's syndrome can have other muscular defects such as ventral hernia and diastasis recti. This association as well as that with Morgagni's hernia suggests a possible muscular deficiency of the ventral paramedian segment of the body in these patients.
  - Pentalogy of Cantrell, Noonan syndrome, Prader–Willi syndrome, and Turner syndrome.
  - Malrotation in up to 30% of patients. This must be kept in mind intraoperatively to obviate the risk of postoperative volvulus.

Diagnosis

- The majority of Morgagni hernias are right sided.
- The most commonly herniated viscera are the colon (70–80%), liver (3–5%), small intestines (2–5%), stomach (2–5%), omentum (10–12%), and spleen.

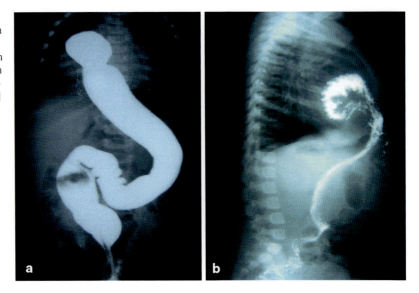

Fig. 48.4 Barium enema showing colonic herniation into a right Morgagni's hernia (**a**) and a lateral film showing colonic herniation (**b**). Note the anterior location of the herniated bowel

- The differential diagnosis includes pleuropericardial cyst, pleural mesothelioma, pericardial fat pad, mediastinal lipoma, tumor or cyst of the diaphragm, thymoma, and anterior chest wall tumors.
- Imaging features vary depending on the herniated contents.
- On chest radiography, they typically appear as a well-defined opacity in the right cardiophrenic angle. Air-containing loops of small or large intestines are occasionally seen (Fig. 48.3).
- The presence of intestines in the sac can be confirmed by barium enema or barium meal and follow-through (Fig. 48.4a).
- A lateral film should be obtained always to confirm the anterior location of the herniated intestines (Fig. 48.4b).
- The diagnosis of Morgagni's hernia can be readily made on CT or MRI. A CT scan can delineate a cardiophrenic mass from the heart and will identify loops of bowel within the chest. The use of CT scan as a diagnostic tool in patients with foramen of Morgagni's hernias has increased the reliability of preoperative diagnosis (Figs. 48.5 and 48.6).

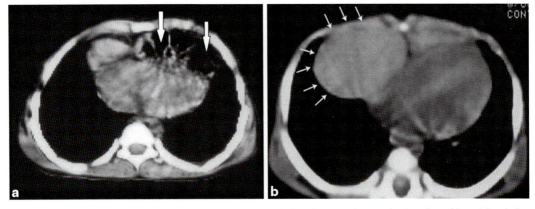

Fig. 48.5 CT scan showing bowel herniation into a Morgagni's hernia. Note the anterior location of bowel herniation and CT scan showing a soft tissue mass into the right side of the chest (**a**). This was shown to be part of the left lobe of liver herniating through a Morgagni's hernia (**b**)

Management 355

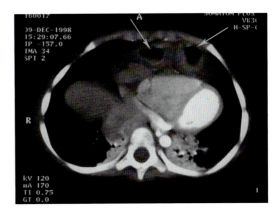

Fig. 48.6 CT scan showing bilateral Morgagni's hernia

Management

- The treatment of Morgagni's hernia is operative repair even in asymptomatic patients. This is to obviate the risk of intestinal obstruction and colonic perforation.
- Conventionally, the treatment of Morgagni's hernia is through an open approach via either thoracotomy or laparotomy. Through laparatomy a bilateral Morgagni's hernia can be repaired easily (Fig. 48.7).
- The recent advances in minimally invasive techniques, thoracoscopy and laparoscopy are being used with increasing frequency to diagnose and treat Morgagni hernias. These minimally invasive surgical techniques have been shown to be superior to and they may replace the more traditional open transabdominal approach.
- Although successful repair can be performed transthoracically, the transabdominal approach whether open or laparoscopically is preferred.
- Considerable controversy exists regarding the need for sac excision and whether prosthetic material should be used. Very rarely a prosthetic patch is needed to repair Morgagni's hernia and where possible the associated hernia sac (>90% of cases) should be excised.
- Currently, the transabdominal approach (laparoscopic or laparoscopic assisted) with interrupted nonabsorbable sutures is the preferred method to repair Morgagni's hernia.

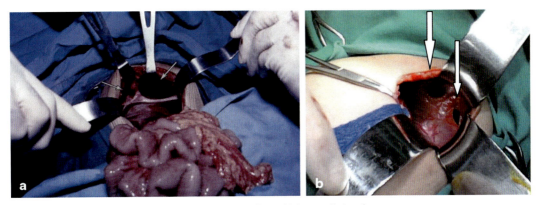

Fig. 48.7 a and b Intraoperative photograph showing bilateral Morgagni's hernia

Recommended Reading

Al-Salem A. Congenital Morgagni's hernia and associated anomalies. J Pediatr Surg Specialities. 2009;3(3):158–72.
Ambrogi V, Forcella D, Gatti A, Vanni G, Mineo TC. Transthoracic repair of Morgagni's hernia: a 20-year experience from open to video-assisted approach. Surg Endosc. 2007;21(4):587–91.

Chapter 49
Congenital Paraesophageal Hernia

Introduction

- Congenital paraesophageal hernia is rare in infants and children.
- Most reported cases are acquired resulting as a complication following Nissen's fundoplication for gastroesophageal reflux.
- By definition, paraesophageal hernia occurs when the stomach protrudes laterally through the esophageal hiatus toward the chest while the gastroesophageal junction remains in its normal anatomic position.
- This however is not the case in the pediatric age group where in most of cases the whole stomach herniates into the thoracic cavity with the gastroesophageal junction lying in the chest. These may represent a combined type of sliding and paraesophageal hernias, or in the pediatric age group congenital paraesophageal hernia is distinct and different from their adult counterpart.
- Another distinguishing feature of pediatric paraesophageal hernia is that it is not uncommon for other intra-abdominal organs to herniate into the chest through the hiatal opening (Figs. 49.1 and 49.2).
- Complications are more prevalent in paraesophageal hernias than in sliding hiatus hernias.
- The defect is within the esophageal hiatus and is lined by a peritoneal sac, usually extending anteriorly and to the right of the esophagus as well as into the posterior mediastinum.
- Acquired paraesophageal hernias are commonly seen in infants under the age of 1, neurologically impaired children, and in those where repair of the crura was not done at the time of fundoplication.
- Congenital paraesophageal hernia on the other hand is relatively rare in the pediatric age group and most of the cases occur sporadically but there are reports of familial paraesophageal hernias.

Etiology

- The exact etiology of congenital paraesophageal hernia is not known.
- It is postulated that congenital paraesophageal hernia is secondary to embryonal developmental defects in the lumbar component of the diaphragm leading to defective right crus of the diaphragm.
- Most reported cases of congenital paraesophageal hernia occur sporadically.
- A familial occurrence of hiatal hernia was first suggested in 1939.
- Since then, there have been several reports documenting the occurrence of hiatal hernia among siblings. This unusual familial occurrence supports a genetic predisposition to the development of congenital paraesophageal hernia and an autosomal dominant mode of inheritance was suggested.

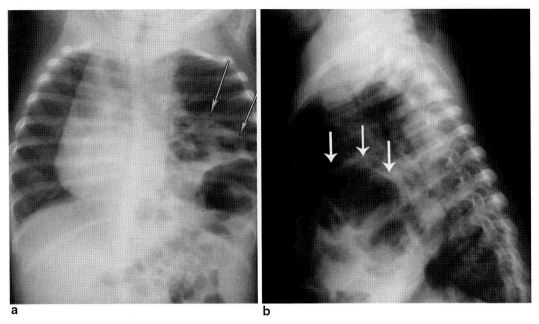

Fig. 49.1 Chest x-ray of a child with a paraesophageal hernia showing herniation of bowel loops in addition to the stomach (**a**) and a lateral chest x-ray showing bowel herniation in a large paraesophageal hernia (**b**)

Fig. 49.2 CT scan showing a large paraesophageal hernia containing stomach and bowel loops

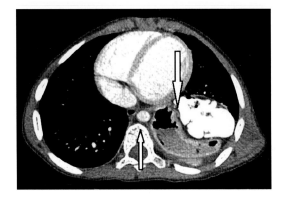

Classification

- Hiatal hernias are classified into two types: a sliding hiatal hernia and a paraesophageal hernia (Figs. 49.3, 49.4, 49.5, 49.6, 49.7, 49.8 and 49.9).
- Paraesophageal hernias constitute about 3.5–5 raesophageal hernias constitute about 3.5s: a sliding F 1:4).

Sliding Hiatal Hernia

- This is the most common type.
- The gastroesophageal junction is displaced superior to the hiatus.
- It is commonly associated with gastroesophageal reflux disease.

Treatment

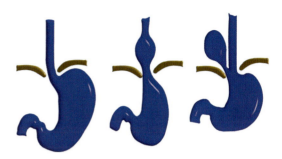

Fig. 49.3 Diagrammatic representation of the different types of hiatal hernias

Paraesophageal Hernia

- The gastroesophageal junction is inferior to the diaphragm, but the fundus and sometimes the whole stomach have migrated alongside the esophagus into the mediastinum.
- Paraesophageal hernia is considered to be a potentially life-threatening condition because of the risk of gastric volvulus, incarceration, or strangulation of the hernia.
- Paraesophageal hernias in the pediatric age group are divided into:
  - Congenital
  - Acquired
- Irrespective of the type, whether congenital or acquired, they are relatively rare.
- The vast majority of paraesophageal hernias are however acquired commonly seen following Nissen's fundoplication for the treatment of gastroesophageal reflux.
- Congenital paraesophageal hernia must also be differentiated from purely intrathoracic stomach, an entity that is known to be associated with a short esophagus.

Clinical Features

- These children usually present with recurrent chest infection or vague gastrointestinal symptoms.
- Awareness of this is important as congenital paraesophageal hernias are known to be associated with potentially lethal complications like gastric volvulus with partial or complete gastric obstruction, strangulation, and perforation (Fig. 49.9).
- It is also of importance to note that large congenital paraesophageal hernia can present at or soon after birth with respiratory distress that can be confused with the more common congenital posterolateral diaphragmatic hernia.

Treatment

- The treatment of congenital paraesophageal hernia is surgical repair (Fig. 49.10).
- This is even for asymptomatic, incidentally discovered cases.
- This is to obviate the risk of gastric volvulus, strangulation, and perforation in spite of its low frequency (Fig. 49.11).
- The addition of an anti-reflux procedure is still controversial.

Fig. 49.4 a and **b** Barium swallow showing sliding hiatal hernia with proximal stricture formation. Note also part of the stomach above the gastroesophageal junction

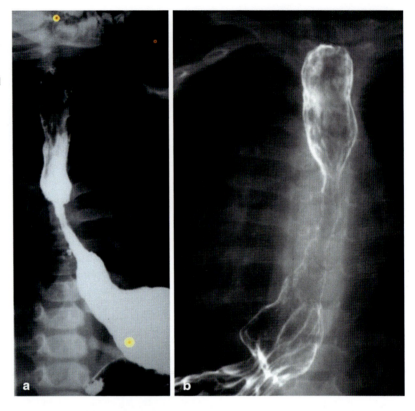

Fig. 49.5 a and **b** Barium meal showing paraesophageal hernia

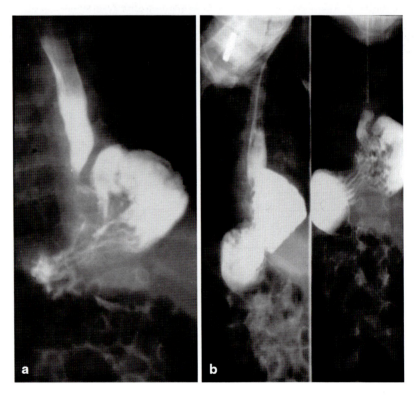

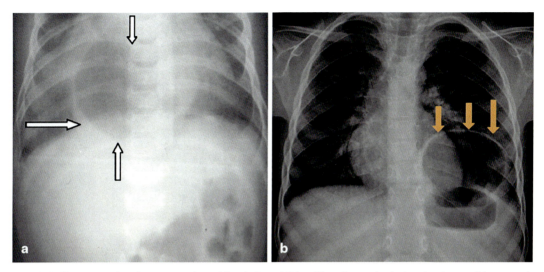

Fig. 49.6 Chest x-ray showing paraesophageal hernia in a child. **a**, Note the gas in the herniated part of the stomach into the chest. **b**, Note the hernia sac containing stomach

Fig. 49.7 Chest x-ray showing paraesophageal hernia. Note the air–fluid level in the herniated part of the stomach

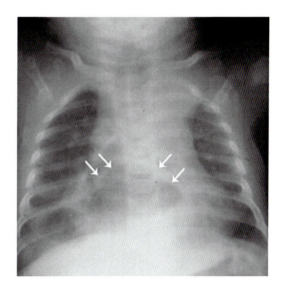

- The rarity of this condition in the pediatric age group makes it difficult to evaluate the true necessity of adding an anti-reflux procedure for these patients.
- Many however advocate adding an anti-reflux procedure at the time of hernia repair. This is to avoid the potential subsequent development of gastroesophageal reflux.
- The principles of repair consist of:
  - Reduction of the hernia content
  - Excision of the hernia sac to prevent recurrence and cyst formation
  - Crural approximation
  - An anti-reflux fundoplication
- The recent advances in minimally invasive surgery have made it feasible and safe to repair paraesophageal hernias laparoscopically in children.

Fig. 49.8 Barium meal showing paraesophageal hernia. Note the position of the stomach above the diaphragm

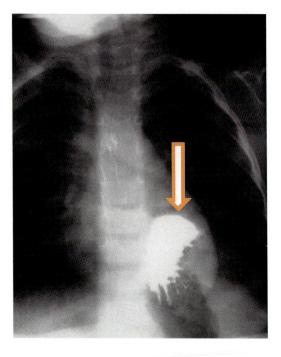

Fig. 49.9 Barium meal showing paraesophageal hernia with intrathoracic gastric volvulus

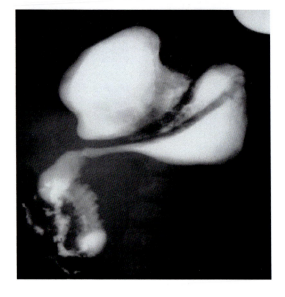

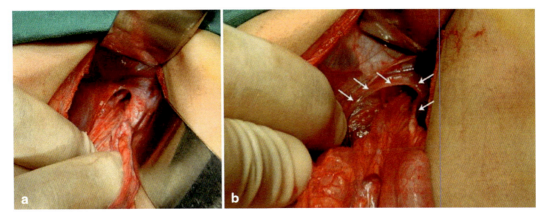

Fig. 49.10 Intraoperative photograph showing the defect through which there was a large paraesophageal hernia after reducing its contents

Fig. 49.11 Barium meal showing a large paraesophageal hernia with almost total herniation of the stomach into the chest and intrathoracic gastric volvulus

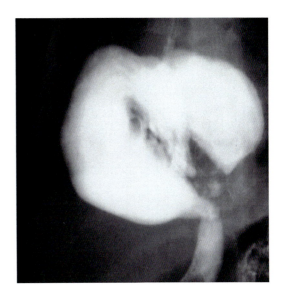

Recommended Reading

Alrabeeah A, Giacomantonio M, Gillis DA. Paraesophageal hernia after Nissen fundoplication: a real complication in pediatric patients. J Pediatr Surg. 1988;23(8):766–8.

Baglaj SM, Noblett HR. Paraoesophageal hernia in children: familial occurrence and review of the literature. Pediatr Surg Int. 1999;15(2):85–7.

Carré IJ, Johnston BT, Thomas PS, Morrison PJ. Familial hiatal hernia in a large five generation family confirming true autosomal dominant inheritance. Gut. 1999;45(5):649–52.

Imamoğlu M, Cay A, Koşucu P, Ozdemir O, Orhan F, Sapan L, Sarihan H. Congenital paraesophageal hiatal hernia: pitfalls in the diagnosis and treatment. J Pediatr Surg. 2005;40(7):1128–33.

Karpelowsky JS, Wieselthaler N, Rode H. Primary paraesophageal hernia in children. J Pediatr Surg. 2006;41(9):1588–93.

Chapter 50
Congenital Lobar Emphysema

Introduction

- Congenital cystic diseases of the lung comprises a group of closely related, rare, but potentially life-threatening anomalies.
- These include:
  - Congenital cystic adenomatoid malformation
  - Pulmonary sequestration
  - Bronchogenic cyst
  - Congenital lobar emphysema (CLE)
- The term emphysema means "swelling" and it is derived from the Greek word emphysan meaning "inflate."
- CLE is a rare developmental anomaly of the lung characterized by lobar hyperinflation.
- CLE is also called infantile lobar emphysema and congenital lobar overinflation.
- In 1954, Gross and Lewis published the first case of CLE.
- It is a potentially reversible though possibly life-threatening cause of respiratory distress in neonates.
- CLE is a rare congenital malformation, with a prevalence of 1 in 20,000 to 1 in 30,000.
- CLE is most often detected in newborns or young infants, but sometimes it remains asymptomatic or in some cases does not become apparent until adulthood.
- CLE is characterized by massive distension and overexpansion of the affected lobe of the lung, usually the left upper lobe or the right middle lobe.
- Overexpansion of the affected lobe as a result of air trapping leads to compression of the surrounding lung as well as the contralateral lung which may cause life-threatening respiratory distress, which if not recognized and treated, may be fatal (Fig. 50.1).
- Congenital cardiac anomalies may be present in as many as 10 % of patients with CLE. All patients with CLE should have adequate preoperative cardiac evaluation by echocardiography.
- CLE commonly occur in whites.
- CLE appears to be more common in males than females. The male-to-female ratio is 3:1.

Sites

CLE primarily involves one lobe of the lung (upper lobes are predominantly involved) as follows:

- Left upper lobe, 40–42 %.
- Right middle lobe, 34–35 %.
- Right upper lobe, 20–21 %.

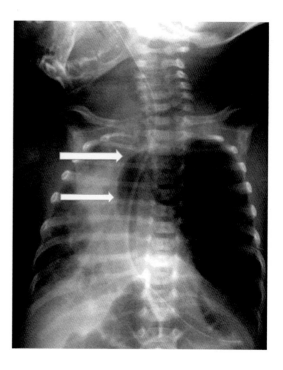

Fig. 50.1 Chest x-ray showing congenital lobar emphysema involving the left upper lobe. Note the mediastinal shift and herniation of the affected lobe to the other side with compression on the contralateral lung

- Involvement of the lower lobes is rare, occurring in fewer than 5 % of patients.
- Bilateral involvement in 20 %.

Pathogenesis

- CLE is characterized by progressive lobar hyperinflation that commonly results from disruption in bronchopulmonary embryological development.
- These result from abnormal embryological interactions between embryonic endodermal and mesodermal components of the lung.
- These disturbances may lead to changes in the number of airways or alveoli or abnormalities in alveolar size. Based on this, CLE is divided into two forms:
  - Hypo alveolar: Characterized by fewer than expected number of alveoli.
  - Polyalveolar: Characterized by greater than expected number of alveoli.
- The exact cause of CLE is not known and several factors have been incriminated. These include:
  - Intrinsic absence or abnormality of cartilaginous rings (deficiency in the cartilage of the bronchial wall). This is seen in 50–60 % of these cases.
  - Extra luminal obstruction and compression of the affected bronchus by abnormal blood vessel (as in the absence of the pulmonary valve) or congenital lung cyst. This leads to emphysema from partial obstruction.
  - Congenital bronchial stenosis and redundant bronchial mucosal flaps.
  - Polyalveolar lobe (the alveolar size may be normal, but the alveolar number is increased three- to fivefold). This leads to hyperexpansion of the affected pulmonary lobe.
- All of these factors lead to a ball-valve effect that permits inflation of the affected lobe during periods of negative intrathoracic pressure, but collapses and obstructs the affected bronchus with expiration. Ultimately, this leads to air trapping and overexpansion of the affected lobe of the lung.

- CLE should be differentiated from the Swyer–James syndrome (i.e., acquired pulmonary abnormality secondary to infection leading to small but hyperlucent lung).
- A mucous plug which can obstruct a bronchus, creating a "check-valve" phenomenon that partially obstructs an airway should be excluded.

Associated Malformations

- Associated congenital malformations are seen in 14–21% of patients with CLE.
- Congenital heart disease (PDA, VSD) is the commonest.
- Of those with congenital heart disease, 10% have additional anomalies including:
  - Rib cage defects
  - Renal anomalies

Clinical Features

- Most patients with CLE present before 6 months of life with recurrent respiratory distress. Half of the cases of CLE present within the first 4 weeks of life and three-quarters are seen in infants less than 6 months of life.
- The presentation of CLE in relation to age is as follows:
  - At birth: 33%
  - By 1 month of age: 50%
  - After 6 months of age: 5%
- Although the majority of patients with CLE present early as an acute neonatal respiratory distress, a small group of them may be asymptomatic or present at a later age with recurrent chest infection.
- Neonates commonly present with mild-to-moderate respiratory distress.
- This is associated with mediastinal shift, hyperresonance, and decreased breath sounds on the affected side.
- Infants usually present with cough, wheezing, respiratory distress, and cyanosis.
- Older children with CLE may present with recurrent chest infections.
- The severity of CLE is variable as follows:
  - Most patients present with moderate respiratory distress.
  - Cyanosis in half of the patients.
  - Less than half present with mild respiratory distress.
  - CLE can be asymptomatic discovered incidentally on chest x-ray.
  - Rarely, CLE presents with severe life-threatening respiratory distress.

Diagnosis

- CLE is most often detected in neonates or identified during in utero ultrasound which shows the affected lobe as an overinflated, fluid-filled lobe associated with mediastinal herniation.
- In neonates, the affected lobe may be slightly opacified, rather than lucent, because it is still filled with fluids. This is important during the initial chest x-ray.

Fig. 50.2 Chest x-ray showing herniation of the emphysematous right upper lobe. Note also the herniation of the affected lobe to the other side

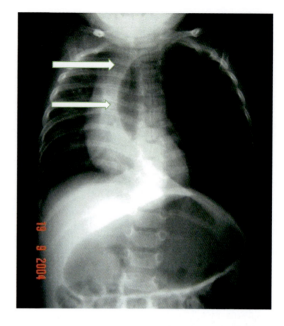

Fig. 50.3 Chest x-ray showing congenital lobar emphysema affecting the left and right upper lobes. Note the compressed collapsed right lower and left lobes (Sail sign)

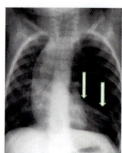

Fig. 50.4 Chest x-ray showing congenital lobar emphysema affecting the left and right upper lobes. Note the compressed collapsed right lower and left lobes (Sail sign)

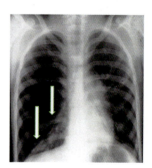

- Radiography of the chest in anteroposterior and lateral films identifies the affected lobe (Figs. 50.2, 50.3, 50.4, and 50.5).
    - This appears as a large, hyperlucent, emphysematous lobe with attenuated but defined vascularity. This is important to differentiate CLE from tension pneumothorax. This is specially so in an infant presenting with acute respiratory distress.
    - This hyperexpanded lobe herniates across the anterior midline to the other side.
    - There is also compression of the remaining lung on that side, flattened hemidiaphragm, and widened intercostal spaces.

Diagnosis

Fig. 50.5 A lateral chest x-ray showing the emphysematous lobe

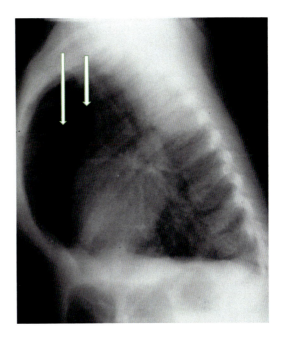

Fig. 50.6 CT-scan of the chest showing herniation of the affected emphysematous lobe. Note also the preserved broncho-vascular markings and mediastinal shift

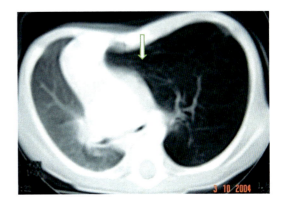

- Collapse of the remaining ipsilateral lung.
- Widening of the rib spaces.
- It is important to exclude a mucous plug which can obstruct a bronchus, creating a "check-valve" phenomenon that partially obstructs an airway.
- Extrinsic causes such as a congenitally large pulmonary artery although rare should be also excluded.
- Hypoplasia or agenesis of the contralateral lung may result in a marked compensatory hyperexpansion of the lung, which can closely resemble CLE.
- The early age onset of CLE precludes the possibility of aspiration a foreign body as an etiological factor. In addition, aspiration usually affects the lower lobe. When bronchoscopy is considered necessary, it should be performed in the operating room. The possibility of air trapping and progressive respiratory distress during the procedure must always be kept in mind and preparations should be made for emergency thoracotomy if necessary.
- Computed tomography scanning can provide details about the involved lobe and its vascularity, as well as information about the remaining lung (Figs. 50.6 and 50.7). This usually shows:

Fig. 50.7 CT-scan of the chest in a patient with congenital lobar emphysema. Note the emphysematous lobe as well as the collapsed ipsilateral lower lobe

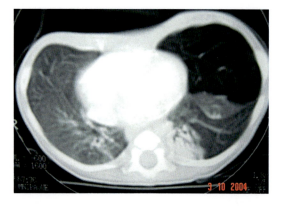

Fig. 50.8 An intraoperative photograph showing the overinflated emphysematous lobe which herniated through the thoracotomy incision

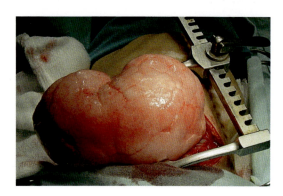

- A hyperlucent, hyperexpanded lobe with attenuated but intact vascularity pattern.
- Midline sub sternal herniation of the affected lobe.
- Compression of the remaining lung.
- The mediastinum is significantly shifted away from the side of the affected lobe.
- Substernal lobar herniation and compression of the remaining lung.
- The cause of obstruction especially extrinsic causes.

- Magnetic resonance imaging (MRI) is not routinely used but can be an adjunct modality to evaluate the vascular supply to the affected lobe. MRI is useful to rule out associated anomalous vascular slings.
- Ventilation–perfusion scan: Ventilation is initially diminished in the affected lobe, but ultimately, isotope retention is seen because of delayed emptying of alveoli in the emphysematous lobe. This can be used also during follow-ups. The markedly attenuated vascularity of the involved lobe results in decreased perfusion of the enlarged lobe.

Treatment and Outcome

- The management of CLE has traditionally been surgical.
- Surgical treatment of CLE is total lobectomy which must be performed early to overcome the potentially life-threatening acute respiratory distress and reduce the possibility of subsequent infection.
- In severely affected patients, the lung is overinflated and will immediately herniate through the surgical incision (Figs. 50.8 and 50.9).

Treatment and Outcome

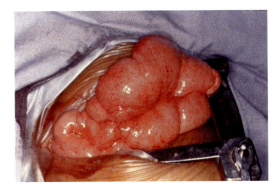

Fig. 50.9 A clinical intraoperative photograph showing the emphysematous lobe herniating through the wound. Note the air filled lobe which is not compressible

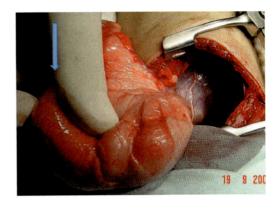

Fig. 50.10 An intraoperative clinical photograph showing the emphysematous lobe. Note the hyper inflated lobe when compared to the normal lobe in the upper part

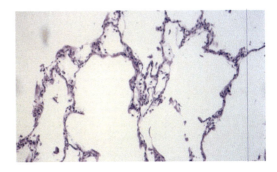

Fig. 50.11 A histological photograph in a patient with congenital lobar emphysema. Note the markedly over distended alveolar spaces

- The increased use of diagnostic imaging resulted in the discovery of asymptomatic and mildly symptomatic infants. This leads to a more conservative approach to these patients.
- Conservative management can be adopted for patients who are stable, asymptomatic, and can be followed-up closely or those with mild or intermittent symptoms.
- For more serious cases of CLE, surgery is necessary, usually a lobectomy to remove the affected lobe.
- Emergency lobectomy may become necessary for neonates with severe respiratory distress.
- Histological examination of the resected lobe shows large, markedly overdistended alveolar spaces without tissue destruction (Figs. 50.10 and 50.11).
- The importance of careful anesthetic induction cannot be overemphasized as these patients may not tolerate positive pressure ventilation which can lead to air trapping with rapid and massive enlargement of the affected lobe, mediastinal shift, and cardiac arrest.

- Total lobectomy is tolerated well in infants and children as growth and expansion of the remaining lung tissue is known to occur in children up to the age of 5 years with subsequent total lung volume and function ultimately returning to normal.
- Some patients have persistent abnormalities in perfusion. Most patients however show little or no abnormalities in pulmonary function after lobectomy or long-term conservative treatment.

Recommended Reading

Al-Salem AH. Congenital lobar emphysema. Saudi Med J. 2002;23(3):335–7.

Azizkhan RG, Cromblehome TM. Congenital cystic lung disease: contemporary antenatal and postnatal management. Pediatr Surg Int. 2008;24(60):643–57.

Colon N, Schlegel C, Pietsch J, Chung DH, Jackson GP. Congenital lung anomalies: can we postpone resection? J Pediatr Surg. 2012;47(1):87–92.

Tander B, Yalçin M, Yilmaz B, Ali Karadağ C, Bulut M. Congenital lobar emphysema: a clinicopathologic evaluation of 14 cases. Eur J Pediatr Surg. 2003;13:108.

Thakral CL, Maji DC, Sajwani MJ. Congenital lobar emphysema: experience with 21 cases. Pediatr Surg Int. 2001;17(2–3):88–91.

Chapter 51
Congenital Cystic Adenomatoid Malformation

Introduction

- Congenital cystic adenomatoid malformation (CCAM) is a rare developmental abnormality of the lung.
- CCAM is considered as a hamartomatous abnormality of the lung (abnormal tissue with an excess of one or more tissue components), which results from adenomatoid proliferation of the terminal bronchioles resulting in the formation of cysts with a consequent reduction in alveolar growth.
- CCAM represents approximately 25 % of all congenital lung malformations.
- CCAM generally communicates with the bronchial tree and derives its blood supply from the pulmonary circulation, in contrast to pulmonary sequestration, which derives its blood supply from the aorta.
- Ch'in and Tang first described CCAM as a distinct entity in 1949.
- Polyhydramnios has also been associated with CCAM. This develops as a result of elevated intrathoracic pressure that leads to esophageal compression and inability to swallow.
- The estimated incidence of CCAM is 1:25,000 to 1:35,000.
- With the increasing use of prenatal ultrasonography as well as improvement in technology and skill, most cases of CCAMs are prenatally diagnosed. CCAMs are typically identified prenatally by routine ultrasonography screening.
- Most postnatally identified cases present in the newborn period.
- CCAM may present in the older child and adults as an incidental finding or discovered secondary to repeated chest infections.
- This lesion occurs more often in males than females (1.8:1).
- CCAMs can affect both side of the lung and any lobe.
- CCAMs commonly involve only one lobe, rarely multiple, but in 15 %, involve two or more lobes on either ipsilateral or contralateral sides.

Classification

- In 1977, Stocker classified CCAM into three types based mostly on cyst size.
    1. Type I CCAM (65 %; Fig. 51.1): This includes
        - Multiple large cysts (>2 cm in diameter).
        - A single large cyst surrounded by numerous smaller cysts.
        - Type I is the most common type of CCAM and is associated with an excellent prognosis.

Fig. 51.1 Diagramatic representation of type I CCAM

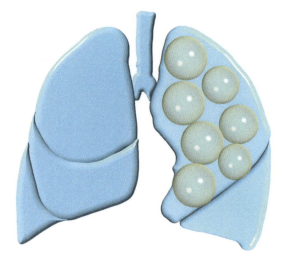

Fig. 51.2 Diagramatic representation of type II CCAM

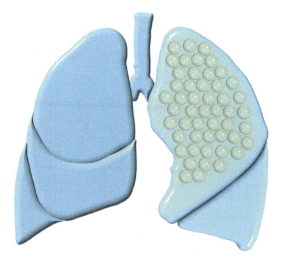

 – The cysts are frequently lined by pseudostratified columnar epithelial cells, which occasionally produce mucin.
2. Type II CCAM (25 %; Fig. 51.2):
 – This is characterized by multiple small cysts, usually <1 cm in diameter.
 – Accounts for >25 % of cases of CCAM.
 – They are characterized by small, relatively uniform cysts resembling bronchioles.
 – As many as 60 % of type II lesions are associated with other congenital anomalies that may affect prognosis, specifically renal agenesis.
 – The cysts generally measure 0.5–2 cm in diameter.
 – These cysts are lined by cuboid-to-columnar epithelium and have a thin fibromuscular wall.
3. Type III CCAM (10 %; Fig. 51.3):
 – These are large and grossly a solid mass without obvious cyst formation.
 – They account for <5–10 % of all cases of CCAM.
 – Microscopically, they consist of multiple microcysts, measuring <0.5 cm in diameter.

Fig. 51.3 Diagramatic representation of type III CCAM

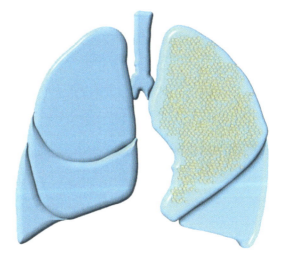

Fig. 51.4 CT scan of the chest showing type I CCAM. Note the large cyst and multiple smaller cysts

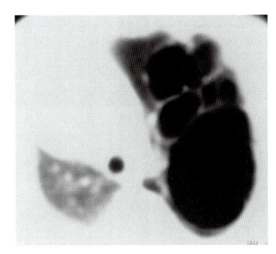

- In 1993, Adzick reported his classification of CCAM into two types.
    1. Microcystic CCAM (Figs. 51.4 and 51.5):
        - Cysts measuring <5 mm in diameter
        - Usually associated with fetal hydrops
        - Have a poor prognosis
    2. Macrocystic CCAM:
        - Cysts measuring >5 mm in diameter
        - Usually not associated with hydrops
        - Have a good prognosis
- CCAM receives its blood supply from the pulmonary circulation and is not sequestered from the tracheobronchial tree.
- Microscopically, the lesions are not true cysts, but communicate with the surrounding lung parenchyma.
- However, type II and III lesions can occasionally coexist with extralobar sequestration, and in such cases, they may receive systemic arterial blood supply.

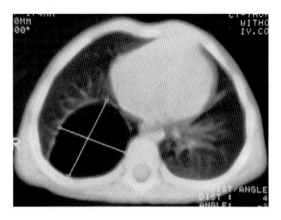

Fig. 51.5 CT scan of the chest showing a large cyst (type I CCAM)

- CCAM may also occur in association with a polyalveolar lobe.
- A polyalveolar lobe is a form of congenital emphysema with increased number of alveoli with normal bronchi and pulmonary vasculature.
- CCAM usually occurs early in fetal life, whereas polyalveolar lobe occurs late.
- The pathophysiologic effects of CCAM may be divided into prenatal and postnatal effects.
- Large lesions may be associated with the development of hydrops fetalis in as many as 40 % of cases and is a poor prognostic sign.
- Hydrops is thought to arise from compression of the inferior vena cava, which compromises venous return and leads to a decrease in cardiac output and the development of effusions. Fetal demise may result; premature delivery is attempted in order to salvage the fetus.
- The other main prenatal event is compromised pulmonary growth. This results in pulmonary hypoplasia which may lead to postnatal respiratory distress.

Presentation

- The usual postnatal presentation of CCAM is a respiratory distress in the newborn period.
- This may be due to:
    - Pulmonary hypoplasia
    - Mediastinal shift
    - Spontaneous pneumothorax
    - Air trapping within the cyst leading to compression of functional pulmonary tissue
    - Pleural effusion secondary to hydrops
- It may range in severity from grunting, tachypnea, and a mild oxygen requirement to fulminant respiratory failure requiring aggressive ventilator support or extracorporeal membrane oxygenation (ECMO).
- CCAM may also remain undiagnosed until it is discovered as an incidental finding later in life.
- Recurrent chest infections due to bronchial compression, air trapping, and inability to clear secretions may be the presenting feature in those presenting later in life.
- A risk of malignant transformation in later years is also noted.
- Hemoptysis has occasionally been described as a manifestation of CCAM in older children.
- Cough, fever, and failure to thrive have all been reported in association with the presentation of CCAM.
- Prenatal regression and complete resolution of CCAM have also been described.

Differential Diagnosis

The differential diagnosis includes:

- Congenital diaphragmatic hernia. This is especially so for CCAM affecting the left lower lobe of the lung.
- Congenital pneumonia.
- Hemothorax.
- Pleural effusion.
- Pneumatocele.
- Pneumothorax.
- Pulmonary sequestration.
- Pneumatoceles that form subsequent to bacterial pneumonia (e.g., streptococcal, staphylococcal) can be mistaken for CCAM, particularly in the older child.
- Congenital lobar emphysema refers to overexpansion of one lobe of the lung, typically an upper lobe or right middle lobe that leads to mass effect and respiratory distress. Although this entity could potentially be confused with CCAM, typical features of overexpanded but normal parenchyma can be observed and confirmed with computed tomography (CT) scan if necessary.
- Pulmonary interstitial emphysema may resemble CCAM when it is complicated by large air collections. However, these are also typically associated with linear collections and preceded by high-pressure ventilation and barotrauma. The air collections are located in the interstitial lymphatics.
- On plain radiographs, intrapulmonary sequestration with infection and abscess formation can be difficult to differentiate from CCAM.
- Bronchogenic cysts are usually fluid filled and well circumscribed.
- Neuroenteric cysts are posterior mediastinal soft tissue masses that are usually associated with vertebral anomalies.
- CCAM is differentiated from other congenital cystic disease of the lung by five characteristics:
  - Absence of bronchial cartilage (unless it is trapped within the lesion)
  - Absence of bronchial tubular glands
  - Presence of tall columnar mucinous epithelium
  - Overproduction of terminal bronchiolar structures without alveolar differentiation, except in the subpleural areas
  - Massive enlargement of the affected lobe that displaces other thoracic structures

Investigations

- Prenatal ultrasonography:
  - With increasing use of prenatal ultrasonography, most cases of CCAMs are prenatally diagnosed.
  - Ultrasonography may also demonstrate evidence of hydrops, such as fetal ascites or pleural effusions.
  - Type I lesions appear as multiple large cystic areas in the lung.
  - Type II lesions appear as multiple small cysts in the lung.
  - Type III lesions and because of the extremely small size of the cysts they appear as a homogenous mass.
- Prenatal ultrasonography is accurate in diagnosing CCAM.
- Prenatally diagnosed lesions may be asymptomatic at birth (71%), and they may have normal radiographic findings (57%).

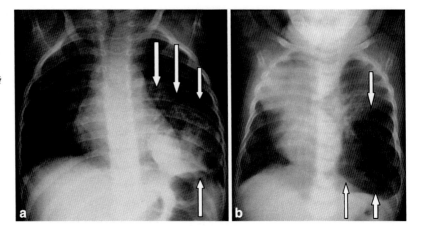

Fig. 51.6 Chest x-ray showing a large cyst in the *left lower lobe* (type I CCAM) (**a**) and another chest x-ray showing multiple cysts affecting the *left lower lobe* (**b**)

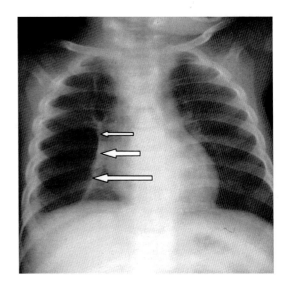

Fig. 51.7 Chest x-ray showing a large cyst in the *right lower lobe*

- Prenatal magnetic resonance imaging (MRI):
  - In CCAM, prenatal MRI findings on T2-weighted images have been reported, such as the following:
    - CCAM appear as intrapulmonary mass with increased signal intensity on T2-weighted images.
    - Type I or type II CCAM lesions have very high signal intensity almost equal to that of amniotic fluid and markedly higher than that of the surrounding unaffected lung tissue.
    - With increasing numbers of microcysts or macrocysts, discrete cystic components may be seen within the mass lesion; cysts larger than 3 mm are visualized easily.
    - Type III CCAM lesions have moderately high signal intensity; the signal intensity is higher than that of unaffected lung tissue but not as high as that of amniotic fluid; type III lesions are relatively homogeneous.
    - Prenatal MRI was less accurate than postnatal CT scan, which remains the most reliable diagnostic modality to specify the location, extent, and type of lesions.
- Chest radiography (Figs. 51.6 and 51.7):
  - The usual appearance is that of multiple cysts or a large cyst with or without adjacent smaller cysts or a mass containing air-filled cysts.

Investigations

Fig. 51.8 Chest x-ray showing left-sided CCAM with air–fluid level

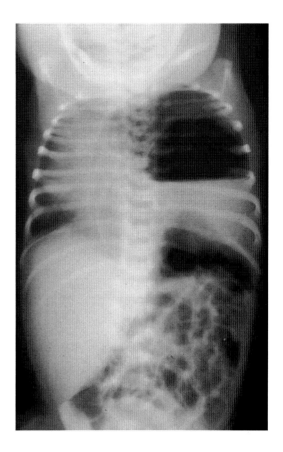

- Other radiological signs include mediastinal shift, pleural and pericardial effusions, and pneumothoraces.
- The diagnosis may not be clear from chest radiography alone. Chest radiography may reveal a mass without any evidence of cysts.
- The presence of superimposed infection may complicate the appearance. An air–fluid level may be evident (Fig. 51.8).

- CT scan of the chest:
    - CT scanning is necessary to determine the type and extent of the lesions.
    - The typical appearance is a multilocular cystic lesion with thin walls surrounded by normal lung parenchyma.
    - CT findings correlate with the pathologic findings (Figs. 51.9 and 51.10).
    - Multiple large cystic lesions (>2 cm in diameter) are seen alone or with other abnormalities (areas of small cysts, consolidation, or low attenuation). Low-attenuation areas are clusters of microcysts.
    - Air–fluid levels can be seen in some cysts. These lesions may be predominantly type I, type II, or a combination of both.
    - CCAM may completely resolve but persistent abnormalities are well demonstrated on CT examination.
    - Approximately 25 % of lesions diagnosed as CCAM may be either pulmonary sequestration or bronchogenic cysts. Overlapping CT features can also exist among other foregut malformations.
    - CT scanning of the chest may outline additional coexisting lesions.

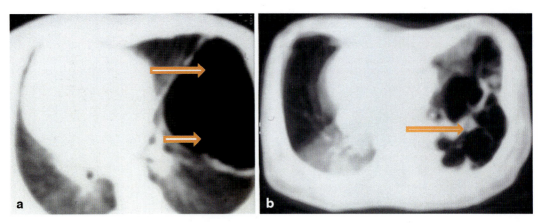

Fig. 51.9 CT scan of the chest showing a large cyst (type I CCAM) (**a**) and CT scan of the chest showing multiple cysts (**b**)

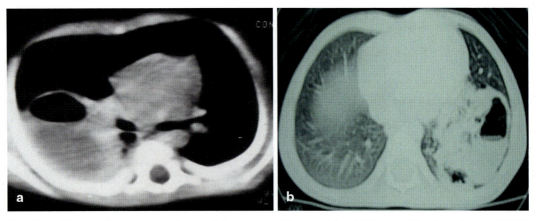

Fig. 51.10 CT scan of the chest showing a soft tissue mass with a cyst (**a**) and CT scan of the chest showing CCAM with superimposed infection (**b**)

- Magnetic resonance imaging:
  - MRI permits increased definition and accurately diagnoses CCAM.
  - MRI may be useful particularly in distinguishing CCAM from congenital diaphragmatic hernia.
- Other imaging studies:
  - Renal and cerebral ultrasonography to exclude coexisting renal and CNS anomalies.
  - Echocardiography to rule out any coexisting cardiac lesions.
  - Furthermore, in infants with respiratory distress, echocardiography may provide evidence of persistent pulmonary hypertension (e.g., right-to-left shunting, increased pulmonary artery pressures).

Treatment and Outcome

- Patients with CCAM complicated by pneumonia should be treated with antibiotics and supportive care, ranging from oxygen supplementation to mechanical ventilation. This is more commonly seen in older children.

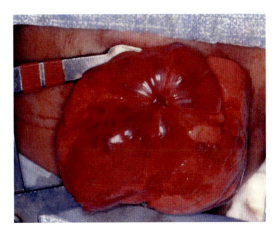

Fig. 51.11 Intraoperative photograph showing type I CCAM

- Surgical intervention is the mainstay of therapy for CCAM including fetal surgery and postnatal surgical resection (Figs. 51.11 and 51.12).
- A fetus diagnosed with CCAM should be monitored closely during pregnancy and the CCAM is excised surgically after birth.
- Fetuses diagnosed with CCAM and hydrops should be referred to a facility with expertise in fetal surgery.
- If fetal surgery is not indicated, close collaboration with a pediatric surgeon is essential because postnatal resection of the CCAM is necessary.
- A few fetuses may develop fluid collections within the chest cavity and, in those situations, a Harrison catheter shunt can be used to drain this into the amniotic fluid.
- Very large CCAMs might pose a danger during birth because of airway compression. In this situation, an EXIT procedure may be necessary.
- In rare extreme cases, where fetus's heart is in danger, fetal surgery can be performed to remove the CCAM.
- Fetal surgery should be considered in patients with large CCAMs and in cases complicated by hydrops, in which the prognosis is poor.
- Thoracocentesis allows drainage of a large cyst with immediate decompression of the CCAM. This, however, is not a very useful procedure as the fluid rapidly reaccumulates.
- Another option is to place a thoracoamniotic shunt that continually drains fluid from the CCAM to the amniotic space. This is most beneficial when the CCAM consists of a large fluid-filled cyst. Complications such as obstruction and shunt dislodgement may occur.
- Resection of the affected lobe (lobectomy) is an alternative procedure for cases with no dominant cyst available for draining.
- Complications included intraoperative bradycardia, the development of preterm labor and maternal mirror syndrome requiring early delivery, and postoperative intrauterine death. Survivors demonstrate residual lung growth and normal development.
- Fetal surgery can improve the survival percentage up to 50–60% in these cases.
- Recently, several studies found that a single course of prenatal steroids (betamethasone) may increase survival in hydropic fetuses with microcystic CCAMs to 75–100%. These studies indicate that large, macrocystic lesions may be treated prenatally without surgical intervention.
- Most series report a mortality rate of 25–30% of all children who present in the newborn period with CCAM; however, these figures do not include asymptomatic children who present later in life. Furthermore, the use of elective abortion may lead to an underestimation of perinatal mortality by preferentially terminating fetuses with a higher risk of mortality.
- The reported mortality rate of prenatally diagnosed CCAMs ranges from 9 to 49%.

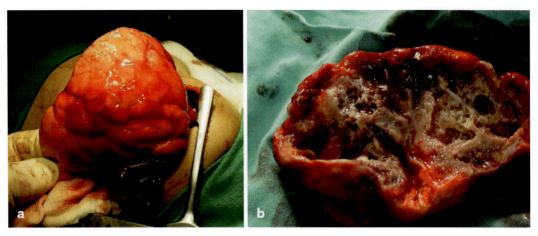

Fig. 51.12 Intraoperative photograph showing multiple cysts of varying sizes (type I CCAM) (**a**) and a clinical photograph showing a resected lobe of the lung affected by CCAM (**b**). Note the varying sizes of the cysts

- Risk factors for a poor outcome include:
  - Hydrops fetalis
  - Microcystic CCAM
  - Pulmonary hypoplasia
- The overall size of the lesion has also been reported as being an important predictor of survival, however, this index may be compromised by the fact that CCAM may decrease in size or even resolve over time in utero.
- The major morbidity is related to pulmonary compromise. A large lesion may be associated with pulmonary hypoplasia. This can cause respiratory distress at birth.
- Rarely, respiratory failure resulting from CCAM may be severe enough to require treatment with ECMO.
- Regardless of whether fetal surgery has been performed, delivery of the affected fetus in a tertiary level facility is essential to optimize outcome and minimize complications arising as a result of CCAM.
- It has been suggested that the presence of bilateral lesions is associated with a worse outcome.
- More controversially, left-sided lesions may be associated with a greater mortality rate than right-sided lesions.
- One study suggested that polyhydramnios is also associated with a poorer outcome.
- Potential for malignant transformation:
  - Mucinous bronchioloalveolar carcinoma
  - Rhabdomyosarcoma

These are recognized in all cases of CCAM. Whether or not complete resection of the affected area completely removes this risk is not known.

- Other complications that have been described in association with CCAM include:
  - Recurrent chest infection
  - Spontaneous pneumothorax
  - Hemopneumothorax
  - Hemoptysis

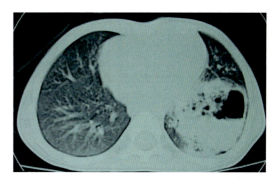

Fig. 51.13 CT scan of the chest showing CCAM complicated by infection. This may necessities resection of more segments of the lung

- Resection of CCAM in all children is recommended to remove the risk of direct complications, such as recurrent infection and pneumothorax. Add to this the risk of malignant potential of CCAM in later life.
- In one-third of cases, the presence of pneumonia may necessitate more extensive pulmonary resection (Fig. 51.13).

Recommended Reading

Adzick NS. Management of fetal lung lesions. Clin Perinatol. 2009;36(2):363–76.
Adzick NS, Harrison MR, Crombleholme TM, Flake AW, Howell LJ. Fetal lung lesions: management and outcome. Am J Obstet Gynecol. 1998;179:884–9.
Giubergia V, Barrenechea M, Siminovich M, Pena HG, Murtagh P. Congenital cystic adenomatoid malformation: clinical features, pathological concepts and management in 172 cases. J Pediatr (Rio J). 2012;88(2):143–8.
Sapin E, Lejeune V, Barbet JP, Carricaburu E, Lewin F, Baron JM, et al. Congenital adenomatoid disease of the lung: prenatal diagnosis and perinatal management. Pediatr Surg Int. 1997;12:126–9.
Stocker JT, Madewell JE, Drake RM. Congenital cystic adenomatoid malformation of the lung: classification and morphologic spectrum. Hum Pathol. 1977;8:155–71.

Chapter 52
Bronchogenic Cyst

Introduction

- Bronchogenic cysts are congenital lesions derived from the primitive foregut.
- They are part of a spectrum of congenital abnormalities of the lung, including pulmonary sequestration, congenital cystic adenomatoid malformation, and congenital lobar emphysema.
- The frequency of bronchogenic cysts is unknown, presumably because most patients are asymptomatic. The estimated prevalence ranges from one in 42,000 to one in 68,000.
- Bronchogenic cysts, while relatively rare, are the most common congenital intrathoracic cyst and account for 18 % of all primary mediastinal masses.
- Most bronchogenic cysts originate in the mediastinum, while 15–20 % occur in the lung parenchyma. The lower lobes are most commonly involved.
- The cysts are typically unilocular, a few centimeters in size, round or oval, and filled with serous or proteinaceous fluid and less commonly hemorrhagic secretions or air.
- Pathology:
  - The wall of bronchogenic cyst contains cartilage, smooth muscles, fibrous tissues, and sometimes seromucinous glands.
  - They are lined by respiratory epithelium.
  - On rare occasions they calcify (Fig. 52.1).

Embryology

- Bronchogenic cysts result from an abnormal budding of the tracheobronchial tree.
- During embryonic development, the primitive foregut arises in the third week of gestation and divides into dorsal portion, which elongates to form the esophagus and ventral portion, which differentiates into the tracheobronchial tree.
- Errors in the development of the ventral foregut will give rise to bronchogenic cysts.
- Lesions arising before or during the separation of the embryonic foregut are situated in the mediastinum (30 %; Fig. 52.2).
- Most of these cysts are located close to the trachea near the carina or main stem bronchi and often are attached by a stalk or share a common wall with one of the major airways. Rarely, there is communication of the cyst with the tracheobronchial tree (Fig. 52.2B).

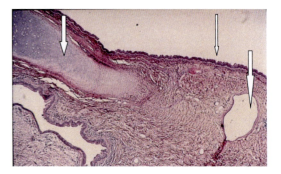

Fig. 52.1 Histological picture of excised bronchogenic cyst. Note the respiratory epithelial lining, seromucinous glands, and cartilage in the wall

- Lesions arising after separations are frequently situated within the lungs (70%). They are thought to result from abnormal airway branching secondary to defective epithelial/mesenchymal cell interaction during the fourth to seventh weeks of gestation (Fig. 52.3).
- These intrapulmonary bronchogenic cysts will often communicate with the bronchial tree and about two-thirds of them will be aerated (Fig. 52.4).
- Intraparenchymal cysts have been consistently reported to be lined by respiratory epithelium and cartilage.
- It is possible that accessory buds from the tracheobronchial tree/primitive foregut may get excluded from the thorax and migrates in an unusual manner to lie in abnormal locations.

Sites and Pathology of Bronchogenic Cysts

- Bronchogenic cysts are developmental abnormalities of the primitive foregut.
- They arise from an abnormal budding of the tracheobronchial anlage of the primitive foregut during the third to seventh weeks of development.
- When attachment to the primitive foregut persists, the cyst is usually associated with the tracheobronchial tree or the esophagus (mediastinal and intrapulmonary bronchogenic cysts).

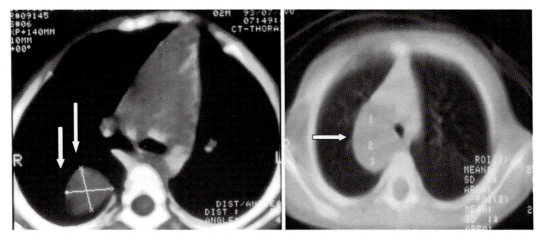

Fig. 52.2 CT scan of the chest showing an intrathoracic bronchogenic cyst and note its relation to the trachea in the second one

Fig. 52.3 CT scan of the chest showing an intrapulmonary bronchogenic cyst

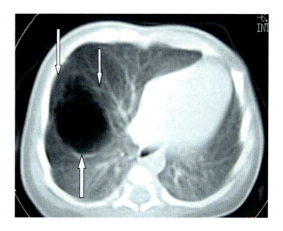

Fig. 52.4 Chest x-ray showing a bronchogenic cyst in the left upper lobe. Note that the cyst is aerated suggesting a communication to the tracheobronchial tree

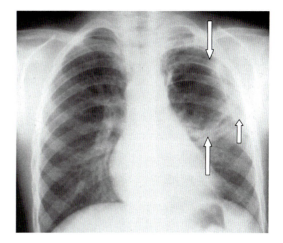

- If complete separation occurs, the cyst may occur in other unusual locations, presumably by migration. These unusual and remote sites include:
  - Inter-atrial septum.
  - Neck.
  - Esophageal wall.
  - Intrapericardial.
  - Abdomen.
  - Cutaneous and subcutaneous tissues.
  - Scapular region.
  - Retroperitoneal space.
  - Bronchogenic cysts have also been reported to extend from the mediastinum through the diaphragm into the abdomen as dumbbell cysts.
- Bronchogenic cysts are usually single but rarely may be multiple.
- They are lined by columnar ciliated epithelium, and their walls often contain cartilage, smooth muscles, fibrous tissue, and bronchial mucous glands. Occasionally, cysts may contain gastric mucosa (Fig. 52.5).
- It is unusual for them to have a patent connection with the airway, but when present, such a communication may promote infection of the cyst by allowing bacterial entry (Fig. 52.6).

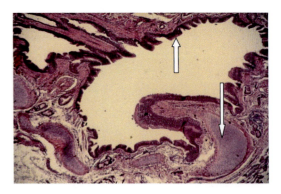

Fig. 52.5 Histological photograph the respiratory epithelial lining and cartilage in the wall

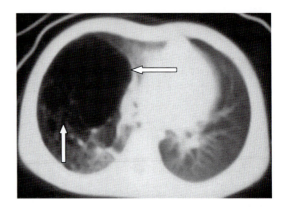

Fig. 52.6 CT scan of the chest showing intrapulmonary bronchogenic cyst. Note the aeration of the cyst suggesting tracheobronchial communication

- Malignant degeneration has been reported in these cysts on rare occasions. Both adenocarcinoma and *rhabdomyosarcoma* have been reported to arise in bronchogenic cysts.

Clinical Presentation

- No clinical presentation is specifically suggestive of bronchogenic cyst because these lesions are frequently asymptomatic.
- They are usually discovered incidentally on chest x-ray. This is specially so for mediastinal bronchogenic cysts.
- The intrapulmonary cysts may have communication with the airway and become infected and are therefore more often symptomatic.
- In infants, the initial presentation may be respiratory distress (Fig. 52.7).
- The diagnosis of bronchogenic cyst should be considered in patients with recurrent chest infections.
- Chest pain, cough, dyspnea, and dysphagia are possible clinical manifestations of bronchogenic cyst.
- These result from compression of the esophagus and/or major airways by the adjacent bronchogenic cyst.
- Bronchogenic cysts located within the abdomen may also produce symptoms because of infection or compression of adjacent structures and hemorrhage has been reported in cysts with ectopic gastric mucosa.

Investigations

Fig. 52.7 Chest x-ray showing a large bronchogenic cyst in an infant who presented with respiratory distress

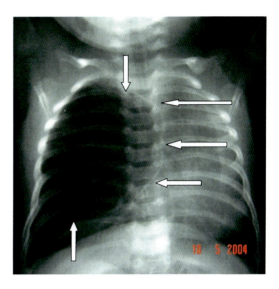

Fig. 52.8 Chest x-ray showing a bronchogenic cyst in the right side of the chest. Note the smooth and demarcated outline

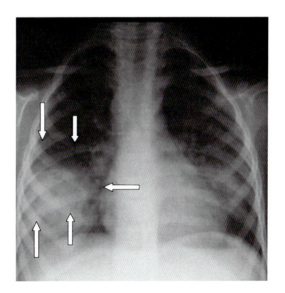

Investigations

- Bronchogenic cysts are prenatally identified in 70% of cases using ultrasonography.
- Bronchogenic cysts are usually an incidental finding and differentiating them from other pathologic conditions is important.
- Chest radiography:
    - This typically shows a sharply demarcated spherical mass of variable size.
    - Most commonly located in the middle mediastinum just in front of the trachea or main stem bronchi at the carinal level.
    - When the cyst communicates with the tracheobronchial tree, an air–fluid level may be seen within the cyst (Figs. 52.8 and 52.9).

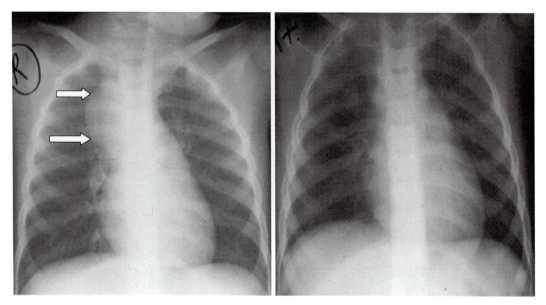

Fig. 52.9 Chest x-ray pre- and postoperative showing a bronchogenic cyst. Note its location close to the trachea

Fig. 52.10 CT scan of the chest showing a large bronchogenic cyst

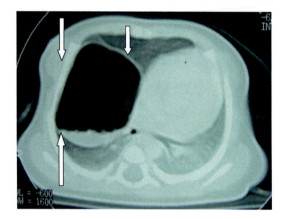

- When the cyst is infected or contains secretions, it may appear as a solid tumor or may demonstrate an air–fluid level.
- Esophagography: A barium swallow may be useful in assessing the degree of extrinsic compression of the esophagus.
- Chest computed tomography (CT) scan:
    - CT scan is useful in localizing bronchogenic cysts and their precise relationships to mediastinal structures.
    - Bronchogenic cysts appear as cysts with smooth borders and thin walls and may contain secretions, pus, air, or rarely blood.
    - Calcifications may also be observed (Fig. 52.10).
- Magnetic resonance imaging (MRI):
    - This usually shows a homogeneous cyst of moderate-to-bright intensity on T2-weighted MRI.
    - On T1-weighted images, bronchogenic cysts may vary in their intensity because of their protein content.

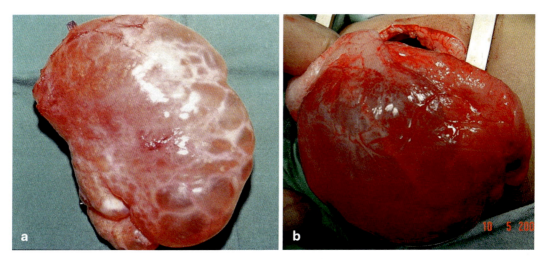

Fig. 52.11 A clinical photograph of a completely resected bronchogenic cyst and a clinical photograph of a patient with bronchogenic cyst being removed by a posterolateral thoracotomy

Fig. 52.12 A clinical photograph of a large bronchogenic cyst resected by a formal lobectomy

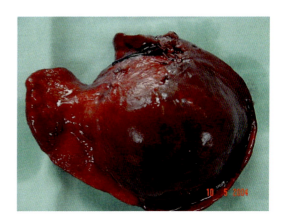

Treatment

- A definitive diagnosis of bronchogenic cysts is not always possible preoperatively.
- Surgical resection is the treatment of all suspected bronchogenic cysts.
- This is to obviate cyst-related complications such as infection, rupture, bleeding, compression, and malignant degeneration (adenocarcinoma and rhabdomyosarcoma).
- Treatment consists of complete surgical resection. This can be accomplished by a posterolateral thoracotomy, thoracoscopy, and at times a median sternotomy may be required (Fig. 52.11).
- In patients with intrapulmonary bronchogenic cysts, lobectomy may be necessary (Fig. 52.12).
- Palliative procedures such as mediastinal puncture and aspiration can be considered in symptomatic patients who are not fit to undergo complete resection.
- The prognosis after complete excision is excellent in all patients with bronchogenic cysts.

Recommended Reading

Díaz Nieto R, Naranjo Torres A, Gómez Alvarez M, Ruiz Rabelo JF, Pérez Manrique MC, Ciria Bru R, et al. Intraabdominal bronchogenic cyst. J Gastrointest Surg. 2010;14(4):756–8. [Epub 2009 May 28].

Gursoy S, Ucvet A, Ozturk AA, Erbaycu AE, Basok O, Yucel N. Seven years experience of bronchogenic cysts. Saudi Med J. 2009;30(2):238–42.

Kosar A, Tezel C, Orki A, Kiral H, Arman B. Bronchogenic cysts of the lung: report of 29 cases. Heart Lung Circ. 2009;18(3):214–8. [Epub 2008 Dec 31].

Chapter 53
Pulmonary Sequestration

Introduction

- A pulmonary sequestration (also known as a bronchopulmonary sequestration) is a rare congenital malformation characterized by:
  - A nonfunctioning mass of normal lung tissue.
  - That lacks normal communication with the tracheobronchial tree.
  - Receives its arterial blood supply from the systemic circulation.
- Pulmonary sequestration is estimated to comprise 0.15–6.4 % of all congenital pulmonary malformations.
- In general, the arterial supply of extralobar pulmonary sequestration comes from an aberrant vessel arising from the thoracic aorta. It usually drains via the systemic venous system to the right atrium, vena cava, or azygous systems.
- The arterial supply typically enters the lung via the pulmonary ligament if the artery originates above the diaphragm. Arteries originating below the diaphragm reach the sequestration by piercing the diaphragm or via the aortic or esophageal hiatus.
- The arterial supply is usually composed of a single vessel that is disproportionately large. This vessel is typically 0.5–2.0 cm in diameter, and multiple arteries are present in 15–20 % of cases in which the arteries are 3 mm or smaller (Fig. 53.1).
- Pulmonary sequestrations usually get their blood supply from the thoracic aorta.
- Intrapulmonary sequestration drains via pulmonary veins while extra pulmonary sequestration drains to the IVC.
- Intrapulmonary sequestrations are the most common form, and 60 % of these are found in the posterior basal segment of the left lower lobe.
- Overall, 98 % of pulmonary sequestrations occur in the lower lobes.
- The left lower lobe is the most common site.
- Bilateral involvement is uncommon.
- About 10 % of cases may be associated with other congenital anomalies.
- In the extrapulmonary sequestration, males are affected approximately four times more often than females.
- The incidence is equal in males and females in intrapulmonary sequestration.

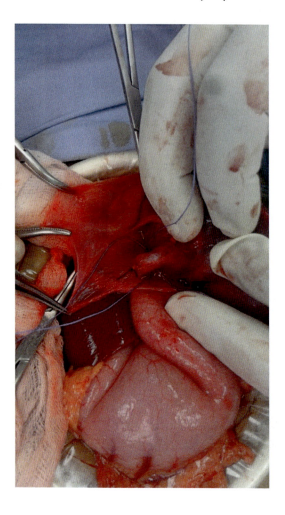

Fig. 53.1 Intraoperative photograph showing a large feeding vessel for extralobar pulmonary sequestration associated with a large para-esophageal hernia

Embryology

- The most commonly accepted theory of pulmonary sequestration formation is based on an accessory lung bud that develops from the ventral aspect of the primitive foregut.
- The pluripotential tissue from this additional lung bud migrates in a caudal direction with the normally developing lung.
- It receives its blood supply from vessels that connect to the aorta and cover the primitive foregut.
- These attachments to the aorta remain and subsequently form the systemic arterial supply of the sequestration.
- Early embryologic development of the accessory lung bud results in formation of the sequestration within normal lung tissue (intrapulmonary sequestration).
- The intrapulmonary sequestration is encased within the same pleural covering.
- In contrast, later development of the accessory lung bud results in the development of extrapulmonary sequestration that may give rise to communication with the gastrointestinal tract.
- The extrapulmonary sequestration is encased with its own pleura.
- Both types of sequestration usually have arterial supply from the thoracic or abdominal aorta.
- Rarely, the celiac axis, internal mammary, subclavian, or renal artery may be involved.
- Intrapulmonary sequestration occurs within the visceral pleura of normal lung tissue and usually has no communication with the tracheobronchial tree.

- The most common location of intrapulmonary sequestration is in the posterior basal segment, and nearly two-thirds of pulmonary sequestrations appear in the left lung.
- Venous drainage for intrapulmonary sequestration is usually via the pulmonary veins, foregut communication is very rare, and associated anomalies are uncommon.
- Extrapulmonary sequestration is completely enclosed in its own pleural sac.
- Extrapulmonary sequestration may occur above, within, or below the diaphragm, and nearly all appear on the left side.
- No communication with the tracheobronchial tree occurs in extrapulmonary sequestration.
- Venous drainage for extrapulmonary sequestration is usually via the systemic venous system and foregut communication and associated anomalies, such as diaphragmatic hernia, are more common.

Classification

Sequestrations are classified anatomically into two types.

Intralobar Sequestration

- Intralobar sequestration is located within a normal lobe and lacks its own visceral pleura as it lies within the same visceral pleura as the lobe in which it occurs.
- The arterial supply is derived from the descending thoracic aorta (75%), upper abdominal aorta or celiac axis (21%), or the intercostal arteries (4%).
- The venous drainage is usually to the left atrium via pulmonary veins (95%) or via the inferior vena cava, superior vena cava, or azygous vein (5%).
- Intralobar sequestration accounts for 75% of all sequestrations.
- Males and females are equally affected.
- Intralobar sequestration is usually located in the paravertebral region in the posterior segment of the left lower lobe.
- Intralobar sequestration is rarely associated with other developmental abnormalities.
- Patients with Intralobar sequestration usually present late in adolescence or adulthood with recurrent chest infection.

Extralobar Sequestration (Figs. 53.2 and 53.3):

- Extralobar sequestration is located outside the normal lung and has its own visceral pleura.
- Extralobar sequestration accounts for 25% of all sequestrations.
- Extralobar sequestration develops as an accessory lung contained within its own pleura.
- Extralobar sequestration is more common in males (80%).
- It is commonly related to the left hemidiaphragm in 80–90% of cases.
- Of the sequestrations, 80% lie between the lower lobe and the diaphragm. Lesions are usually located in the region of the posterior basal segments of the lower lobes. Left-sided lesions are more common than right-sided lesions.
- The mass may be closely associated with the esophagus, and fistulae may develop.
- It may present as a subdiaphragmatic or retroperitoneal mass (10%).

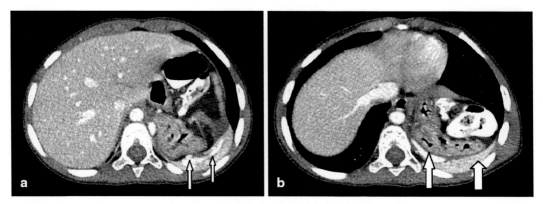

Fig. 53.2 a and **b** CT scan showing pulmonary sequestration involving the left lower lobe associated with a large paraesophageal hernia and CT scan showing pulmonary sequestration (*thick arrow*) associated with a large paraesophageal hernia. Note the large blood vessel supplying the sequestration (*thin arrows*)

- The arterial supply of extralobar sequestration is from an aberrant vessel arising from the thoracic aorta or abdominal aorta (80%). In rare cases, the arterial supply may be from anomalous vessels arising from the splenic, gastric, subclavian, and intercostal vessels (20%).
- It usually drains via the systemic venous system to the right atrium, commonly the inferior vena cava, or azygous systems (75%) and rarely via the pulmonary veins (25%).
- It is more common in males (4:1).
- Congenital anomalies occur more frequently in patients with extralobar sequestration (65%).
- Associated congenital anomalies include:
  - Congenital cystic adenomatoid malformation (CCAM)
  - Congenital diaphragmatic hernia
  - Vertebral anomalies
  - An accessory spleen
  - Congenital heart disease
  - Pulmonary hypoplasia
  - Colonic duplication
- Extralobar sequestration is enveloped in its own pleural and rarely gets infected.
- The usual presentation is in infancy with respiratory distress or as a homogeneous soft tissue mass.

Diagnosis

Ultrasonography

- Ultrasonography is useful in the prenatal diagnosis of pulmonary sequestration.
- The typical sonographic appearance of pulmonary sequestration is an echogenic homogeneous mass that may be well defined or irregular.
- Some lesions have a cystic or more complex appearance.
- Doppler studies are helpful to identify aberrant systemic artery that arises from the aorta and to delineate venous drainage.

Fig. 53.3 Intraoperative photograph showing extralobar pulmonary sequestration

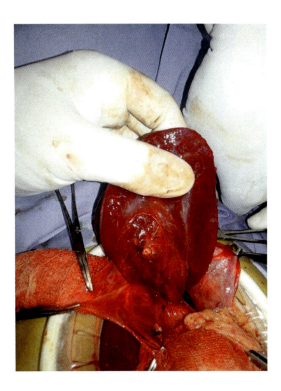

- Detection by color flow Doppler of a systemic artery from the aorta to the fetal lung lesion is a pathognomonic feature of pulmonary sequestration.

Chest Radiography

- It is difficult to distinguish an intrapulmonary sequestration from extrapulmonary sequestration on plain chest x-ray.
- Intrapulmonary sequestrations appear as a heterogeneous and ill-defined mass.
- Extrapulmonary sequestrations appear as solid, well-defined, and retrocardiac mass.
- A mass in the posterobasal segment of the lung in a young patient with recurrent, localized pulmonary infections is suggestive of intralobar pulmonary sequestration. Such a lesion usually resolves incompletely with appropriate medical treatment.
- Extralobar pulmonary sequestrations are more often solid and are associated with elevation of the ipsilateral diaphragm.
- Intralobar pulmonary sequestration appears more cystic and may show air if a pulmonary communication exists.

Chest Computed Tomography

- Computed tomography (CT) scans have 90 % accuracy in diagnosing pulmonary sequestration.
- The diagnosis of an intralobar pulmonary sequestration can be confirmed by enhanced contrast helical CT scanning with three-dimensional reconstruction.

- Volumetric slip-ring scanning (either spiral or multisection) can define the vascular supply and venous drainage of intralobar and extralobar sequestrations with a much higher degree of certainty.

Arteriography

- An arteriogram has been considered essential in documenting the systemic blood supply of pulmonary sequestration, allowing definitive diagnosis as well as preoperative planning.
- Diagnosis with arteriography is based on the demonstration of systemic arterial blood supply to the lung sequestration, but arteriography is invasive, and its findings are nonspecific.
- Arteriography is helpful in differentiating pulmonary sequestration from other abnormalities of the lung, such as pulmonary arteriovenous fistulae, but the CT scans should be correlated with clinical presentation and chest radiographs.
- Demonstration of a systemic artery supplying lung tissue is not pathognomonic of sequestration, because a congenital, anomalous, systemic arterial supply to normal segments of the lung is rare but well known.
- The definitive diagnosis is made by using angiography (conventional, CT angiography, or magnetic resonance angiography, MRA), which delineates the feeding vessel to the sequestration along with its venous system.

Magnetic Resonance Imaging

- Magnetic resonance imaging (MRI) and MRA can provide information similar to that of CT scans without the need for ionizing radiation.
- The most common appearance is a solid mass that may be homogeneous or heterogeneous, sometimes with cystic changes.
- MRI is less accessible, takes longer time to perform, is subject to motion artifacts, and requires sedation in infants and small children.

Treatment

- Surgical resection is the treatment of choice for patients with sequestration whether symptomatic or not.
- Surgical resection is the treatment of choice for patients who present with infection or symptoms resulting from compression of normal lung tissue.
- Management of an asymptomatic pulmonary sequestration with no connection to the surrounding lung is controversial; however, most surgeons advocate resection of these lesions because of the likelihood of recurrent lung infection, the need for larger resection if the sequestration becomes chronically infected, and the possibility of hemorrhage from arteriovenous anastomoses.
- The treatment of pulmonary sequestration is a segmentectomy via a thoracotomy or thoracoscopy.
- Extrapulmonary sequestration can usually be excised without loss of normal lung tissue.
- Intrapulmonary sequestrations often require lobectomy because the margins of the sequestration may not be clearly defined.
- Complete thoracoscopic resection of pulmonary lobes in infants and children with sequestration has been described with low mortality and morbidity.

Recommended Reading

Boubnova J, Peycelon M, Garbi O, David M, Bonnard A, De Lagausie P. Thoracoscopy in the management of congenital lung diseases in infancy. Surg Endosc. 2011;25(2):593–6.

Wei Y, Li F. Pulmonary sequestration: a retrospective analysis of 2625 cases in China. Eur J Cardiothorac Surg. 2011;40(1):e39–42.

Chapter 54
Anorectal Malformations

Introduction

- Anorectal malformations occur in approximately 1 per 4000–5000 live births.
- Anorectal malformations affect boys and girls with similar frequency. However, imperforate anus will present as the low type 90% of the time in females and 50% of the time in males.
- Additional congenital defects are frequently associated with anorectal malformations, ranging from 40 to 70%, with the urinary tract being the most commonly involved.
- Although the etiology remains unknown, a slight genetic predisposition appears to exist.
- Anorectal malformations comprise a wide spectrum of anomalies that affect boys and girls and can involve malformations of the distal anus and rectum as well as the urinary and genital tracts.
- Malformations range from minor, easily treated defects that carry an excellent functional prognosis to complex defects that are difficult to treat, are often associated with other anomalies, and carry a poor functional prognosis.

Associated Anomalies

- The more severe the anorectal malformation, the more likely the presence of associated abnormalities.
- Genitourinary defects:
  - Approximately 30–50% of all patients with anorectal malformations have an associated urogenital anomaly. The frequency of this varies with the type of anorectal defect as follows:
    - Persistent cloaca: 90%
    - Recto-bladder neck fistula: 84%
    - Rectoprostatic urethral fistula: 63%
    - Rectovestibular fistula: 47%
    - Rectobulbar urethral fistula: 46%
    - Rectoperineal fistula: 26%
    - Imperforate anus without fistula: 31%
  - Urinary anomalies include:
    - Renal agenesis
    - Vesicoureteral reflux
    - Neurogenic bladder
    - Renal dysplasia

- Megaureter
- Hydronephrosis
- Ectopic ureter
— Gynecological malformations are particularly important in cloaca malformation. About 35% of newborns with cloacae have hydrocolpos and 50% have duplicated Müllerian structures.

- Tethered cord:
  - A tethered spinal cord refers to the intravertebral fixation of the phylum terminale.
  - Approximately 25% of patients with anorectal malformation have a tethered spinal cord.
  - The prevalence of this anomaly increases with increasing height and complexity of the anorectal anomaly.
  - Patients with a hypodeveloped sacrum and associated urologic problems are more likely to have a tethered cord.
  - A tethered cord may cause motor and sensory disturbances of the lower extremities.
  - Patients with anorectal malformations and tethered cord have a poorer prognosis for bowel and urinary function.

- Sacral and spinal defects (30%):
  - The sacrum is the most commonly affected bony structure.
  - Currently, calculating the sacral ratio is more important than the number of sacral vertebrae.
  - About 25% of those with high anomalies and 10% of those with low anomalies have sacral defects.
  - Assessment of sacral hypodevelopment (sacral ratio) correlates with the patient's functional prognosis. Normal sacra have a calculated sacral ratio >0.7.
  - Hemisacrum is almost always associated with a presacral mass (teratomas or anterior meningoceles).
  - Hemivertebrae may also affect the lumbar and thoracic spine.
  - Patients may have spinal anomalies other than tethered cord, such as syringomyelia and myelomeningocele.

- Chromosomal abnormalities: particularly Down's syndrome.
- Gastrointestinal abnormalities include:
  - Tracheoesophageal abnormality (10%)
  - Duodenal atresia (1–2%)
  - Malrotation
  - Hirschsprung's disease (0.2%)
  - Vertebral, anorectal, cardiac, tracheoesophageal, renal and radial agenesis, and limb (VACTERL) association

- Cardiovascular anomalies: 12–22% of anorectal malformations have cardiac anomalies particularly tetralogy of Fallot and ventricular septal defect (VSD)

Clinical Features

- Patients with anorectal malformations are usually discovered because there is no anal opening or the anal opening is abnormal.

Investigations 403

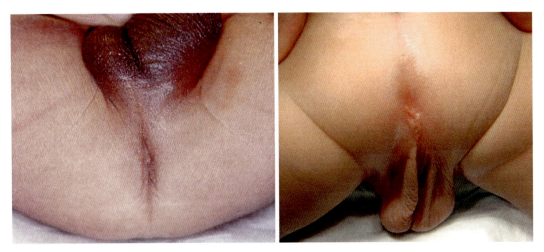

Fig. 54.1 Clinical photograph of two patients with high anorectal malformations. Note the flat perineum and absence of fistula

- Clinical inspection of the buttocks is important. A flat bottom or flat perineum, as evidenced by the lack of a midline fold and the absence of an anal dimple, indicates that the patient has poor muscles in the perineum. These findings are associated with a high anorectal malformation (Fig. 54.1).
- Perineal signs found in patients with low malformations include (Figs. 54.2 and 54.3):
  - The presence of meconium at the perineum
  - A bucket-handle malformation (a prominent skin tag located at the anal dimple, below which an instrument can be passed)
  - An anal membrane (through which meconium is visible)
- The presence of a single perineal orifice in a patient is clinical evidence of a persistent cloaca.
- In 80–90 % of newborn boys, clinical evaluation and urinalysis provide enough information for the surgeon to decide whether a colostomy is required.
- Meconium is not usually observed at the perineum in a newborn with rectoperineal fistula until at least 16–24 h of life.
- Abdominal distension does not develop during the first few hours of life but is required to force meconium through a rectoperineal fistula, as well as through a urinary fistula (Fig. 54.4).
- It is also important to note whether there is meconium in the urine.

Investigations

- Imaging studies performed in the newborn period include the following:
  - Abdominal ultrasonography to evaluate urologic anomalies.
  - Plain radiography of the spine may reveal spinal anomalies, such as spina bifida and spinal hemivertebrae.
  - Plain radiography of the sacrum in the anterior-posterior and lateral projections may demonstrate sacral anomalies, such as a hemisacrum and sacral hemivertebrae. In addition, the degree

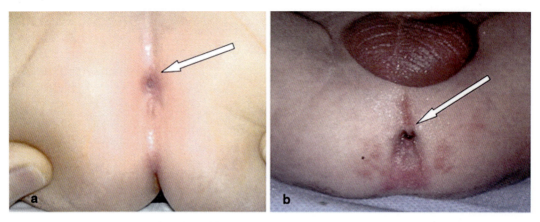

Fig. 54.2 A clinical photograph of a patient with low anorectal agenesis. Note the perineal fistula (**a**) and the meconium passing through a perineal fistula (**b**)

Fig. 54.3 A clinical photograph showing the bucket-handle deformity

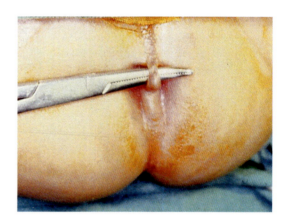

Fig. 54.4 A clinical photograph showing abdominal distension in a newborn with high anorectal agenesis

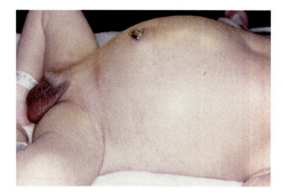

of sacral hypodevelopment may be assessed and a sacral ratio can be calculated (the distance from the coccyx to the sacroiliac joint divided by the distance from the sacroiliac joint to the top of the pelvis; Fig. 54.5).
- Spinal ultrasonography in the newborn to find evidence of a tethered spinal cord and other spinal anomalies.

Investigations

Fig. 54.5 Diagrammatic representation of calculating the sacral ratio

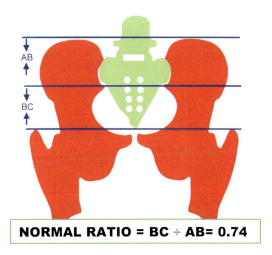

Fig. 54.6 A lateral radiograph of a patient with anorectal agenesis. Note the air column in the distal rectum

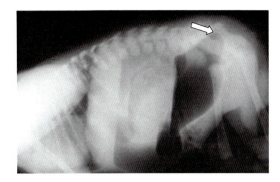

Fig. 54.7 A lateral radiograph showing the air column in the distal rectum. Note the distance between the distal air and site of the marked anus

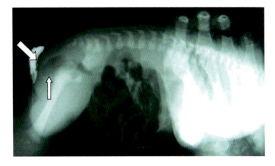

- Cross-table lateral radiography may help demonstrate the air column in the distal rectum (Fig. 54.6).
- Obtain cross-table lateral radiographs with the newborn prone, with the pelvis elevated, and with a radiopaque marker placed on the perineum. This is done 16–24 h post delivery.
  - Rarely, radiography reveals the column of air in the distal rectum to be within 1 cm of the perineum; in these instances, treatment is similar to that for rectoperineal fistula and a newborn perineal operation may be performed.
  - If the air column is more than 1 cm from the perineum, a colostomy is indicated (Fig. 54.7).

Table 54.1 Classification of anorectal malformations

Sex	Male	Female
Type of anomaly	Rectoperineal fistula	Rectoperineal fistula
	Rectourethral fistula	Rectovestibular fistula
	Rectobulbar fistula	
	Rectoprostatic fistula	
	Rectovesical fistula (bladder neck)	Persistent cloaca
		<3 cm common channel
		>3 cm common channel
	Imperforate anus without fistula	Imperforate anus without fistula
	Rectal atresia	Rectal atresia
	Complex defects	Complex defects

Classification

- The traditional classification of anorectal malformations divides them into:
  - High
  - Intermediate
  - Low
- This was based on the relation of the terminal end of the bowel remaining above (high), within (intermediate), or below the levator ani muscle (pelvic floor) which is the main muscle of continence.
- Invertogram in a dead lateral position with the hips slightly flexed gives accurate information regarding the nature of the anomaly.
- The radiological landmarks used for this purpose are the pubococcygeal line (PC line; a line between the pubis and the coccyx) and the I point (tip of the ischium) to which the air shadow of the terminal end of the bowel is correlated. The measurements used are:
  - If the air shadow crosses the (I) point, it is a low anomaly.
  - If it crosses the PC line but stops short of the (I) point, it is an intermediate anomaly.
  - If the air shadow of the terminal end of the bowel stops above the PC line, it is a high anomaly.
  - This was replaced by a simpler measurement depending on the distance between the end of the gas shadow in the terminal end of the colon and the mark placed at the site of the future anal opening. In high defects, the distance is more than 1 cm while in low defects the distance is less than 1 cm.
- Subsequently, anorectal malformations were classified anatomically as shown in Table 54.1.
- In boys, 85% have a rectourinary fistula and 35% have a rectoperineal fistula, while 93% of girls have an external fistula (Figs. 54.8 and 54.9).
- The most common defect in females is rectovestibular fistula (Fig. 54.10).
- Table 54.1 lists the classifications of anorectal malformations. Figures 54.11, 54.12, 54.13, 54.14, 54.15, 54.16, 54.17, and 54.18 illustrate these malformations.
- Most high anomalies in girls are cloacae; a high anomaly with a rectovaginal fistula is exceedingly rare.

Treatment

- The surgeon's primary concern in correcting these anomalies is bowel control. Problems with urinary control and sexual function must also be considered.

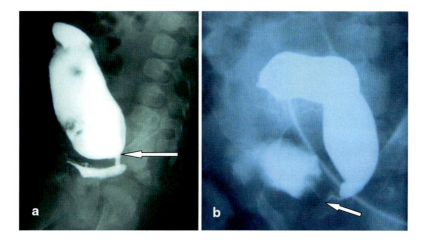

Fig. 54.8 a and **b**, A loopogram showing a rectovesical fistula in two patients with high anorectal fistula

- Early diagnosis, treatment of associated anomalies, and efficient and meticulous surgical repair provide the best chance for a good functional outcome.
- Some patients experience fecal and occasional urinary incontinence despite excellent anatomic repair.
- Associated anomalies such as a poorly developed sacrum and tethered cord and/or myelomeningocele contribute to an inability to achieve continence.
- For patients with fecal incontinence, an effective bowel management program was designed to improve quality of life.

Diagnosis and Early Treatment

- During the first 24–48 h of life in a newborn with an anorectal malformation, the following two questions should be answered:
  - Does the newborn have any associated anomalies that need to be treated?
  - Should the neonate undergo a primary definitive procedure without a protective colostomy or should he or she undergo a protective colostomy with definitive repair at a later date?
- During the first 24 h of life, the newborn should receive intravenous fluids, antibiotics, and be evaluated for associated anomalies that may represent a risk to the baby's life, mainly cardiac malformations, esophageal atresia, and urologic defects.
- A nasogastric or orogastric tube should be passed to protect the baby from aspiration.
- If the baby has signs of a perineal fistula, an anoplasty can be performed without a protective colostomy. This can be done during the first 48 h of life or delayed depending on the baby's condition (Figs. 54.19 and 54.20).
- If, after 24 h, there is no meconium on the perineum, a cross-table lateral x-ray with the baby in prone position is done. If air in the rectum is seen located below the coccyx, less than 1 cm from the skin, and the baby is in good condition with no significant associated defects, consider performing local exploration without a protective colostomy (Fig. 54.21).
- Conversely, if the rectal gas does not extend beyond the coccyx, the distance between the gas and skin is more than 1 cm, the patient has meconium in the urine, an abnormal sacrum, or a flat bottom, a colostomy is made.
- This allows for a future distal colostogram which will precisely delineate the anatomy. A posterior sagittal anorectoplasty is performed within the first few months of life (Fig. 54.22).

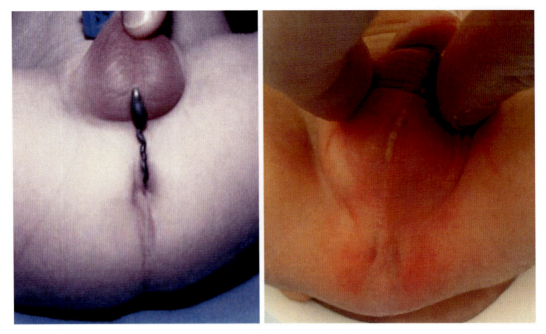

Fig. 54.9 Clinical photographs showing rectoperineal fistula in males. Note the meconium passing subcutaneously to the scrotum

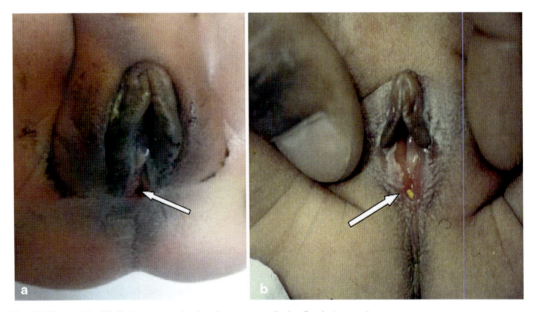

Fig. 54.10 a and **b**, Clinical photographs showing rectovestibular fistula (arrows)

- The indications for colostomy compared with anoplasty based on the sex of the newborn are as follows:
  - Male newborns:
    - Rectoperineal fistula: anoplasty
    - Rectobulbar urethral fistula, rectoprostatic urethral fistula, recto-bladder neck fistula, imperforated anus without fistula, and rectal atresia: colostomy
  - Female newborns:
    - Rectoperineal fistula and rectovestibular fistula: anoplasty.
    - Imperforated anus without fistula, persistent cloaca, rectal atresia, and rectovaginal fistula: colostomy.
    - For rectovestibular fistula, some surgeons will perform a colostomy followed by minimal posterior sagittal anorectoplasty or dilatation of the fistula followed by minimal posterior sagittal anorectoplasty.

Colostomy in anorectal malformations:

- A descending colon colostomy with separated stomas (double-barrel colostomy) is recommended (Fig. 54.23). The advantages of this type of colostomy include the following:
  - Only a small portion of distal colon is defunctionalized, but with an adequate amount of rectosigmoid for the future pull-through. This leaves a longer segment of the colon for water absorption and so at the end the stools are well formed. This also reduces skin excoriations.
  - Washing and cleaning the portion of the colon distal to the colostomy is relatively easy.
  - Distal colostography is easy to perform.
  - The separated stomas prevent spillage of stool from the proximal to distal bowel. This avoids stool impaction distally and avoids urinary tract infections in the presence of a fistula between the rectum and urinary system.
  - Prolapse is uncommon with a sigmoid colostomy.
- When performing a colostomy in the newborn, the distal bowel should be irrigated to remove all the meconium. This prevents formation of dried meconium distally which may be difficult to clean subsequently and also avoid a megasigmoid, which may lead to constipation after the colostomy ultimately gets closed.
- Colostomy errors include the following:
  - Too-distal sigmoidostomy: The colostomy is placed too distal and interferes with the subsequent pull-through procedure.
  - Right upper quadrant sigmoidostomy: Instances of inadvertent sigmoid colostomy placed in the right upper quadrant during an attempt to perform a transverse colostomy which interferes with the subsequent pull-through procedure.
  - Incomplete diversion of stool: A loop colostomy does not divert the stool completely and allows for distal stool impaction and urinary tract infections.
  - Megarectum: Transverse colon colostomies may produce megarectum due to passage and accumulation of mucous distally.

Definitive repair:

- Performing the definitive repair within the first 6 months of life has important advantages including:
  - Less time with an abdominal stoma.
  - Less size discrepancy between proximal and distal bowel at the time of colostomy closure.
  - Easier anal dilations.
  - Placing the rectum in the right location early in life may represent an advantage in terms of the potential for acquired local sensation.

Fig. 54.11 A clinical photograph of a male child with low anorectal malformation and rectoperineal fistula. Note the good anal dimple and the meconium passing from the fistula subcutaneously to the base of scrotum

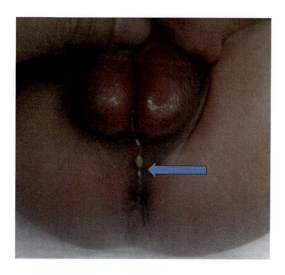

Fig. 54.12 Diagrammatic representation of a male with rectoperineal fistula

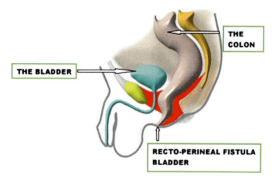

Fig. 54.13 Diagrammatic representation of a female with rectoperineal fistula

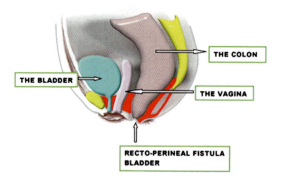

Fig. 54.14 Diagramatic representation of a female with rectovestibular fistula

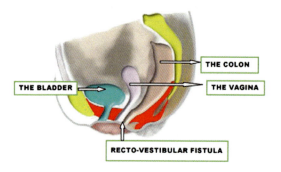

Diagnosis and Early Treatment

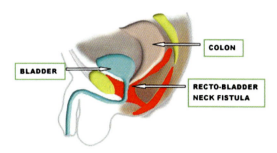
Fig. 54.15 Diagrammatic representation of a male with recto-bladder neck fistula

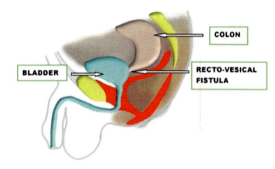
Fig. 54.16 Diagrammatic representation of a male with rectovesical fistula

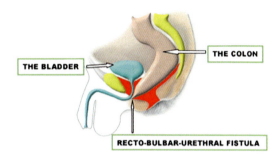
Fig. 54.17 Diagramatic representation of a male with rectobulbar urethral fistula

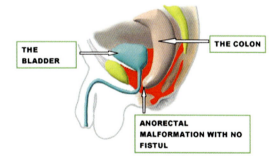
Fig. 54.18 Diagrammatic representation of an anorectal malformation without fistula

- Once the patient recovers from colostomy and demonstrates good growth and development, the definitive operation can be planned for 4–12 weeks later.
- Definitive repair involves a posterior sagittal approach. The most delicate part of this operation in females is the separation of the rectum and vagina, which share a common wall.
- A distal colostogram showing the terminal end of the bowel extending below the second sacral vertebra indicates that posterior sagittal anorectoplasty can be performed (Fig. 54.24).

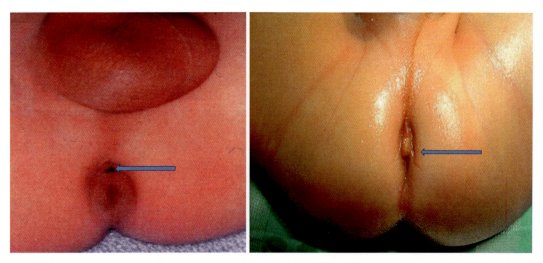

Fig. 54.19 Clinical photograph of two patients with low anorectal malformations. Note the rectoperineal fistula in the first one and well-formed anal dimple with a bulge in the second one

Fig. 54.20 A clinical photograph showing an anoplasty for a low anorectal malformation

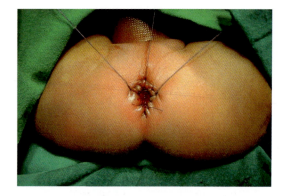

Fig. 54.21 A lateral x-ray showing the air column in the terminal part of the rectum. Note its relation to the coccyx

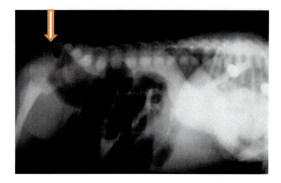

- Alternatively, in higher lesions one can combine the abdominal and the posterior sagittal approaches.
- Exposure through the posterior sagittal approach enables the accurate placement of the bowel through the levator ani and the striated muscle complex leading to better chances of continence.
- Besides this, the delineation and closure of a fistula is greatly facilitated.

Fig. 54.22 A distal loopogram in a patient with high anorectal agenesis. Note the distance between the terminal part of the rectum and the site of the normal anal opening which is more than 1 cm

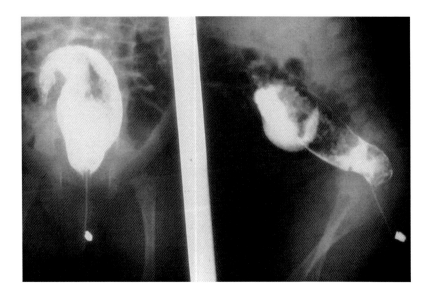

- Anorectal abnormalities in 90% of newborn boys may be repaired solely with a posterior sagittal approach, whereas 10% require an additional abdominal component (with laparotomy or laparoscopy) to mobilize a very high rectum.
- Perineal fistulas are repaired with a minimal posterior sagittal incision that is large enough to divide the external sphincter and to mobilize the anus back to the center of the sphincter complex. The sphincter mechanism is always located posterior to the fistula site. This operation may be performed in the neonatal period without a protective colostomy.
- An electrical stimulator helps reveal the location of the sphincteric mechanism (Fig. 54.25).
- In 10% of newborn boys with this defect, the rectum enters the urinary tract at the bladder neck level. The repair of this malformation involves a posterior sagittal incision and an abdominal component (via laparoscopy or laparotomy). The distal rectum is separated from the urinary tract, mobilized, and pulled through to lie within the sphincteric muscles.
- In patients with rectovestibular fistula, the rectum and posterior vagina share a common wall; this separation is the most difficult part of the operation.
- Rectal atresia:
  - A rare malformation, rectal atresia, occurs in 1% of patients.
  - The anal canal is normal, and, externally, the anus appears typical.
  - However, a blockage exists 1–2 cm from the anal skin.
  - These babies should undergo colostomy at birth; definitive repair involves a posterior sagittal approach and an anastomosis between the posterior rectum and the anal canal.
- At 2 weeks post surgery, anal calibration is performed, followed by a program of anal dilatations. The anus must be dilated twice daily and the size of the dilator is increased every week. The final size to be reached depends on the patient's age.
- Once the desired size is reached, the colostomy may be closed.
- Dilatations are continued afterward according to a protocol.
- Dilatations are a vital part of postoperative treatment to avoid an anoplasty stricture.

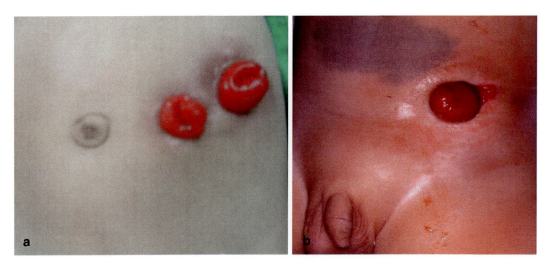

Fig. 54.23 Clinical photographs showing an ideal double barrel sigmoid colostomy (**a**) and a loop sigmoid colostomy (**b**)

Fig. 54.24 A distal loopogram in a patient with high anorectal agenesis. Note the mark at the anal opening site and contrast at the end of the rectum. The distance between the two is more than 1 cm denoting a high type of anomaly

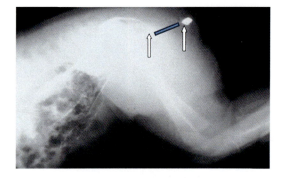

Fig. 54.25 Clinical photograph showing a muscle stimulator

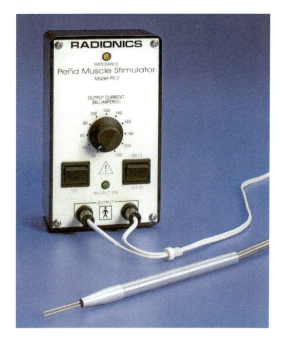

Postoperative Functional Disorders

- Constipation is the most common problem encountered after treatment for imperforated anus. This appears to be a hypomotility disorder secondary to chronic bowel dilatation.
- Failure to avoid constipation may result in megarectum and megasigmoid and can lead to fecal impaction and overflow incontinence.
- Those with the most benign defects (i.e., the least amount of perirectal dissection) experienced the worst constipation.
- Occasionally, constipation becomes so severe that patients develop chronic fecal impaction and constant soiling. Once the constipation is treated, the patient regains continence.
- When constipation is severe and the patient has a megasigmoid and the patient is fecally continent, resection of the sigmoid has been found to dramatically reduce the patient's laxative requirements.
- Complications of surgery include dehiscence and infection, which may be avoided with colostomy before the main repair. These complications may compromise the chance of achieving normal bowel function.

Prognosis

- Apart from the anorectal anomaly, the status of the sacrum, spine, and muscles greatly affects a patient's fecal continence. Even with a perfect reconstruction, a patient with a poor sacrum or spine may not achieve bowel control.
- The sacrum is a good predictor of outcome. Patients with a normal sacrum are much more likely to have fecal continence. Patients with a hypodeveloped sacrum are much more likely to be incontinent. A sacral ratio has been developed to allow for a more objective assessment of the sacrum. Patients with a sacral ratio < 0.3 only rarely achieve continence. A hypodeveloped sacrum is also a good predictor of associated spinal problems, such as tethered cord.
- Approximately 75% of all patients with anorectal malformations have voluntary bowel movements.
- Approximately 50% have occasional soiling.
- Episodes of soiling are usually related to constipation; when constipation is treated properly, the soiling usually disappears.
- Approximately 40% of all patients have voluntary bowel movements and no soiling.
- About 25% of patients with anorectal malformations have fecal incontinence and must have a bowel-management program with a daily enema to keep them clean.
- Bowel control must be evaluated when the child is older than 3 years.
- Patients with low defects (e.g., rectoperineal fistula, rectal atresia) have excellent outcomes.
- Girls with rectovestibular fistulas have very good outcomes, except for a tendency to develop constipation.
- Approximately 60% of boys with rectourethral fistulae and normal sacra have good outcomes.
- Patients with very high malformations (e.g., recto-bladder neck fistula in boys) have poor outcomes.
- If a given defect carries a good prognosis, such as rectovestibular fistula, rectoperineal fistula, rectal atresia, rectourethral bulbar fistula, or imperforate anus without fistula, expect the child to have voluntary bowel movements by age 3 years. Such children require supervision to avoid fecal impaction, constipation, and soiling.
- Certain defects indicate a poor prognosis, such as a high cloaca (common channel >3 cm) or a recto-bladder neck fistula.

- Patients with rectoprostatic fistulas carry an almost equal chance of voluntary bowel movements or incontinence. Toilet training should be attempted at age 3 years and if unsuccessful, a bowel-management program should be initiated. Each year, during vacation, bowel control should be attempted and if unsuccessful, the bowel management should be restarted. As the child grows older and more cooperative, the likelihood of achieving bowel control improves.
- Once it is determined that a daily enema is needed, those can be given antegrade via a Malone appendicostomy.
- Urinary incontinence occurs in boys with anorectal malformations only when they have an extremely defective or absent sacrum, an abnormal spine, or when the basic principles of surgical repair are not followed and important nerves are damaged during the operation.

Recommended Reading

Hedlund H, Peña A, Rodriguez G, Maza J. Long-term anorectal function in imperforate anus, treated by a posterior sagittal anorectoplasty: manometric investigation. J Pediatr Surg. 1992;27:906–9.

Peña A. Results in the management of 322 cases of anorectal malformations. Pediatr Surg Int. 1988;3:94–104.

Peña A. Surgical management of anorectal malformations: a unified concept. Pediatr Surg Int. 1988;3:82–93.

Peña A. Surgical treatment of high imperforate anus. World J Surg. 1985;9:236–45.

Peña A, deVries PA. Posterior sagittal anorectoplasty: important technical considerations and new applications. J Pediatr Surg. 1982;17:796–811.

Chapter 55
Cloacal Anomalies

Introduction

- Cloacal malformation is a very rare abnormality found in 1 of every 40,000–50,000 newborn females.
- Persistent cloacae occur exclusively in girls and are the most complex and technically challenging defects in the spectrum of anorectal malformations.
- Cloacae represent a spectrum of defects, but the common denominator is the presence of a single perineal orifice and the rectum, vagina, and urethra open into a single common channel (Figs. 55.1 and 55.2).
- The length of the common channel varies from 1 to 10 cm, with an average of approximately 3 cm (Fig. 55.3).
- It is important to correctly diagnose persistent cloaca in the neonatal period because 90 % of babies with this malformation have an associated urologic problem, and 40 % have hydrocolpos.
- About 30 % of these patients have a hydrocolpos. The hydrocolpos may produce two important complications:
  - It may compress the trigone of the bladder, producing ureterovesical obstruction, megaureter, and hydronephrosis.
  - The hydrocolpos if left undrained may become infected, leading to a pyocolpos.
- Approximately 40 % of these patients have a double Mullerian system consisting of two hemiuteri and two hemivaginas. This septation disorder may be partial or total and symmetric or asymmetric.
- The urinary tract and the distended vagina may both need to be managed within the newborn period to avoid serious complications.
- The goals of treatment include:
  - Early diagnosis
  - Immediate neonatal management
  - An anatomic reconstruction to achieve bowel and urinary control, as well as normal sexual function

Clinical Features

- Persistent cloaca is a clinical diagnosis.
- The presence of a single perineal orifice provides clinical evidence of persistent cloaca (Fig. 55.4).
- The external genitalia often appear small.

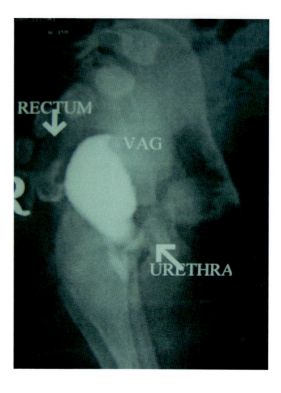

Fig. 55.1 Contrast study showing a classic cloaca where the rectum, vagina, and urethra join together and open in a single perineal opening

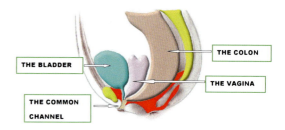

Fig. 55.2 Diagrammatic representation of a cloaca showing the urethra, vagina, and rectum joining together in a common channel

- Examination of the abdomen may reveal an abdominal mass (hydrocolpos).
- The distended vagina is a common cause of an obstructed urinary tract because of its pressure on the trigone; therefore, once the vagina is decompressed, the urinary tract may no longer be obstructed. If the hydrocolpos is not drained during the newborn period, it can become infected forming pyocolpos.
- A hemisacrum is almost always associated with a presacral mass, commonly teratomas, or anterior meningoceles.
- The Currarino triad includes an anorectal malformation, a hemisacrum, and a presacral mass.

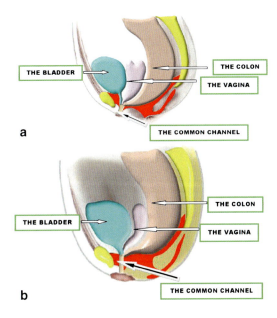

Fig. 55.3 a and **b** Diagrammatic representation of cloaca. Note the length of the common channel which is variable, ranging from 1 to 10 cm but commonly around 3 cm

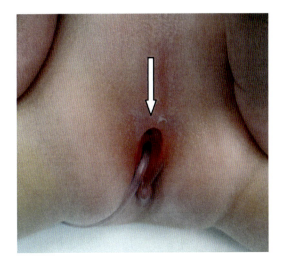

Fig. 55.4 Clinical photograph showing a single perineal opening in a patient with cloaca

Associated Anomalies

- Associated defects are common with cloaca.
- Most vital to recognize are the urological abnormalities.
- More than 80% of all patients with a cloaca have an associated urogenital anomaly.
- These include absent kidney, vesicoureteral reflux, horseshoe kidney, ectopic ureters, double ureters, hydronephrosis, and megaureters as a result of vesicoureteral reflux or ureterovesical obstruction.
- A tethered spinal cord: an intravertebral fixation of the phylum terminale.
- Patients with anorectal malformations and tethered cord have a worse functional prognosis regarding bowel and urinary function.

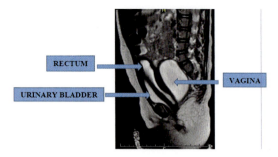

Fig. 55.5 MRI of a patient with cloaca showing the rectum, urethra, and vagina joining distally together in a common channel

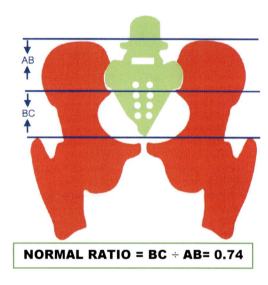

Fig. 55.6 Diagrammatic representation of calculating the sacral ratio

- Sacrum and spine anomalies. The sacrum is the most frequently affected bony structure. Anomalies of the sacrum include hypodevelopment, sacral hemivertebrae, and hemisacra.
- Hemivertebrae may also affect the lumbar and thoracic spine, leading to scoliosis.
- Patients with cloaca may have spinal anomalies other than tethered cord, such as syringomyelia and myelomeningocele.

Investigations

- Plain radiography of the spine can show spinal anomalies, such as spina bifida and spinal hemivertebrae.
- Plain radiography of the sacrum in the anterior–posterior and lateral projections can reveal sacral anomalies, such as a hemisacrum and sacral hemivertebrae.
- Abdominal ultrasonography to evaluate for urologic anomalies and a distended vagina (hydrocolpos).
- Spinal ultrasonography in the first 3 months of life.
- Magnetic resonance imaging (MRI) to evaluate the anomalies of the cloaca, the presence of tethered cord and sacrum and spine (Figs. 55.5 and 55.6).
- Traditionally, to evaluate the degree of sacral deficiency, the number of sacral vertebral bodies was counted.

- A more objective assessment of the sacrum can be obtained by calculating a sacral ratio (the distance from the coccyx to the sacroiliac joint divided by the distance from the sacroiliac joint to the top of the pelvis).
- Normal sacra have a ratio of >0.7.
- Bowel control has rarely been observed in patients with ratios <0.3.
- Lateral radiography is more accurate than the anteroposterior view because its calculation is not affected by the tilt of the pelvis.
- The assessment of the hypodevelopment of the sacrum correlates with the patient's subsequent functional prognosis.
- Echocardiography to detect associated cardiac anomalies.

Classification

- Cloacae represent a wide spectrum of defects.
- In all, the rectum, vagina, and urethra open together and share a common channel.
- The length of this common channel is variable and ranges from 1 to 10 cm.
- The length of this common channel is important for both management and prognosis.
- Based on the length of the common channel, cloacae are divided into two main groups (Fig. 55.3):

    1. Short common channel: <3 cm.
    2. Long common channel: >3 cm.

Management

- The goals of early management are:

    - Detect associated anomalies
    - Diversion of the gastrointestinal tract
    - Drainage of hydrocolpos
    - Divert the urinary tract when necessary

- The management of cloaca is performed in stages.
- The first stage consists of fecal diversion and urinary and vaginal diversion if necessary (Figs. 55.7, 55.8, and 55.9).
- The definitive repair is performed at a later date, followed by colostomy closure. The definitive operation is called the posterior sagittal anorectovaginourethroplasty (PSARVUP).
- It consists mainly of:

    - Separating the rectum from the urogenital tract
    - Followed by separation of the vagina from the urethra and bladder
    - Reconstruction of the common channel as a neo-urethra
    - Mobilization and dissection of the vagina so that it could be pulled down to be placed posterior to the urethra
    - Performance of a pull-through of the rectum placing it within the limits of the sphincter

- Total diversion of the gastrointestinal tract with a colostomy placed in the descending colon and with a mucous fistula is recommended.

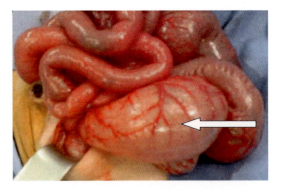

Fig. 55.7 Intraoperative photograph showing dilated sigmoid colon in a patient with cloaca

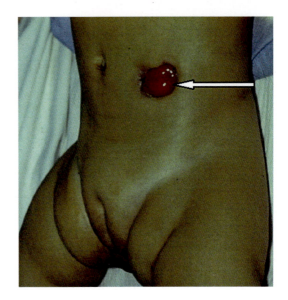

Fig. 55.8 A clinical photograph showing sigmoid colostomy for fecal diversion

- Total diversion of the fecal stream is necessary to prevent urinary infections.
- The defunctionalized colon is used for the future rectal pull-through; thus, adequate length must be ensured when the colostomy site is chosen.
- The patient must be left with a good length of distal colon long enough for the future pull-through, and even for a vaginal replacement if needed.
- The mucous fistula is also important for radiologic evaluation.
- Patients with cloaca have no contraindications to definitive surgery when future fecal or urinary incontinence is a concern.
- Even for patients with incontinence, a bowel management program is almost always successful in keeping a patient clean and dry.
- In patients in whom bowel management is unsuccessful (<3%), a permanent colostomy may be the best option to ensure good quality of life.
- In patients with urinary incontinence, many options are available for keeping a patient clean.
- Urinary diversions, such as the Mitrofanoff procedure and the use of intermittent catheterization, are usually successful in keeping the patient dry of urine.
- The repair of persistent cloaca represents a technical challenge and should be performed in specialized centers by pediatric surgeons dedicated to the care of these patients.

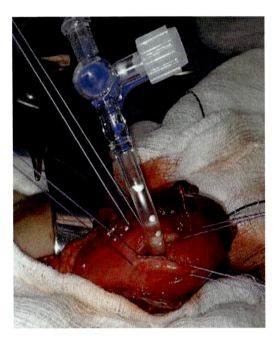

Fig. 55.9 An intraoperative photograph showing pyocolpos in a patient with cloaca which is being drained

- Cystoscopy and vaginoscopy are essential components for evaluation of the patient with persistent cloaca. This is important to define the anatomy and plan surgical reconstruction. It is important to determine the length of the common channel, the presence of vagina or a bifid vagina, the presence of one cervix or more, and the site of rectal fistula.
- Prognostic factors include:
  - The quality of the sacrum and spine
  - The quality of the sphincter muscles
  - The length of the common channel
- Repair in patients with a common channel shorter than 3 cm is feasible through the posterior sagittal approach without an abdominal approach (total urogenital mobilization). This allows mobilization of the urethra and vagina as one structure.
- In patients with a common channel longer than 3 cm, a laparotomy is usually required (transabdominal extended total urogenital mobilization).
- Complex vaginal mobilizations are often required, and vaginal replacement (with colon or small intestine) is frequently necessary.
- Approximately 50 % of patients have various degrees of vaginal or uterine septation. These can be totally or partially repaired during the main operation.
- The Foley catheter remains in place for approximately 10–14 days.
- Anal calibration is performed 2 weeks after the operation, followed by a program of anal dilatations. Once the desired size is reached, the colostomy can be closed.
- Cystoscopy and vaginoscopy should be performed before colostomy closure to ensure that no urethrovaginal fistula is present, which would necessitate a reoperation which should be done with the colostomy still in place.
- Dilatations are continued afterward according to a prescribed protocol. They are a vital part of the postoperative management to avoid a stricture at the anoplasty site.

Recommended Reading

Hendren WH. Management of cloacal malformations. *Semin Pediatr Surg.* 1997;6(4):217–27.

Hendren WH. Cloaca, the most severe degree of imperforate anus: experience with 195 cases. *Ann Surg.* 1998;228(3):331–46.

Levitt MA, Peña A. Cloacal malformations: lessons learned from 490 cases. *Semin Pediatr Surg.* 2010;19:128–38.

Levitt MA, Mak GA, Falcone RA, Peña A. Cloacal exstrophy—pull through or permanent stoma? A review of 53 patients. *J Pediatr Surg.* 2008;43:164–70.

Levitt MA, Bischoff A, Peña A. Pitfalls and challenges of cloaca repair; how to reduce the need for reoperations. *J Pediatr Surg.* 2011;46:1250–5.

Peña A. The surgical management of persistent cloaca: results in 54 patients treated with a posterior sagittal approach. J Pediatr Surg. 1989;24:590–8.

Chapter 56
Cloacal Extrophy

Introduction

- Cloacal extrophy is a very rare and complex malformation characterized classically by:

  - Omphalocele
  - Extrophy of the two hemi bladders
  - Extrophied ileocecal region which presents between the two hemi bladders
  - Imperforate anus
  - Ambiguous genitalia (Figs. 56.1 and 56.2)

- Cloacal extrophy, which is also called vesico-intestinal fissure, is one of the rare and complex malformations with a reported incidence between 1 in 200,000 and 1 in 400,000 live births.
- Classically, cloacal extrophy consists of five components:

  - Omphalocele.
  - Extrophy of the two hemi bladders.
  - Lateral cecal fissure which presents between the two hemi bladders.
  - Imperforate anus.
  - Ambiguous genitalia.
  - Many other variants have also been described.

Embryology

- The exact embryogenesis of cloacal extrophy is not known, and many theories have been suggested; however, no single theory can adequately explain all the abnormalities seen in cloacal extrophy.
- The most accepted theory is that cloacal extrophy results from premature rupture of the cloacal membrane prior to caudal migration of the urorectal septum, and fusion of the genital tubercles.
- Embryologically, the urorectal septum divides the cloaca after the fourth week of intra-uterine life into an anterior urogenital sinus and a posterior anorectal canal.
- The cloacal membrane is invaded by lateral mesodermal folds at approximately 4 weeks of gestation.
- It is postulated that if this mesodermal invasion does not occur, the infraumbilical cloacal membrane persists leading to poor lower abdominal wall development.
- The cloacal membrane eventually ruptures but if this happens prior to the descent of the urorectal septum, which happens at 6–8 weeks of gestation, then cloacal extrophy results.

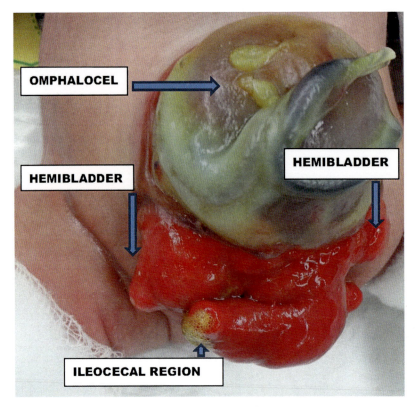

Fig. 56.1 Clinical photograph showing the components of the cloacal extrophy

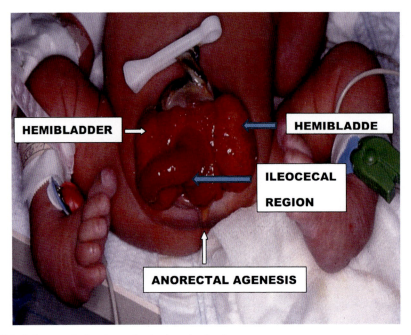

Fig. 56.2 Clinical photograph showing a classic cloacal extrophy

Fig. 56.3 Clinical photograph of a newborn with cloacal extrophy. Note also the bilateral talipes equinovarus

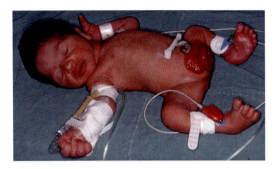

- So cloacal extrophy occurs due to the failure of two concomitant mesodermal migrations. First, the urorectal septum fails to develop and divide the urogenital sinus from the rectum; second, the mesodermal proliferation forming the infraumbilical abdominal wall and genital tubercle fails to develop.
- Failure of these two events to occur results in extrophy of both bladder and intestine.
- Classically, cloacal extrophy is made up of omphalocele, extrophied ileocecal region of bowel, extrophied hemi bladders each with its ipsilateral ureter, and anorectal agenesis.
- The pubic bones are widely separated, and spinal dysraphism is common in these patients.

Associated Anomalies

- Cloacal extrophy is commonly associated with other anomalies including cardiovascular and central nervous system anomalies.
- Omphalocele (70–90%).
- Vertebral anomalies (46%).
- Upper urinary tract (42%). Upper urinary tract anomalies include pelvic kidney, horseshoe kidney, hypoplastic kidney, and solitary kidney.
- Malrotation (30%).
- Lower extremity anomalies (30%) (Fig. 56.3).
- Double appendix (30%).
- Absent appendix (21%).
- Short small bowel (19%).
- Small bowel atresia (5%).
- Abdominal musculature deficiency (1%).
- Vertebral malformations include sacralization of L5, congenital scoliosis, sacral agenesis, and interpedicular widening (Fig. 56.4).

Clinical Features and Management

- Cloacal extrophy is a very rare and complex anomaly of the urogenital tract and intestinal tract resulting in extrophy of both bowel and bladder (Fig. 56.5).
- It is more common in males (with a male–female sex ratio of 2:1).
- It is also called OEIS Complex, (Omphalocele, Extrophy of the cloaca, Imperforate Anus, and Spinal Defects).

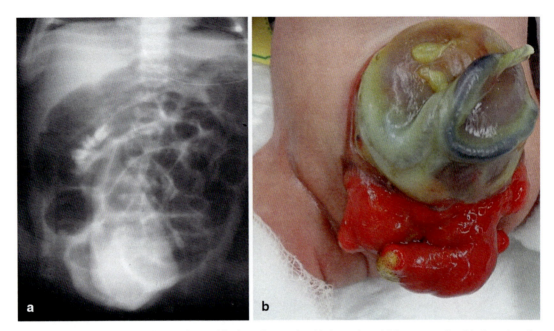

Fig. 56.4 Abdominal x-ray of a newborn with cloacal extrophy (**a**) (note the widely separated pubic bones) and a clinical photograph showing cloacal extrophy (**b**). Note the omphalocele, the urinary bladder into two halves and the prolapsed ileocecal region with the terminal ileum open with meconium passing from it

Fig. 56.5 A clinical photograph showing cloacal extrophy. Note the prolapsing ileum in the middle between the two halves of the urinary bladder

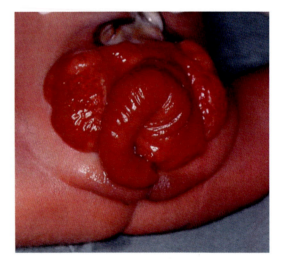

- Commonly in cloacal extrophy, the extrophied bowel is the ileocecal region with little or no large bowel distally, but there are cases where there is colonic extrophy with enough large bowel length (Fig. 56.6).
- Its clinical features include omphalocele, imperforate anus, and extrophy of two hemi bladders, between which lies the everted cecum. A small colon ends blindly in the pelvis, and the terminal ileum often prolapses out of the exposed cecum.
- The presence of enough large bowel is advantageous from the reconstruction point of view, because, normally, the extrophied ileocecal region and the presence of short large bowel should be preserved for reconstruction of the anorectal malformation, and not to be used for urinary bladder augmentation (Fig. 56.6).

Clinical Features and Management

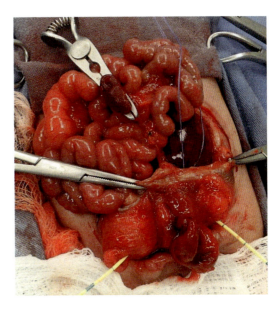

Fig. 56.6 An intraoperative photograph showing the urinary bladder open into two halves with part of the intestine in the middle. Note also the two ureteric catheters passed into the ureters

- Every effort must be made to preserve all large intestines because it can not only be used for bladder augmentation, which is necessary in the majority of these patients to increase the bladder compliance, but also for vaginal reconstruction in those who had gender reassignment.
- Add to this the valuable absorptive function of the large bowel.
- Augmentation of the urinary bladder may be performed using the hindgut if enough length is available in the ileum or part of the stomach. In the absence of large intestine, both small bowel and stomach can be used for bladder augmentation but gastrocytoplasty was shown to be superior.
- Gender assignment is one of the difficult tasks in the management of newborns with cloacal extrophy.
- Genetic females should not raise a problem as they will be raised as females.
- In genetic males with cloacal extrophy, the phallic structures are usually small and completely bifid with insufficient phallic tissue to reconstruct an adequate penis.
- There is now general consensus that genetic males with insufficient phallus be gender reassigned as phenotypic females, and to minimize testosterone imprinting on the nervous system, this should be done in the immediate newborn period with early orchidectomy.
- Males with adequate bilateral or unilateral phallic structures should, however, be raised as males.
- In the classic repair of cloacal extrophy in males an epispadias is created initially after urinary bladder closure.
- The management of newborns with cloacal extrophy has progressed over the years, and now a very reasonable outcome is expected in most cases. This, however, requires a team approach including neonatologists, pediatric surgeons, pediatric urologist, neurosurgeons, geneticists, and social workers.
- Although there are general guidelines in managing newborns with cloacal extrophy, after thorough evaluation of the anatomical abnormalities, the management should be individualized.
- Immediate management is directed to the medical stabilization of the infant.
- Evaluation and appropriate management of associated malformations should be undertaken.
- For infants who have few other associated malformations and are medically stable, staged closure can be considered.
- The bowel should be moistened with saline and covered with protective plastic dressing.
- Evaluation of the genitalia and gender assignment should be made by a gender assignment team, including a pediatric urologist, pediatric surgeon, pediatrician, and pediatric endocrinologist.

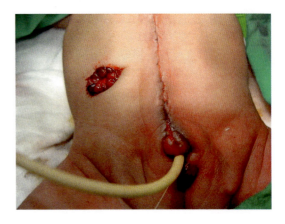

Fig. 56.7 A clinical postoperative photograph showing a diverting ileostomy and a urinary catheter in the already closed urinary bladder

- Consultation of social worker, pediatric orthopedic surgeon, and other disciplines should be obtained.
- The initial operation consists of separating the bowel from the bladder to create an intestinal stoma; closing the omphalocele; and reapproximating, closing, or leaving the extrophied bladder undisturbed (Fig. 56.7).
- The importance of creating a colostomy instead of an ileostomy to prevent problems with diarrhea, dehydration, and acidosis is emphasized.

Recommended Reading

Lund DP, Hendren WH. Cloacal extrophy: experience with 20 cases. J Pediatr Surg. 1993;28:1360–9.

Manzoni GA, Ransley PG, Hurwitz RS. Cloacal extrophy and cloacal extrophy variants: a proposed system of classification. J Urol. 1987;138:1065–8.

Ricketts RR, Woodard JR, Zwiren GT, Andrews HG, Broeker BH. Modern treatment of cloacal extrophy. J Pediatr Surg. 1991;26:444–50.

Stolar CJH, Randolph JG, Flanigan LP. Cloacal extrophy: individualized management through a staged surgical approach. J Pediatr Surg. 1990;25:505–7.

Chapter 57
Hepatoblastoma

Introduction

- Hepatoblastoma is a malignant embryonal liver tumor that occurs almost exclusively in infants and very young children.
- Hepatoblastoma is the most common primary liver tumor in children.
- It originates from immature liver precursor cells and usually affect the right lobe of the liver more often than the left lobe.
- Hepatoblastoma accounts for 79% of all liver tumors in children and almost two-thirds of primary malignant liver tumors in the pediatric age group.
- The annual incidence of hepatoblastoma in infants younger than 1 year is 11.2 cases per million.
- The annual incidence in children overall was 1.5 cases per million.
- White children are affected almost five times more frequently than black children. Black patients tend to have worse outcomes.
- Males are typically affected more frequently than females; the male-to-female ratio is 1.7:1.
- Hepatoblastoma usually affects children younger than 3 years, and the median age at diagnosis is 1 year.
- The right lobe is involved three times more commonly than the left, with bilobar involvement seen in 20–30% and multicentric involvement in 15%.

Etiology

- The etiology of hepatoblastoma is unknown but it has been associated with a number of genetic conditions that are associated with an increased risk for developing hepatoblastoma. They include:
  1. Beckwith-Wiedemann syndrome
     - Beckwith–Wiedemann syndrome (BWS) an overgrowth syndrome characterized by a combination of:
     - Large birth weight and length
     - Hypoglycemia
     - Macroglossia
     - Omphalocele
     - Hemihypertrophy
     - Nevus flammeus
     - Genitourinary malformations.

- Children with BWS are much more likely than other children to develop certain childhood cancers, particularly Wilms' tumor and hepatoblastoma.
- In addition to Wilms' tumor and hepatoblastoma, children with BWS are also at increased risk of developing adrenal cortical carcinoma, neuroblastoma, and *rhabdomyosarc*oma.
- The relative risk for the development of hepatoblastoma in BWS is 22.80.
- The incidence of hepatoblastoma has increased 1000–10,000-fold in infants and children with BWS.

  2. Familial adenomatous polyposis:
     ◦ This is a group of rare inherited diseases of the gastrointestinal tract.
     ◦ It is a syndrome characterized by early-onset colonic polyps and adenocarcinoma and frequently develop hepatoblastomas.
     ◦ The relative risk for the development of hepatoblastoma in familial adenomatous polyposis is 12.20.
     ◦ There is an association between hepatoblastoma and familial adenomatous polyposis (FAP); children in families that carry the adenomatous polyposis coli (APC) gene are at an 800-fold increased risk for hepatoblastoma. However, hepatoblastoma occurs in < 1% of FAP family members.
  3. Hemihypertrophy: This condition is the improper growth of one limb on one side of the body in comparison with the other side.
  4. Low birth weight: There is also an association of prematurity/low birth weight and hepatoblastoma. The relative risk for hepatoblastoma for children who weighed less than 1000 g at birth was 15.64 compared with 2.53 for those weighing 1000–1499 g and 1.21 for 2000–2499 g.
  5. Loss of heterozygosity (LOH) of chromosome at location 11p occurs commonly in hepatoblastoma. These are identified in association with BWS and hemihypertrophy.
  6. Isochromosome 8q is seen in mixed hepatoblastomas.
  7. Trisomy 20 is seen in pure epithelial hepatoblastomas.
  8. Associated factors also include young maternal age, maternal smoking during pregnancy, high maternal pregnancy weight, and maternal use of oral contraceptives.
  9. Cases of hepatoblastoma have been associated with total parenteral nutrition-related cholestasis and type I glycogen storage disease.

Clinical Features

- Most patients present with an abdominal mass (Fig. 57.1).
- Less common symptoms are: decreased appetite, anorexia, weight loss, nausea, vomiting, back pain, early puberty in boys, fever, and abdominal pain.
- Rarely, they present with acute abdomen due to tumor rupture.

Investigations

- Complete blood count, liver function tests, electrolytes, blood urea, and creatinine.
- Alpha-fetoprotein (AFP) test: AFP levels in the blood can be used both to diagnose hepatoblastoma and to monitor its response to treatment and follow-up. AFP levels of less than 100 μg/mL is a poor prognostic factor.

Investigations

Fig. 57.1 Clinical photograph of a patient with hepatoblastoma showing a large abdominal mass

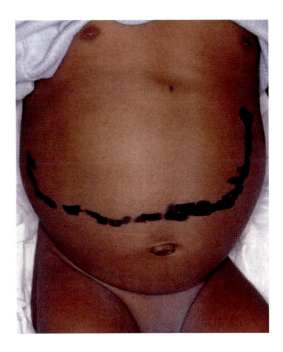

Fig. 57.2 Chest x-ray of a patient with hepatoblastoma showing a large right-sided upper abdominal soft-tissue mass pushing the diaphragm upwards

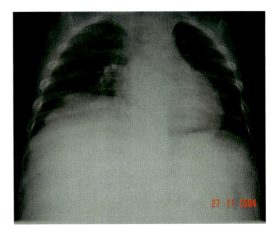

- Abdominal and chest x-rays: This reveals a right upper quadrant abdominal soft-tissue mass. Calcification is seen in approximately 6% of hepatoblastomas (Fig. 57.2).
- Abdominal ultrasound: This is valuable in detecting the organ of origin of the tumor, its size, and nature as well as vascular involvement.
- Chest and abdominal computed tomography (CT scan): This allows more accurate assessment of site and size of the tumor as well as involvement of nearby structures particularly regional lymph nodes. CT scanning of the chest is important to assess for pulmonary metastases (Fig. 57.3).
- Magnetic resonance imaging (MRI): This is superior to CT scan and allows more and accurate outlines of the tumor and feasibility of resection (Fig. 57.4).
- Technetium-99 m sulfur-colloid liver scintigraphy (Fig. 57.5): Hepatoblastomas usually demonstrate hypervascularity, with prominent tracer avidity at the site of the tumor within a few seconds

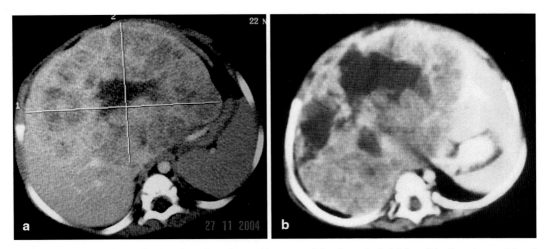

Fig. 57.3 Abdominal CT scans showing a large hepatoblastoma arising from the left lobe of the liver in one (**a**) and from the right lobe of liver in (**b**)

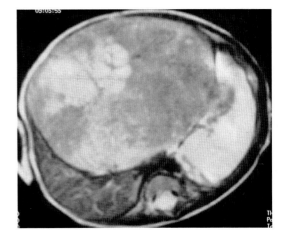

Fig. 57.4 Magnetic resonance imaging (MRI) of the abdomen showing a large hepatoblastoma

of the appearance of the bolus in the abdominal aorta. This increased activity persists into the venous phase. Delayed images typically demonstrate a photopenic defect at the tumor site.
- Bone scans: This is recommended to evaluate for bone metastases when the patient is symptomatic.
- Positron emission tomography (PET) CT: Most hepatoblastomas are positive on fludeoxyglucose PET before therapy and therefore this nuclear scan may be helpful for detection of metastasis and assessment of tumor viability.

Staging

- Stage I: Hepatoblastoma that is completely removed with surgery.
- Stage II: Hepatoblastoma that is mostly removed by surgery but very small amounts of the cancer are left in the liver.

Pathology 435

Fig. 57.5 Isotope scan showing a hepatoblastoma arising from the right lobe of the liver

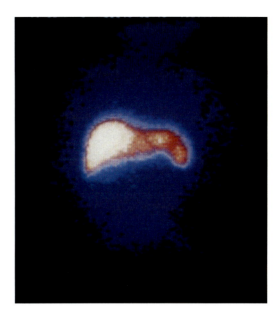

Fig. 57.6 Stage 1: Tumor involves only one quadrant; three adjoining liver quadrants are free of tumor

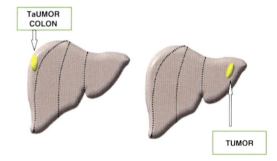

- Stage III: Hepatoblastoma that cannot be completely removed and the cancer cells are found in the lymph nodes.
- Stage IV: Hepatoblastoma that has spread (metastasized) to other parts of the body.
- Recurrent: The disease has returned after it has been treated. It may come back in the liver or in another parts of the body.
- Metastases at diagnoses occur in 10–20 % of patients, with the lung being the predominant site of metastases both at presentation and relapse. Other sites of distant metastases, including brain and bone, are rare and usually occur in the setting of relapsed disease.

The PRETEXT staging system for hepatoblastoma (Figs. 57.6, 57.7, 57.8, and 57.9):

Pathology

- Histologically, hepatoblastoma is composed of epithelial and mesenchymal elements in varying proportions and at various stages of differentiation (Figs. 57.10 and 57.11)
- The epithelial element is variable from the primitive blastema through embryonal hepatocytes to fetal hepatocytes and because of this hepatoblastoma is classified by histology as:

Fig. 57.7 Stage 2: Tumor involves one or two quadrants; two adjoining quadrants are free of tumor

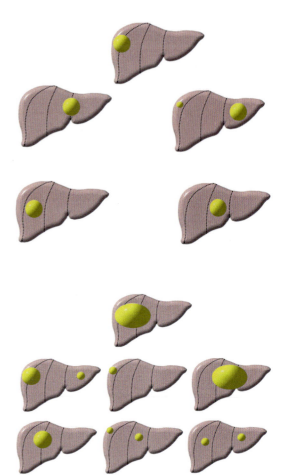

Fig. 57.8 Stage 3: Tumor involves three quadrants and one quadrant is free of tumor or tumor involves two quadrants and two nonadjoining quadrants are free of tumor

- Epithelial (56 %)
- Mixed epithelial/mesenchymal (44 %)

- Epithelial hepatoblastoma is further subdivided into:

  - Pure fetal (31 %)
  - Embryonal (19 %)
  - Macrotrabecular (3 %)
  - Small-cell undifferentiated (3 %)

- The pure fetal pattern is composed of small, round, uniform cells with abundant cytoplasm and distinct cytoplasmic membranes. The cells are arranged into thin trabeculae, usually two to three cells thick, with alternating light and dark areas.
- The embryonal pattern is composed of fetal cells as well as cells arranged into sheets of irregular, angulated cells with a high nucleocytoplasmic ratio, increased nuclear chromatin, and indistinct cytoplasmic membranes. Pseudorosette and acinar formation are also common.
- Foci of extramedullary hematopoiesis are seen in both the fetal and embryonal areas.
- The macrotrabecular hepatoblastoma refers to a growth pattern in which fetal or embryonal cells numbered 10 cells or more in thickness are present as a repetitive pattern within the tumor within a cord or cluster, as opposed to the usual 2–6-cell-thick cords or plates.

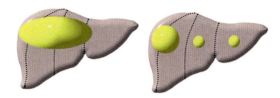

Fig. 57.9 Stage 4: Tumor involves all four quadrants; there is no quadrant free of tumor

- "Undifferentiated" or "anaplastic" hepatoblastomas are composed of small round cells with scanty cytoplasm and hyperchromatic nuclei. There is nuclear enlargement to three times those of typical tumor cells, hyperchromasia, and atypical mitoses.
- Approximately 44% of hepatoblastoma contain both mixed epithelial and mesenchymal components.
- The most common mesenchymal elements are osteoid and cartilage.
- The mixed pattern of epithelial and mesenchymal hepatoblastoma accounts for 44% of the cases and further subdivided into those without teratoid features (34%) and 10% with teratoid features such components as squamous epithelium and striated muscle. The highly cellular primitive mesenchyme consists of elongated, spindle-shaped cells with a scanty cytoplasm, and elongated plump nuclei with rounded ends, resembling fibroblastoid/myofibroblastoid tissue.
- Approximately 20% of the mixed types of hepatoblastomas contain a variety of tissues, including stratified squamous epithelium, melanin pigment, mucinous epithelium, cartilage, bone, and striated muscle in addition to the epithelial cells, fibrous tissue, and osteoid-like material. These tumors have been termed "teratoid hepatoblastomas".
- Because these histologic types tend to be randomly intermingled, both fine-needle aspiration and biopsies may capture a nonrepresentative sample of tumor.
- Of the histologic subtypes (pure fetal, embryonal, mixed epithelial–mesenchymal, macrotrabecular, and small cell undifferentiated), the fetal subtype carries the most favorable prognosis, and small cell undifferentiated the worst with macrotrabecular histology probably having an intermediate prognosis.

Histological Classification of Hepatoblastoma

1. Hepatoblastoma, wholly epithelial type (56%):

    a. Fetal subtype (31%)
    b. Mixed embryonal/fetal subtype (19%)
    c. Macrotrabcular subtype (3%)
    d. Small cell undifferentiated subtype (3%)

2. Hepatoblastoma, mixed epithelial, and mesenchymal type (44%):

    a. Without teratoid features (34%)
    b. With teratoid features (10%)

3. Hepatoblastom, not otherwise specified

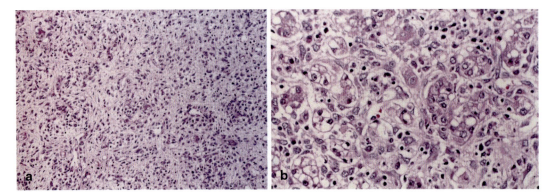

Fig. 57.10 a and **b** Histological picture of hepatoblastoma. Note the epithelial and mesenchymal components and the large hyperchromatic nuclei

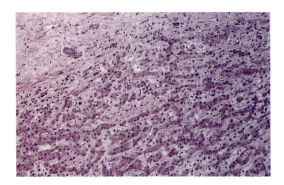

Fig. 57.11 Histological picture of hepatoblastoma. Note the epithelial and mesenchymal components as well as the arrangements of the epithelial cells into thin trabeculae (Fetal type)

Treatment and Prognosis

- Surgery remains the mainstay in the treatment of hepatoblastoma and the prognosis is directly related to tumor stage (Fig. 57.12).
- Surgery and adjuvant chemotherapy have markedly improved the prognosis of children with hepatoblastoma.
- Complete surgical resection of the tumor at the time of diagnosis, followed by adjuvant chemotherapy, is associated with nearly 100% survival rates.
- The prognosis however remains poor in children with residual tumor after initial surgical resection, even if they receive aggressive adjuvant chemotherapy.
- Significant data now support a role for preoperative neoadjuvant chemotherapy if the tumor is inoperable or if the tumor is unlikely to achieve gross total resection at initial diagnosis (Figs. 57.13 and 57.14).
- Liver transplantation is also playing an increasing role in cases in which the tumor is unresectable after chemotherapy or in "rescue" transplantation when initial surgery and chemotherapy are not successful.
- Contraindications to immediate resection include (Fig. 57.15):
    - Extensive bilateral liver involvement
    - Presence of vascular invasion of major hepatic veins or inferior vena cava
    - Diffuse multifocal disease
    - Distant metastasis

Treatment and Prognosis

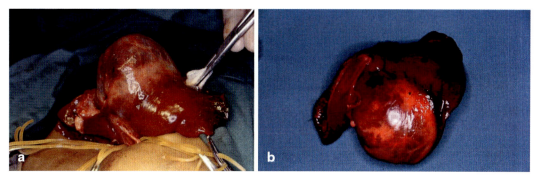

Fig. 57.12 Intraoperative photograph showing hepatoblastoma (**a**) that was resected (**b**)

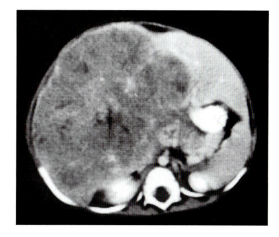

Fig. 57.13 Abdominal CT scan showing a large unresectable hepatoblastoma arising from the right lobe of the liver

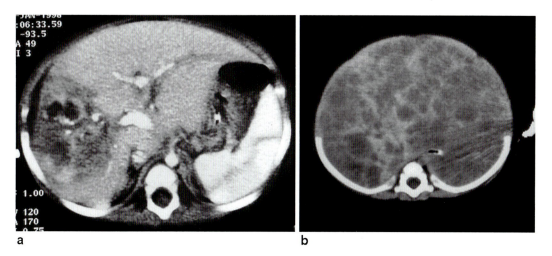

Fig. 57.14 Abdominal CT scan showing a large hepatoblastoma arising from the right lobe of the liver that is not resectable (**a**) and CT scan of the same patient following preoperative chemotherapy (**b**). Note the good response and marked reduction in the size of the tumor

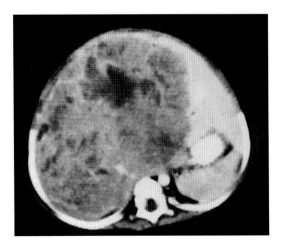

Fig. 57.15 Abdominal CT scan of a patient with widespread hepatoblastoma involving both lobes of the liver

- At the time of diagnosis, 40–60% of hepatoblastomas are considered to be unresectable and 10–20% of patients are found to have pulmonary metastases.
- Preoperative chemotherapy converts nearly 85% of these "unresectable" lesions to ones that can be entirely grossly removed, that is, to stage I or II lesions with subsequent long-term survival.
- Preoperative chemotherapy has increased the resectability of hepatoblastoma from 40 to 60% to 90%, with the more extensive tumors requiring transplantation to remove the involved portions of liver.
- Tumor stage at the time of initial resection is the key prognostic factor in determining the survival of children with hepatoblastoma.
- The 3-year event-free survival for stage I–II is 90%, 50% for stage III, and only 20% for stage IV.
- Neoadjuvant chemotherapy followed by resection has become the mainstay in the treatment of hepatoblastoma.
- Treatment strategies currently combine surgery, chemotherapy (adjuvant and neoadjuvant), and transplantation as defined by the stage of the tumor.
- The 5-year survival rates based on the COG staging system are as follows:

    1. Stage I (favorable histology): 100%
    2. Stage I (unfavorable histology): 98%
    3. Stage II: 100%
    4. Stage III: 69%
    5. Stage IV: 37%

- The 5-year survival rates based on the Société Internationale d'Oncologie Pédiatrique—Epithelial Liver Tumor Study Group (SIOPEL) staging are as follows:

    1. Stage I: 100%
    2. Stage II: 91%
    3. Stage III: 68%

Recommended Reading

Ang JP, Heath JA, Donath S, Khurana S, Auldist A. Treatment outcomes for hepatoblastoma: an institution's experience over two decades. Pediatr Surg Int. 2007;23(2):103–9.

Recommended Reading

Czauderna P, Otte JB, Aronson DC, Gauthier F, Mackinlay G, Roebuck D, et al. Guidelines for surgical treatment of hepatoblastoma in the modern era—recommendations from the Childhood Liver Tumour Strategy Group of the International Society of Paediatric Oncology (SIOPEL). Eur J Cancer. 2005;41(7):1031–6.

De Ioris M, Brugieres L, Zimmermann A, Keeling J, Brock P, Maibach R, Pritchard J, Shafford L, Zsiros J, Czauderna P, Perilongo G. Hepatoblastoma with a low serum alpha-fetoprotein level at diagnosis: the SIOPEL group experience. Eur J Cancer. 2007;44(4):545.

Otte JB, Pritchard J, Aronson DC, Czauderna P, Maibach R, Perilongo G, et al. Liver transplantation for hepatoblastoma: results from the International Society of Pediatric Oncology (SIOP) study SIOPEL-1 and review of the world experience. Pediatr Blood Cancer. 2004;42(1):74–83.

Perilongo G, Shafford E, Maibach R, Aronson D, Brugières L, Brock P, et al. Risk-adapted treatment for childhood hepatoblastoma. Final report of the second study of the International Society of Paediatric Oncology—SIOPEL 2. Eur J Cancer. 2004;40(3):411–2.

Schnater JM, Aronson DC, Plaschkes J, Perilongo G, Brown J, Otte JB, et al. Surgical view of the treatment of patients with hepatoblastoma: results from the first prospective trial of the International Society of Pediatric Oncology Liver Tumor Study Group. Cancer. 2002;94:1111–20.

Zsiros J, Maibach R, Shafford E, Brugieres L, Brock P, Czauderna P, et al. Successful treatment of childhood high-risk hepatoblastoma with dose-intensive multiagent chemotherapy and surgery: final results of the SIOPEL-3HR study. J Clin Oncol. 2010;28(15):2584–90.

Chapter 58
Hodgkin's and Non-Hodgkin's Lymphoma

Introduction

- Hodgkin's lymphoma was named after Thomas Hodgkin, who first described abnormalities in the lymph system in 1832.
- It accounts for 5 % of cancers in the pediatric age group.
- Overall, it is more common in males, except for the nodular sclerosis variant, which is slightly more common in females.
- The annual incidence of Hodgkin's lymphoma is about 1 in 25,000 people.
- Hodgkin's lymphoma is rarely diagnosed before the age of 5years. The number of cases increases significantly in the second decade of life.
- Hodgkin's lymphoma is characterized by the orderly spread from one group of lymph nodes to another and by the development of systemic symptoms with advanced disease.
- Microscopically, Hodgkin's lymphoma is characterized by the presence of multinucleated Reed–Sternberg cells (Fig. 58.1).
- Hodgkin's lymphoma occurs at two peaks: the first in young adulthood (age 15–35) and the second in those over 55 years.
- Hodgkin's lymphoma may be treated with radiation therapy, chemotherapy, or hematopoietic stem cell transplantation. The choice of treatment depends on the age and sex of the patient and the stage, bulk, and histological subtype of the disease.
- Patients with a history of infectious mononucleosis due to Epstein–Barr virus may have an increased risk of Hodgkin's lymphoma, but the precise contribution of Epstein–Barr virus remains largely unknown.

Classification

- Classical Hodgkin's lymphoma (excluding nodular lymphocyte predominant Hodgkin's lymphoma) can be subclassified into four pathologic subtypes based upon Reed–Sternberg cell morphology and the composition of the reactive cell infiltrate seen in the lymph node biopsy specimen.
- Nodular sclerosing Hodgkin's lymphoma:
  - The most common subtype.
  - It is composed of large tumor nodules showing scattered lacunar classical Reed–Sternberg cells set in a background of reactive lymphocytes, eosinophils, and plasma cells with varying degrees of collagen fibrosis/sclerosis.

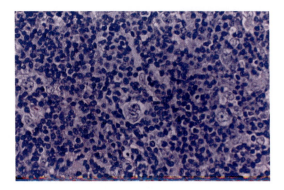

Fig. 58.1 Histological picture showing features of Hodgkin's lymphoma including the multinucleated Reed–Sternberg cells

- Mixed-cellularity Hodgkin's lymphoma:
  - It is the second most common subtype.
  - It is composed of numerous classic Reed–Sternberg cells admixed with numerous inflammatory cells including lymphocytes, histiocytes, eosinophils, and plasma cells without sclerosis.
  - This type is most often associated with Epstein–Barr virus infection.
- Lymphocytic predominance Hodgkin's lymphoma:
  - This is a rare subtype.
  - Shows many features which may cause diagnostic confusion with nodular lymphocyte predominant B cell non-Hodgkin's lymphoma (NHL).
  - This subtype has the most favorable prognosis.
- Lymphocyte-depleted Hodgkin's lymphoma:
  - This is a rare subtype.
  - Composed of large numbers of often pleomorphic Reed–Sternberg cells with only few reactive lymphocytes.
  - It may easily be confused with diffuse large-cell lymphoma.
  - Many cases previously classified within this category would now be reclassified under anaplastic large cell lymphoma.
  - Nodular lymphocyte predominant Hodgkin's lymphoma expresses CD20, and is not currently considered a form of classical Hodgkin's.

Staging

- The staging is the same for both Hodgkin's as well as NHLs.
- Lymphangiograms or laparotomies are very rarely performed, having been supplanted by improvements in imaging with the computed tomography (CT) scan and positron emission tomography (PET) scan.
- The Ann Arbor staging classification:
  - Stage I: Involvement of a single lymph node region (I) (mostly the cervical region) or single extra lymphatic site (Ie).
  - Stage II: Involvement of two or more lymph node regions on the same side of the diaphragm (II) or of one lymph node region and a contiguous extra lymphatic site (IIe).

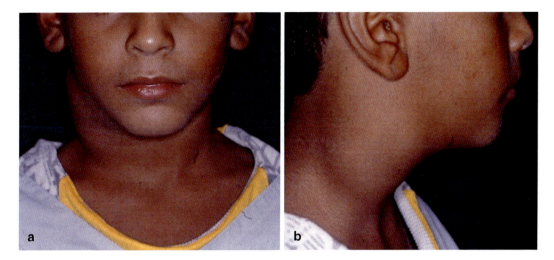

Fig. 58.2 Clinical photograph showing enlarged cervical lymph nodes in a child with Hodgkin's lymphoma

- Stage III: Involvement of lymph node regions on both sides of the diaphragm, which may include the spleen (IIIs) and/or limited contiguous extra lymphatic organ or site (IIIe, IIIes).
- Stage IV: Disseminated involvement of one or more extra lymphatic organs.

- The absence of systemic symptoms is signified by adding "A" to the stage; the presence of systemic symptoms is signified by adding "B" to the stage.
- For localized extra nodal extension from mass of nodes that does not advance the stage, subscript "E" is added.
- Splenic involvement is signified by adding "S" to the stage.

Clinical Features

Patients with Hodgkin's lymphoma may present with the following symptoms:

- Lymph nodes:
  - Painless enlargement of one or more lymph nodes (Fig. 58.2).
  - The nodes may feel rubbery when examined.
  - The cervical and supraclavicular lymph nodes are most frequently involved (80–90%).
  - The lymph nodes of the chest are often affected, and these may be noticed on a chest radiograph.
- Itching.
- Night sweats.
- Weight loss.
- Splenomegaly (30%).
- Hepatomegaly (5%).
- Back pain.
- Red-colored patches on the skin, easy bleeding, and petechiae due to low platelet count.
- Systemic symptoms: About one-third of patients with Hodgkin's disease may also present with systemic symptoms, including low-grade fever; night sweats; unexplained weight loss, pruritus due to increased levels of eosinophils in the bloodstream; or fatigue.

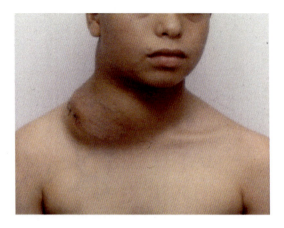

Fig. 58.3 Clinical photograph in a child with Hodgkin's lymphoma. Note the site of excisional biopsy

- Systemic symptoms such as fever, night sweats, and weight loss are known as B symptoms; thus, presence of fever, weight loss, and night sweats indicate that the patient's stage is, for example, 2B instead of 2A.
- Cyclical fever: Patients may also present with a cyclical high-grade fever known as the Pel–Ebstein fever.

Etiology

- The cause is unknown or multifactorial.
- Risk factors for Hodgkin's lymphoma include:
  - Male sex
  - Ages: 15–40 years and over 55 years
  - Family history of Hodgkin's lymphoma
  - History of infectious mononucleosis
  - HIV or the presence of AIDS
  - Prolonged use of human growth hormone
  - Exposure to toxins, such as Agent Orange

Diagnosis

- Definitive diagnosis of Hodgkin's lymphoma is by excisional lymph node biopsy (Figs. 58.3 and 58.4).
- Blood tests including complete blood count (CBC), liver function test (LFT), renal function test (RFT), total protein, and albumin.
- Chest x-ray and CT scan (Fig. 58.5).
- PET is used to detect small deposits that do not show on CT scan.

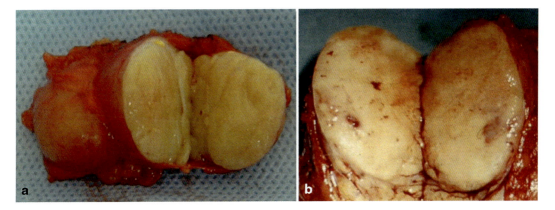

Fig. 58.4 a and **b** Clinical photograph showing an excised lymph node in a child with Hodgkin's lymphoma. The lymph node is replaced by tumor cells

Fig. 58.5 Chest x-ray (**a**) and CT scan (**b**) in a child with mediastinal lymphoma

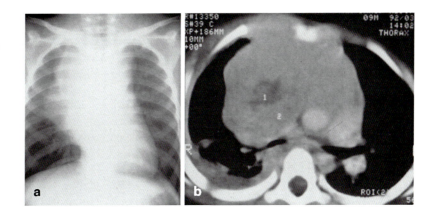

Treatment

- Hodgkin's lymphoma can be subclassified by histological type. The treatment and prognosis in Hodgkin's lymphoma usually depends on the stage of disease rather than the histology type.
- The choice of treatment depends on the age, sex, bulk, and the histological subtype of the disease.
- Patients with early stage disease (IA or IIA) are effectively treated with radiation therapy or chemotherapy.
- Patients with later disease (III, IVA, or IVB) are treated with combination chemotherapy alone.
- Patients of any stage with a large mass in the chest are usually treated with combined chemotherapy and radiation therapy.
- Currently, the adriamycin, bleomycin, vinblastine, and dacarbazine (*ABVD*) chemotherapy regimen is the standard treatment of Hodgkin's disease.
- The Stanford V regimen involves a more intensive chemotherapy and incorporates radiation therapy.
- Bleomycin, etoposide, adriamycin, cyclophosphamide, vincristine, procarbazine, prednisone (BEACOPP) is a form of treatment for stages >II.
- Late adverse effects of treatment include cardiovascular disease and second malignancies such as acute leukemias, lymphomas, and solid tumors within the radiation therapy field.

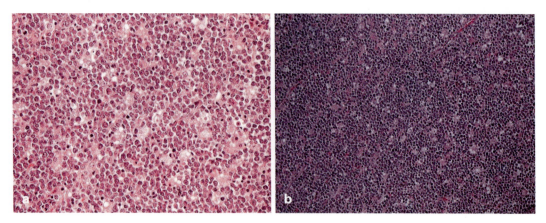

Fig. 58.6 Histology picture of Burkitt's lymphoma. Note the sheets of uniform cells (**a**) and the starry sky appearance (**b**)

- Long-term endocrine adverse effects are a major concern, mainly gonadal dysfunction and growth retardation. Gonadal dysfunction seems to be the most severe endocrine long-term effect, especially after treatment with alkylating agents and/or pelvic radiotherapy.

Non-Hodgkin Lymphoma

- The NHLs are a diverse group of cancers that include any kind of lymphoma except Hodgkin's lymphomas.
- NHLs can occur at any age and are often marked by lymph nodes that are larger than normal, fever, and weight loss.
- The median age at presentation for most subtypes of NHL is older than 50 years. The exceptions are Burkitt's lymphoma, high-grade lymphoblastic and small noncleaved lymphomas, which are the most common types of NHL observed in children and young adults.
- NHL, which includes Burkitt's, accounts for 30–50% of childhood lymphoma.
- Burkitt's lymphoma:
  - Burkitt's lymphoma is named after Denis Parsons Burkitt, a surgeon who first described the disease in 1956 while working in Africa.
  - The tumor consists of sheets of a monotonous (i.e., similar in size and morphology) population of medium-sized lymphoid cells with high proliferative activity and apoptotic activity (the "starry sky" appearance; Fig. 58.6).
  - Currently, Burkitt's lymphoma can be divided into three main clinical variants: the endemic, the sporadic, and the immunodeficiency-associated variants.
  - The endemic variant:
    - Occurs in equatorial Africa.
    - It is the most common malignancy of children in this area.
    - Children affected with the disease often also had chronic malaria, which is believed to have reduced resistance to Epstein–Barr virus.
    - The disease characteristically involves the jaw or other facial bone, distal ileum, cecum, ovaries, kidney, or the breast.
  - The sporadic type of Burkitt's lymphoma (also known as "non-African"). The ileocecal region is the common site of involvement (Figs. 58.7 and 58.8).
  - Immunodeficiency-associated Burkitt's lymphoma is usually associated with HIV infection or occurs in posttransplant patients who are taking immunosuppressive drugs. Burkitt's lymphoma can be one of the initial manifestations of AIDS.

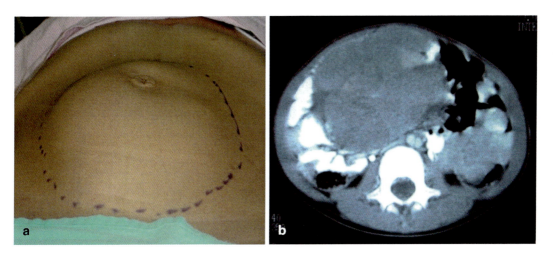

Fig. 58.7 A clinical photograph (**a**) and abdominal CT scan (**b**) of a child with abdominal Burkitt's lymphoma

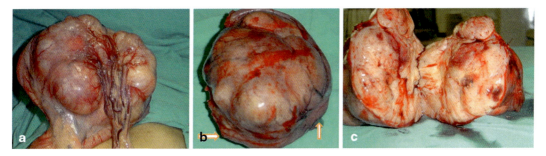

Fig. 58.8 a–c An intraoperative photograph showing a large abdominal Burkitt's lymphoma in the ileocecal region that was excised. Note the attached small intestines which were resected together with the tumor and the resected abdominal Burkitt's lymphoma that was opened

- There are many different types of NHL. These types can be divided into aggressive (fast-growing) and indolent (slow-growing) types, and they can be formed from either B cells or T cells.
- About 85 % of all malignant lymphomas are NHLs.
- Immune suppression is implicated in the pathogenesis of NHL, with a clear correlation between the degree of immune suppression and the risk of developing NHL.
- HIV-infected patients are at an increased risk for developing both Hodgkin's lymphoma and NHL when compared with the general population.
- The relative risk of NHL among HIV-infected patients is 150–250-fold higher than in the general population.
- The t (14; 18) (q32; q21) translocation is the most common chromosomal abnormality associated with NHL. This translocation occurs in 85 % of follicular lymphomas and 28 % of higher grade NHLs.
- Currently, several NHL classifications exist.
- The Working Formulation, originally proposed in 1982, classified and grouped lymphomas by morphology and clinical behavior (i.e., low, intermediate, or high grade).
- In the 1990s, the Revised European–American Lymphoma (REAL) classification attempted to apply immunophenotypic and genetic features in identifying distinct clinicopathologic NHL entities.

- The World Health Organization (WHO) classification. This classification divides NHL into those of B cell origin and those of T cell and natural killer (NK) cell origin. It lists more than 80 different forms of lymphomas in four broad groups.
- The treatment of NHL varies greatly, depending on tumor stage, grade, type, and patient factors (e.g., symptoms, age, performance status).

Recommended Reading

Leechawengwongs E, Shearer WT. Lymphoma complicating primary immunodeficiency syndromes. Curr Opin Hematol. 2012;19(4):305–12.

Ng AK, Mauch PM. Late effects of Hodgkin's disease and its treatment. Cancer J. 2009;15(2):164–8.

Voss SD, Chen L, Constine LS, Chauvenet A, Fitzgerald TJ, Kaste SC, Slovis T, Schwartz CL. Surveillance computed tomography imaging and detection of relapse in intermediate- and advanced-stage pediatric Hodgkin's lymphoma: a report from the Children's Oncology Group. J Clin Oncol. 2012;30(21):2635–40.

Wolden SL, Chen L, Kelly KM, Herzog P, Gilchrist GS, Thomson J, et al. Long-term results of CCG 5942: a randomized comparison of chemotherapy with and without radiotherapy for children with Hodgkin's Lymphoma—a report from the Children's Oncology Group. J Clin Oncol. 2012;30(26):3174–80.

Chapter 59
Neuroblastoma

Introduction

- Neuroblastoma is a malignant embryonal tumor of the sympathetic nervous system arising from neural-crest-derived neuroblasts.
- It is one of the small, blue, round cell tumors of childhood. Other such tumors include:
  - Ewing sarcoma
  - Non-Hodgkin lymphoma
  - Primitive neuroectodermal tumors
  - Rhabdomyosarcoma
- Neuroblastoma is the most common extracranial solid tumor in childhood and the most common intra-abdominal malignancy of infancy.
- It is considered the fourth most common malignancy of childhood, preceded by leukemias, central nervous system (CNS) tumors, and lymphomas.
- The incidence of neuroblastoma is approximately 1 out of 100,000 children and is slightly more common in boys.
- It comprises 6–10 % of all childhood cancers.
- Neuroblastoma is seen commonly in the first year of life, and some neuroblastoma cases are congenital. Only 10 % of neuroblastoma cases occur in children older than 5 years of age.
- A common site of occurrence is in the adrenal glands, but it can also develop in the neck, chest, abdomen, or pelvis.
- Neuroblastomas which arise from primordial neural crest cells (the sympathetic chain and the adrenal medulla) are called the peripheral neuroblastic tumors (a type of neurocristopathies). They have similar origins but show a wide pattern of differentiation ranging from the well-differentiated ganglioneuroma, the moderately differentiated ganglioneuroblastoma, and the malignant neuroblastoma.
- Neuroblastoma is known to demonstrate spontaneous regression from an undifferentiated tumor to a completely benign one.
- Neuroblastoma is a tumor exhibiting extreme heterogeneity and is divided into three risk groups: low, intermediate, and high. Low-risk tumor is most commonly seen in infants and has good prognosis, whereas high-risk tumor is difficult to treat successfully even with the most intensive multimodal therapies available.
- Neuroblastoma often spreads to other parts of the body before any symptoms are apparent (metastasis can be its first presenting symptom) and 50–60 % of all neuroblastomas present with metastases.

Sites of Origin

- Embryologically, during the fifth week of intrauterine life, primitive sympathetic neuroblasts migrate from the neural crest to the adrenal gland and along the entire sympathetic chain. Therefore, neuroblastoma can arise anywhere in the adrenal glands or along the sympathetic chain.
- The most common site for neuroblastoma to originate is in the abdominal cavity (65%). This includes the adrenal gland (40%) and paraspinal sympathetic ganglia (25%).
- Neuroblastoma can also develop anywhere along the sympathetic nervous system chain from the neck to the pelvis.
- Frequencies of neuroblastoma in different locations include:
  - Adrenal gland (40%).
  - Paraspinal sympathetic chain (25%).
  - Chest (15%).
  - Neck (3%).
  - Miscellaneous (12%).
  - Pelvis (5%).
  - In rare cases, no primary tumor can be identified.
- Infants more commonly present with thoracic and cervical neuroblastomas, whereas older children more frequently have abdominal tumors.

Etiology

- The etiology of neuroblastoma is not well understood.
- Some neuroblastomas however do run in families and have been linked genetically. Familial neuroblastoma is caused by a very rare germ line mutation in the anaplastic lymphoma kinase (ALK) gene.
- A deletion of the short arm of chromosome 1 is also found in 70–80% of all patients with neuroblastomas.

Clinical Features

- The signs and symptoms of neuroblastoma vary depending on the site affected.
- Sixty-five percent of primary neuroblastomas occur in the abdomen, with most of these occurring in the adrenal gland (Fig. 59.1).
- As a result, most children present with abdominal symptoms, such as fullness or distension. Typically, children with localized disease are asymptomatic, whereas those with disseminated neuroblastoma are generally sick and may have systemic manifestations, including weight loss, anorexia, and failure to thrive, fever, irritability, and bone pain.
- The most common finding in those with abdominal neuroblastoma is a nontender, firm, irregular abdominal mass that crosses the midline (Fig. 59.2).
- Most neuroblastomas produce catecholamines which result in interesting presentations in children with neuroblastoma.
- Kerner–Morrison syndrome is caused by vasoactive intestinal peptide (VIP) tumor secretion and is more commonly associated with ganglioneuroblastoma or ganglioneuroma. It causes intractable

Clinical Features

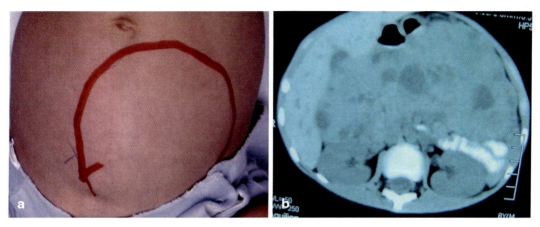

Fig. 59.1 a Clinical photograph in a patient with abdominal neuroblastoma. Note the mass crossing the midline. **b** Abdominal CT scan showing a large abdominal neuroblastoma crossing the midline

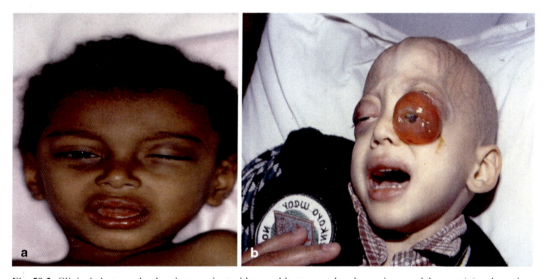

Fig. 59.2 Clinical photographs showing a patient with neuroblastoma and ecchymosis around the eyes (**a**) and a patient with neuroblastoma with metastasis to the retrobulbar area (**b**)

secretory diarrhea, resulting in hypovolemia, hypokalemia, and prostration. This syndrome typically resolves following the complete removal of the tumor.
- William Pepper in 1901 described a localized primary tumor and metastatic disease limited to the skin, liver, and bone marrow in infants. Pepper syndrome has since been associated with stage 4S neuroblastoma, a unique entity that occurs only in infants younger than 1 year. Pepper syndrome generally is associated with spontaneous regression. Some infants with stage 4S neuroblastoma, however, die of massive hepatomegaly, respiratory failure, and overwhelming sepsis.
- "Blueberry muffin" babies are infants in whom neuroblastoma has metastasized to subcutaneous sites. When provoked, the nodules become intensely red and subsequently blanch for several minutes thereafter. The response is probably secondary to the release of vasoconstrictive metabolic tumor by-products.
- Hutchinson syndrome results in bone pain with consequent limping and pathologic fractures. It results from widespread metastasis of neuroblastoma to the bones.

Fig. 59.3 Abdominal x-ray showing a large soft-tissue density occupying most of the abdomen

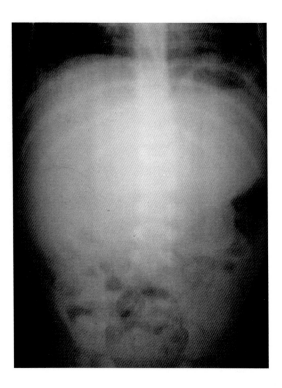

- Neuroblastomas that arise in the paraspinal ganglia may invade through the neural foramina, compress the spinal cord, and subsequently cause paralysis.
- Infrequently, neuroblastoma can become metastatic to the retrobulbar region, leading to rapidly progressive, unilateral, painless proptosis, periorbital edema, and ecchymosis of the upper lid ("raccoon eyes") (Fig. 59.2).

Investigations and Diagnosis

- Abdominal x-ray most commonly reveals a soft-tissue density and finely stippled calcifications (Fig. 59.3).
- Chest x-ray may show a soft-tissue density with fine calcification in the posterior mediastinum in cases of thoracic neuroblastoma (Fig. 59.4).
- Abdominal ultrasound is more informative regarding the site, consistency, and size of the mass.
- Abdominal and thoracic CT scan or MRI (for paraspinal tumors) provides more information about the mass, regional lymph nodes, invasion, and distant metastasis (Fig. 59.5).
- Bone scan and a skeletal survey detect cortical bone disease.
- Another way to detect neuroblastoma is the meta-iodobenzylguanidine (MIBG) scan, which is taken up by 90–95 % of neuroblastomas, often termed "mIBG-avid." MIBG scan which is a labeled isotope derivative of norepinephrine is quite sensitive and specific in the detection of metastasis to bones and soft tissue. MIBG is recommended for reassessment both during and after treatment of neuroblastoma.
- Recently, positron emission tomography (PET) scan has been used for the detection of non-MIBG avid disease and for follow-up of high risk cases.

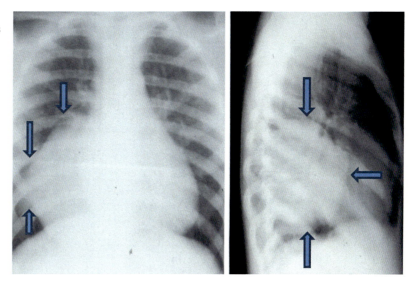

Fig. 59.4 Chest x-ray showing a soft-tissue mass in the posterior mediastinum in a patient with thoracic ganglioneuroma

- Ninety percent of neuroblastomas secrete elevated levels of catecholamines and their metabolites which include dopamine, homovanillic acid (HVA), and/or vanillylmandelic acid (VMA). These are found in the urine or blood.
- This fact becomes clinically relevant because children with undifferentiated tumors excrete higher levels of HVA than VMA. This occurs because undifferentiated tumors have lost the final enzymatic pathway that converts HVA to VMA. A low VMA-to-HVA ratio is consistent with a poorly differentiated tumor and indicative of a poor prognosis. HVA and VMA levels measured prior to treatment serve as markers and if elevated after the treatment indicates persistent disease or recurrence.
- Elevated levels of neuron-specific enolase (NSE), lactic dehydrogenase (LDH > 1000), and ferritin (> 150) are markers useful in the diagnosis of neuroblastoma as well as the prognosis.
- Approximately 96% of patients with metastatic neuroblastomas have an elevated NSE level, which has been associated with a poor prognosis.

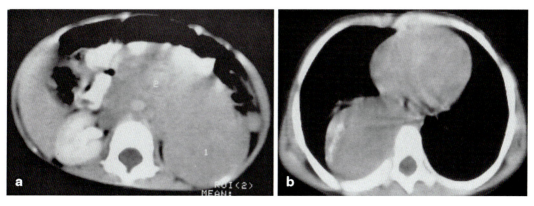

Fig. 59.5 a Abdominal CT scan showing a large abdominal mass arising from the left adrenal gland and crossing the midline. b Thoracic CT scan showing a ganglioneuroma in the posterior mediastinum. Note the presence of calcification in the mass

- Specific requirements to stage neuroblastoma include:
  1. Bilateral bone marrow aspirates and biopsy
  2. Abdominal and chest CT scan
  3. Bone scan
  4. MIBG scan

Recently, an international committee on neuroblastoma staging recommended obtaining two bone marrow aspirates and two biopsies, one from each posterior iliac crest.

- According to the International Neuroblastoma Staging System (INSS), the diagnosis of neuroblastoma is based on either:
  1. Characteristic histopathologic findings of neuroblastoma
  2. The presence of neuroblastoma cells in a bone marrow aspirate or biopsy sample
  3. Elevated levels of urinary catecholamine metabolic by-products
- The pretreatment tumor pathology is an important prognostic factor, along with age at diagnosis and mitosis-karyorrhexis index (MKI).
- The neuroblastoma pathological classification system was established in 1999 and revised in 2003 by the International Neuroblastoma Pathology Committee (INPC, also called Shimada system) which describes "favorable" and "unfavorable" neuroblastoma.

Biological markers and their importance in prognosis of neuroblastoma:

1. Age: The younger the age the better the prognosis.
2. DNA index: The DNA index refers to the amount of DNA within the nucleus when compared to the normal amount (diploid). Hyperdiploidy (DNA index > 1) correlate with a lower stage at presentation, better response to chemotherapy, and improved prognosis.
3. N-myc: This is an oncogene found on chromosome 2p. Amplification and over expression of the gene is associated with poor prognosis.
4. NGF (nerve growth factor) and its receptor tyrosine kinase (TRK): TRK is a transmembrane protein which is involved in cellular differentiation and apoptosis. There are three subtypes: TRK-A, TRK-B, and TRK-C. Expression of TRK-A on the cell correlates with good prognosis, younger age, and tumor regression. TRK-B expression is associated with poor outcome while TRK-C is associated with good prognosis.
5. Chromosome 1p: Loss of heterozygosity and deletion of chromosome 1p is associated with poor prognosis.
6. Chromosome 17: Gain in the region of 17q more specifically in the surviving gene area correlate with poor prognosis.

Staging

The INSS was established in 1986 and revised in 1988. The staging is based on neuroblastoma anatomical presence at diagnosis as follows:

- Stage 1: Localized tumor confined to the area of origin.
- Stage 2A: Unilateral tumor with incomplete gross resection, identifiable ipsilateral, and contralateral lymph node negative for tumor.

- Stage 2B: Unilateral tumor with complete or incomplete gross resection, with ipsilateral lymph node positive for tumor, and identifiable contralateral lymph node negative for tumor.
- Stage 3: Tumor infiltrating across midline with or without regional lymph node involvement or unilateral tumor with contralateral lymph node involvement or midline tumor with bilateral lymph node involvement.
- Stage 4: Dissemination of tumor to distant lymph nodes, bone marrow, bone, liver, or other organs except as defined by stage 4S.
- Stage 4S: Age <1-year-old with localized primary tumor as defined in stage 1 or 2, with dissemination limited to liver, skin, or bone marrow (<10% of nucleated bone marrow cells are tumors). Stage 4S is the most unusual group, comprising approximately 5% of patients with neuroblastoma.

The new International Neuroblastoma Risk Group (INRG) classifies neuroblastoma at diagnosis based on a new International Neuroblastoma Risk Group Staging System (INRGSS):

- Stage L1: Localized disease without image-defined risk factors
- Stage L2: Localized disease with image-defined risk factors
- Stage M: Metastatic disease
- Stage MS: Metastatic disease "special" where MS is equivalent to stage 4 S
- The new risk assignment for neuroblastoma is based on:

  1. The new INRGSS staging system
  2. Age (< or >18 months)
  3. Tumor grade
  4. N-myc amplification
  5. Unbalanced 11q aberration
  6. Ploidy

This divides neuroblastoma into four pretreatment risk groups: very low, intermediate, and high risk.

- There are three distinct histological patterns of the neurocristopathies:
  - Neuroblastoma.
  - Ganglioneuroblastoma.
  - Ganglioneuroma.
- They represent a spectrum of maturation and dedifferentiation. The typical neuroblastoma is characterized by small uniform cells that contain dense hyperchromatic nuclei and scanty cytoplasm.
- A neuritic process called neuropil is pathognomonic of all except the most primitive neuroblastoma.
- Homer-Wright pseudorosettes are clusters of neuroblasts surrounding areas of eosinophilic neuropil and are observed in 15–50% of neuroblastomas. If identified, they are diagnostic of neuroblastoma (Fig. 59.6).

Treatment and Outcome

- The primary goals of surgery are:
  1. To determine an accurate diagnosis
  2. To completely remove the primary tumor
  3. To provide accurate surgical staging
  4. To offer adjuvant therapy for delayed primary surgery
  5. To remove residual disease with second-look surgery

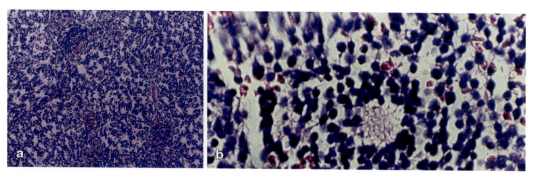

Fig. 59.6 Histopathology of neuroblastoma showing small uniform cells that contain dense hyperchromatic nuclei and scanty cytoplasm (**a**) and also uniform small cells with dense hyperchromatic nuclei (**b**). Note also the pseudorosettes

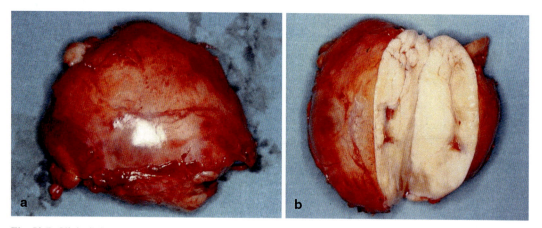

Fig. 59.7 Clinical photograph of a resected ganglioneuroma. Note the fleshy cut section

- Neuroblastoma is a very complex tumor with different types and variable behavior. At one end there are benign tumors that may resolve spontaneously, while at the other end are aggressive tumors with an average survival rate of 40%.
- When the lesion is localized, it is generally curable (Fig. 59.7).
- The long-term survival for children with advanced disease and older than 18 months of age is poor despite aggressive multimodal therapy (intensive chemotherapy, surgery, radiation therapy, stem cell transplant, differentiation agent isotretinoin also called 13-*cis*-retinoic acid, and frequent immunotherapy with anti-GD2 monoclonal antibody therapy) (Fig. 59.8).
- Biologic and genetic characteristics have been identified to classify patients with neuroblastoma into low-, intermediate-, and high-risk groups for planning treatment. These criteria include:

  1. The age of the patient at diagnosis
  2. The extent of disease spread
  3. The microscopic appearance
  4. The genetic features including DNA ploidy
  5. The N-myc oncogene amplification

Fig. 59.8 Abdominal CT scan of a patient with advanced neuroblastoma

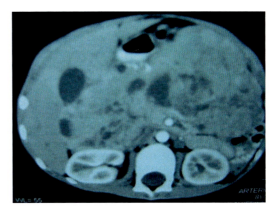

- The therapies for these different risk groups are different.
  1. Low-risk groups can frequently be observed without any treatment at all or cured with surgery alone.
  2. The intermediate-risk group is treated with surgery and chemotherapy.
  3. The high-risk group is treated with intensive chemotherapy, surgery, radiation therapy, bone marrow/hematopoietic stem cell transplantation, biological-based therapy with 13-*cis*-retinoic acid (isotretinoin or Accutane), and antibody therapy usually administered with the cytokines granulocyte macrophage colony-stimulating factor (GM-CSF) and interleukin (IL)-2.
- With current treatments, patients with low- and intermediate-risk disease have an excellent prognosis with cure rates above 90% for low risk and 70–90% for intermediate risk.
- In contrast, therapy for high-risk neuroblastoma resulted in cures in only about 30%.
- The addition of antibody therapy has improved survival rates for high-risk neuroblastoma but they continue to have poor outcomes despite intensive therapy.
- Unfortunately, approximately 70–80% of patients older than 18 months present with metastatic disease, usually in the lymph nodes, liver, bone, and bone marrow. Less than half of these patients are cured, even with the use of intensive therapy followed by autologous bone marrow or stem cell transplant.
- Patients whose tumors have N-myc amplification tend to have rapid tumor progression and a poor prognosis. This is even in those with other favorable factors such as low-stage or 4S neuroblastoma.
- In contrast to N-myc amplification expression of the H-ras oncogene correlates with lower stages of the disease.
- Deletion of the short arm of chromosome 1 is the most common chromosomal abnormality seen in neuroblastoma and carries a poor prognosis.
- DNA index is another factor that correlates with response to therapy in infants. Infants whose neuroblastoma have hyperdiploidy (i.e., DNA index > 1) have a good therapeutic response. In contrast, infants whose tumors have a DNA index of 1 are less responsive and require more aggressive therapy. DNA index does not have any prognostic significance in older children.
- The 5-year survival rate in patients with stage-4S disease is 75%.
- Infants with disseminated neuroblastoma have favorable outcomes when treated with combined chemotherapy and surgery. In contrast, children older than 1 year with high-stage neuroblastoma have very poor survival rates despite intensive multimodal therapy.

Recommended Reading

Brodeur GM, Pritchard J, Berthold F, Carlsen NL, Castel V, Castelberry RP, et al. Revisions of the international criteria for neuroblastoma diagnosis, staging, and response to treatment. J Clin Oncol. 1993;11(8):1466–77.

Haase GM, Perez C, Atkinson JB. Current aspects of biology, risk assessment, and treatment of neuroblastoma. Semin Surg Oncol. 1999;16(2):91–104.

Maris JM, Hogarty MD, Bagatell R, Cohn SL. Neuroblastoma. Lancet. 2007;369(9579):2106–20.

Matthay KK, Villablanca JG, Seeger RC, Stram DO, Harris RE, Ramsay NJ, et al. Treatment of high-risk neuroblastoma with intensive chemotherapy, radiotherapy, autologous bone marrow transplantation, and 13-cis-retinoic acid. Children's Cancer Group. N Engl J Med. 1999;341(16):1165–73.

Matthay KK, Reynolds CP, Seeger RC, Shimada H, Adkins ES, Haas-Kogan D, et al. Long-term results for children with high-risk neuroblastoma treated on a randomized trial of myeloablative therapy followed by 13-cis-retinoic acid: a children's oncology group study. J Clin Oncol. 2009;27(7):1007–13.

Schmidt ML, Lal A, Seeger RC, Maris JM, Shimada H, O'Leary M, et al. Favorable prognosis for patients 12 to 18 months of age with stage 4 nonamplified MYCN neuroblastoma: a Children's Cancer Group Study. J Clin Oncol. 2005;23(27):6474–80.

Chapter 60
Ovarian Cysts and Tumors

Introduction

- Ovarian tumors are relatively rare in the pediatric age group.
- They make up 1.5% of all childhood malignancies.
- Although rare, they can be malignant and lethal.
- They represent a range of pathologies ranging from highly aggressive malignant tumors to benign cysts.
- In the pediatric age group, ovarian tumors may be one of three:

  1. Physiologic cysts
  2. Benign tumors
  3. Malignant neoplasms

- Epithelial cysts and benign teratomas are the most common benign tumors and germ cell tumors are the most common malignant tumors.
- The most common ovarian tumor is the germ cell tumor (60–85% of ovarian neoplasms in the pediatric age group).
- Treatment of all ovarian malignancies involves salpingo-oophorectomy. For complete staging of ovarian malignant tumors, omentectomy, lymph node sampling, and peritoneal washing is recommended.
- Patients with malignant germ cell tumors in addition to surgery are treated with chemotherapy. This is cisplatin-based chemotherapy and proved to be very effective.
- Ovarian tumors are also classified according to the origin of their cellular components into:

  – Germ cell tumors
  – Surface epithelial cell tumors
  – Sex cord stromal tumors

Germ Cell Tumors

- Are the most common type in children and among these, the most common is the teratoma.
- These include:

  1. Teratomas
  2. Dysgerminomas
  3. Yolk sac tumors
  4. Choriocarcinomas

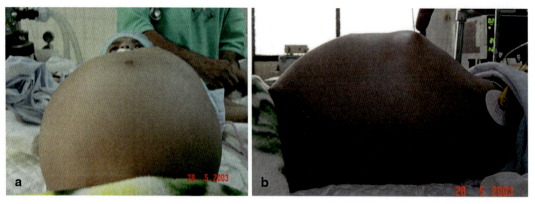

Fig. 60.1 a and **b** Clinical photographs showing a very large ovarian teratoma causing marked abdominal distension

Fig. 60.2 CT scan of the abdomen and pelvis showing a huge mass occupying most of the abdomen

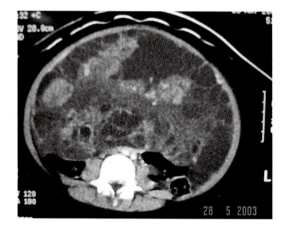

Ovarian Teratoma

- Teratomas are the most common germ cell tumors.
- Ovarian teratomas have a potential for malignancy and this is found more commonly in solid teratomas. Solid teratomas, however, are less common than the cystic variety.
- Teratomas commonly present in adolescent females and usually grow to a large size, large enough to twist and produce abdominal pain (Fig. 60.1).
- Teratomas are usually benign tumors. They have a characteristic appearance and teeth, bone, and hair are found inside the tumor.
- They are subdivided into mature teratomas, which are benign, or immature teratomas which may be either malignant or benign (Figs. 60.2 and 60.3).
- Most benign teratomas are composed of mature cells, but 20–30% also contain immature elements, most often neuroepithelium.
- The tumors may be picked up on plain film due to the presence of calcification in two-thirds of teratomas (Fig. 60.4).

Introduction

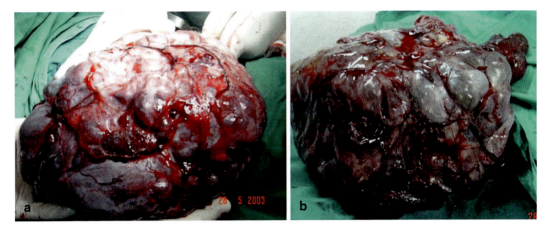

Fig. 60.3 a and b Intraoperative photographs showing a large ovarian tumor which turned out to be an immature ovarian teratoma

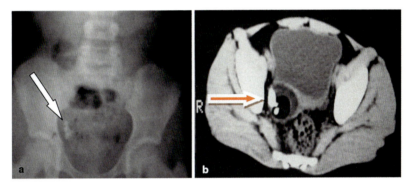

Fig. 60.4 Abdominal x-ray (**a**) and CT scan (**b**) showing pelvic calcification in an ovarian teratoma

Malignant Germ Cell Tumor

These tumors include:

1. Yolk sac tumors
2. Choriocarcinoma
3. Immature tearatomas

Benign Cystic Teratomas (Dermoid Cysts)

- This is the most common benign ovarian tumor in childhood and is composed of mature, well-differentiated tissue.
- Approximately 10% are bilateral (Fig. 60.5).

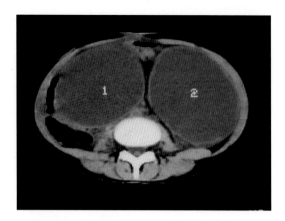

Fig. 60.5 CT scan showing bilateral ovarian cysts

- About 50% will have a calcification visible on x-ray.
- The average age of patients with benign ovarian teratomas is 12 years.
- These teratomas tend to undergo torsion.
- Dermoid cysts are normally treated with oophorectomy.

Dysgerminoma

- The second most common ovarian tumor in children after the teratoma.
- It is the most common malignant ovarian tumor in children and adolescents.
- The tumor is typically low-grade and on imaging it is solid, smooth, and well encapsulated.
- Of the dysgerminomas, 20% are bilateral.
- Usually grow to a large size before diagnosis.
- Dysgerminomas are usually nonfunctioning tumors.
- These tumors can spread locally and are known to be very radiosensitive.
- They have a good prognosis with >90% survival.

Rhabdomyosarcoma

- It is the most common soft tissue sarcoma in children and a frequent cause of death.
- Roughly 10% of all solid tumors in childhood are Rhabdomyosarcomas.
- These tumors are extremely malignant and tend to invade locally and metastases by hematogenous and through lymphatic routes.
- Without treatment, 90% of patients die within 1 year of diagnosis.
- Rhabdomyosarcomas occur equally in males and females and are seen in two age peaks at 4–6 years and 16–18 years of age.
- The different histologic types that can be seen in a rhabdomyosarcoma include alveolar, embryonal, embryonal-botryoid, pleomorphic, and undifferentiated.
- Among these types, the alveolar variety has the worst prognosis.
- The botryoides type has the classic grape-like appearance.
- Rhabdomyosarcomas most commonly originate from the pelvis and genitourinary tract (40%).

Introduction

Ovarian Carcinomas

- Are unusual in pediatric age group. It accounts for only 1 % of all tumors in girls below the age of 17 years.
- Tumor markers: CA 125 serology in these tumors has only 78.1 % sensitivity and 76.8 % specificity but it is useful in identifying recurrent or residual disease.
- Ultrasonography usually shows a solid, cystic, or mixed tumor as well as evidence of metastasis to the liver or retroperitoneal lymph nodes.
- Computed tomography (CT) scan is more useful in showing the extent of tumor, exact origin of tumor, lymph node status, and peritoneal and liver metastasis.
- Bone scan: for detection of metastasis.
- Histopathological classification: serous, mucinous, and undifferentiated.
- Surgery is done to confirm the diagnosis, stage the disease, and achieve tumor clearance in early stages and cytoreduction in late cases.
- Chemotherapy: cisplatin, cyclophosphamide, carboplatin, bleomycin, etoposide, and paclitaxel in various combinations.
- Prognosis depends on stage of the disease and histology, but the prognosis in premenarchal girls appears to be poor.

Ovarian Cysts

- Ovarian cysts are common and frequently seen on prenatal ultrasound examination. They result as a response to maternal and placental hormones, and usually spontaneously involute.
- Up to 30 % of female fetuses have ovarian cysts measuring >1 cm in diameter on prenatal ultrasound, but only 1 in 100,000 female neonates demonstrate ovarian cysts postnatally.
- Approximately half of these simple cysts are follicular cysts and half are lutein cysts. Some are infracted cysts and difficult to classify.
- Ovarian cysts are the most common ovarian mass in adolescents.
- Neonatal ovarian cysts have almost no risk of malignancy.
- Neonatal ovarian cysts are divided depending on:
    1. The size of the cyst (<5 cm vs. >5 cm)
    2. The characterization of the cyst (simple vs. complex)
- Small (<5 cm) simple asymptomatic cysts are treated conservatively.
- Complex cysts of any size and large (>5 cm) simple cysts require intervention (Fig. 60.6).

All complex ovarian cysts, regardless of size, should be surgically removed because of possible torsion or neoplasm.

- The complex cysts often represent an ovarian torsion with hemorrhage or, on rare occasion, are cystic structures that originate from other intrabdominal structures (intestinal duplication, omental cyst).
- The large simple cysts require treatment to avoid the increased risk of ovarian torsion and hemorrhage. Either limited laparotomy or laparoscopy can be used to confirm the diagnosis and decompress the cyst without sacrificing ovarian tissue (Figs. 60.7, 60.8, 60.9, and 60.10).
- Ovarian tissue should be preserved if possible, and sometimes enucleation is possible but at other times oophorectomy or salpingo-oophorectomy is the treatment of choice.
- Ovarian cysts that have twisted or ruptured have been reported to be a cause of neonatal ascites.

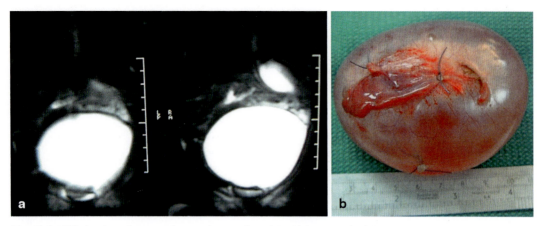

Fig. 60.6 MRI showing a large ovarian cyst in a newborn (**a**) which was excised (**b**)

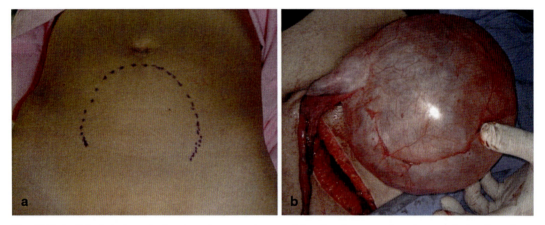

Fig. 60.7 A clinical photograph showing a large ovarian cyst (**a**) and an intraoperative photograph showing a large ovarian cyst (**b**)

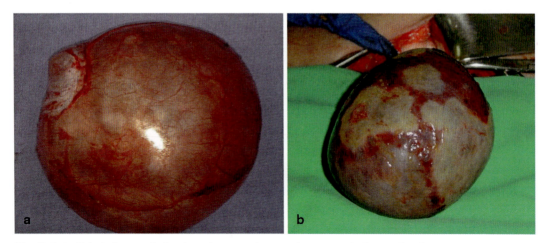

Fig. 60.8 A clinical photograph showing a large ovarian cyst that was excised (**a**) and an intraoperative photograph showing a large ovarian cyst with hemorrhage into it (**b**)

Introduction

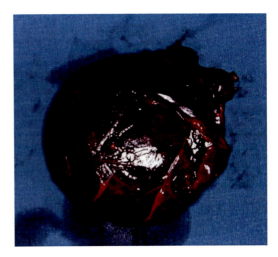

Fig. 60.9 A clinical photograph showing an ovarian cyst with spontaneous hemorrhage that was excised

- Ovarian masses in prepubertal girls must be evaluated and treated as potential malignant lesions. Functional cysts are very uncommon in this age group.
- In the post- and peri-menarchal girls, ovarian cysts are common, and treatment is determined by the size and characterization of the cyst. These cysts are usually either follicular or corpus luteum cysts. Follicular cysts are the most common type, and should be considered abnormal if they are >2 cm in diameter.
- A normal physiologic follicle may be up to 2 cm in size. Corpus luteum cysts develop after ovulation and are lined with lutenized theca and granulose cells. These cysts often have a hemorrhagic appearance.
- In the postmenarchal girl, a unilocular cyst <5 cm in diameter does not require surgical intervention and should be followed-up by ultrasound examination in 6–8 weeks.
- Larger simple cysts and complex cysts should be considered potentially malignant, and evaluated and treated accordingly.

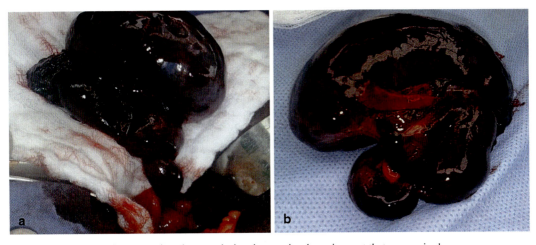

Fig. 60.10 a and b An intraoperative photograph showing a twisted ovarian cyst that was excised

- Epithelial ovarian tumors make up a greater percentage of the ovarian tumors (33%) in girls 15–17 years of age. Prior to surgical excision of ovarian masses in this age range, tumor markers should be measured preoperatively. These include alpha-fetoprotein, beta HCG, and CA 125 levels.
- Other benign ovarian tumors include cyst adenomas, fibromas, thecomas, para-ovarian cysts, infarcted unidentifiable tissue, and lipid cell tumors.

Recommended Reading

Amies Oelschlager AM, Sawin R. Teratomas and ovarian lesions in children. Surg Clin North Am. 2012;92(3):599–613, viii.

Brandt ML, Helmrath MA. Ovarian cysts in infants and children. Semin Pediatr Surg. 2005;14:78–85.

Hayes-Jordan A. Surgical management of the incidentally identified ovarian mass. Semin Pediatr Surg. 2005;14:106–10.

Tajiri T, Souzaki R, Kinoshita Y, Yosue R, Kohashi K, Oda Y, Taguchi T. Surgical intervention strategies for pediatric ovarian tumors: experience with 60 cases at one institution. Pediatr Surg Int. 2012;28(1):27–31.

Templeman CL, Fallat ME. Benign ovarian masses. Semin Pediatr Surg. 2005;14:93–9.

VonAllmen D. Malignant lesions of the ovary in childhood. Semin Pediatr Surg. 2005;14:100–5.

Yang C, Wang S, Li CC, Zhang J, Kong XR, Ouyang J. Ovarian germ cell tumors in children: a 20-year retrospective study in a single institution. Eur J Gynaecol Oncol. 2011;32(3):289–92.

Chapter 61
Pediatric Liver Tumors

Introduction

- Liver tumors may be either benign or malignant.
- The liver is the third most common organ for intra-abdominal tumors in children, following neuroblastoma and Wilms tumor.
- The incidence of primary malignant liver tumors per year is about 1–1.5 per million children.
- Liver tumors account for 1.3 % of all pediatric malignancies.
- Hepatoblastoma and hepatocellular carcinoma are the most common tumors and account for two-thirds of all hepatic neoplasms.
- Benign liver tumors include:
  - Hemangiomas
  - Hemangioendothelioma
  - Mesenchymal hamartomas
  - Hepatic adenoma
  - Focal nodular hyperplasia

Presentation of liver tumors:

- Abdominal distension
- A palpable abdominal mass
- Anemia
- Thrombocytopenia
- Leukocytosis
- Weight loss
- Fever
- Anorexia

Investigations

- Complete blood count (CBC), electrolytes, liver function tests, and alpha-fetoprotein levels
- Alpha-fetoprotein is a valuable marker in children
- Alpha-fetoprotein levels are elevated in 50–70 % of children with hepatic neoplasms
- Abdominal ultrasound to determine the site and consistency of the tumor

- Computed tomography (CT) scan and magnetic resonance imaging (MRI) of the chest and abdomen
  - These are valuable to localize the site, extent, consistency, and multiplicity of the lesions
  - To detect metastases
  - To facilitate surgical planning and determine resectability
- The definitive diagnosis of liver tumors can be proven only by a biopsy

Classification

Benign Tumors

- They represent 30% of hepatic tumors and include:
  - Hemangiomas
  - Hemangioendotheliomas
  - Mesenchymal hamartomas
  - Focal nodular hyperplasia
  - Hepatic adenoma

Malignant Tumors

- Malignant tumors represent 70% of hepatic tumors and include:
  - Hepatoblastoma: The most common primary malignant hepatic tumor in childhood, accounting for 43% of all pediatric liver tumors
  - Hepatocellular carcinoma: Accounts for 23% of pediatric hepatic malignancies
  - Other primary liver tumors include:
    - Undifferentiated sarcoma
    - Biliary rhabdomyosarcoma
    - Angiosarcoma
    - Rhabdoid tumors

Hepatic Hemangiomas

- Hemangiomas are the most common benign liver tumors in children.
- Commonly, they occur within the first 6 months of life.
- They are made up of endothelial-lined vascular spaces and vary from small, incidentally found masses to large cavernous hemangiomas.
- Hemangioendothelioma is considered a subtype of hemangioma that is typically found in infants.
- Hemangioendothelioma is more common in females, with a female-to-male ratio of 4.3:1 to 2:1.

Clinical Features

- Most hepatic hemangiomas are discovered incidentally during radiological evaluation.
- Infants generally present with abdominal distension.

- Associated cutaneous hemangiomas are present in 10% of hepatic hemangioma cases.
- About 50% of infants with hepatic hemangiomas have high-output cardiac failure at their initial presentation.
- Large hepatic hemangiomas may lead to consumptive coagulopathy (Kasabach–Merritt syndrome). They may present with hemorrhage and respiratory distress.

Investigations

- Abdominal ultrasound, CT scan, or magnetic resonance imaging (MRI) is used to localize the site and size of the tumor.
- CBC may reveal anemia.
- Liver function tests may show elevated aspartate transaminase levels and hyperbilirubinemia.
- Occasionally, alpha-fetoprotein level is elevated.
- Low platelet count suggests consumptive coagulopathy (Kasabach–Merritt syndrome).
- Hypothyroidism has been observed in large tumors secondary to antibodies to thyroid-stimulating hormone.

Treatment

- The natural history for hemangiomas is spontaneous regression in the first 2 years of life; however, treatment is required if cardiac failure or platelet consumption occurs.
- Several treatment options are available:
  - High-dose corticosteroids (3–5 mg/kg/d) are administered for 3–5 weeks
  - Diuretics and digitalis to improve the cardiac function in cases of heart failure
  - Correction of anemia and thrombocytopenia
  - Daily subcutaneous administration of α-interferon (3 million U/m^2/kg) may lead to involution of hemangiomas
- Other treatment options include:
  - Aminocaproic acid
  - Vincristine
  - Cyclophosphamide
  - Aminocaproic acid may be used in addition to cryoprecipitate to ameliorate the coagulopathy associated with Kasabach–Merritt syndrome

Surgical Therapy

- Focal hemangiomas can be treated with complete surgical excision or with selective hepatic artery embolization.
- Operative ligation of the hepatic artery can also be used to decrease shunting through the hemangioma, with subsequent improvement in cardiac output.
  - Radiation therapy is usually avoided because angiosarcomatous degeneration of benign hemangiomas following radiation has been reported.
  - Rarely, liver transplantation may be indicated for diffuse hemangioma that is unresponsive to steroid and interferon therapy.

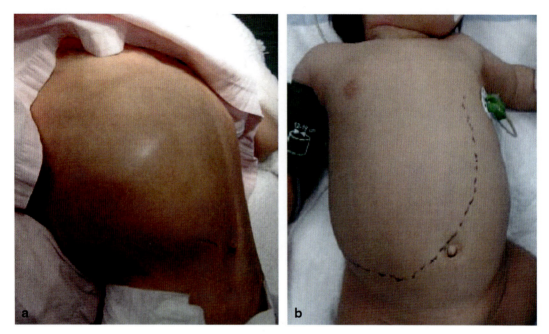

Fig. 61.1 a and **b** Clinical photographs showing large abdominal mass due to mesenchymal hamartoma

Mesenchymal Hamartomas

- Mesenchymal hamartomas are rare, comprising about 6% of liver tumors in children.
- They are typically diagnosed in children younger than 2 years of age.
- They usually grow during the first few months of life, then may stabilize, grow, or regress.
- Mesenchymal hamartomas are more commonly seen in the right lobe of the liver.
- They are often multicystic, heterogeneous, and confined to one lobe of the liver, more commonly the right lobe.

Presentation, Investigation, and Treatment

- Mesenchymal hamartomas are usually asymptomatic.
- They present as a palpable abdominal mass (Fig. 61.1).
- Alpha-fetoprotein level may be elevated.
- Abdominal X-ray may show calcification (Fig. 61.2).
- Abdominal CT scan and MRI reveal a well-circumscribed, multilocular cystic mass with solid septae and stroma (Fig. 61.3).
- Enucleation and marsupialization of the mass are treatment options.
- Complete surgical excision with a rim of normal liver tissue is the treatment of choice (Figs. 61.4 and 61.5).
- There are reports of sarcoma and hepatoblastoma arising from mesenchymal hamartoma.
- Mesenchymal hamartomas have a tendency to recur, which makes complete excision the treatment of choice.

Classification

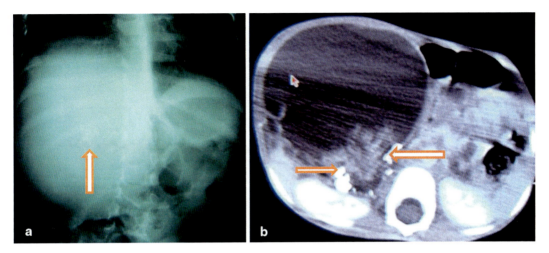

Fig. 61.2 Abdominal X-ray showing a soft tissue density mass with calcification (**a**) and abdominal CT scan showing a large liver tumor with calcification (**b**)

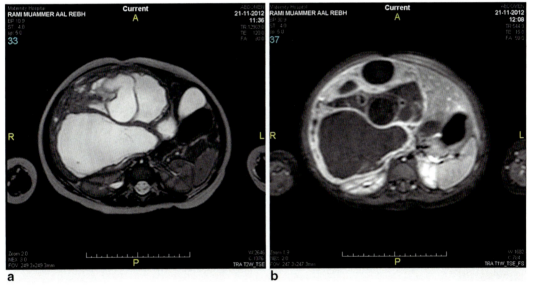

Fig. 61.3 **a** and **b** Abdominal MRI showing multicystic liver tumor

Focal Nodular Hyperplasia and Hepatic Adenomas

- Focal nodular hyperplasia and hepatic adenomas are rarely seen in children.
- Both of these benign tumors have an association with high estrogen and frequently occur in adolescent girls.
- Hepatic adenomas are associated with oral contraceptive use.
- Usually, they are asymptomatic or cause nonspecific symptoms including abdominal pain and mass (Fig. 61.6).
- A characteristic central scar on CT scan is pathognomonic for focal nodular hyperplasia.

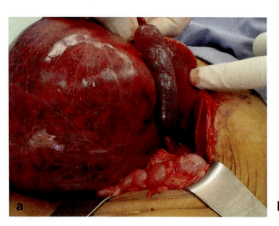 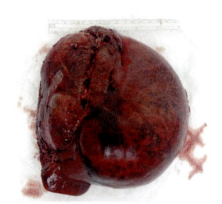

Fig. 61.4 Intraoperative photograph showing a large liver tumor arising from the right lobe of the liver (**a**) and a clinical photograph showing a large mesenchymal hamartoma after total excision (**b**)

Fig. 61.5 A clinical photograph showing a large liver mesenchymal hamartoma. Note the multiple cysts

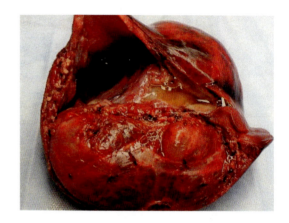

- A three-phase CT scan is the investigation of choice to make the diagnosis of focal nodular hyperplasia.
- A technetium sulfur colloid scan is used to differentiate focal nodular hyperplasia from adenomas. This reveals uniform uptake by focal nodular hyperplasia.
- Open liver biopsy may be required for definitive diagnosis.
- Focal nodular hyperplasia has no malignant potential and is often asymptomatic.
- Many surgeons advocate elective resection of focal nodular hyperplasia to prevent spontaneous rupture and hemorrhage (Fig. 61.6).
- Other surgeons advocate follow-up of these patients with serial ultrasounds.
- If the lesions are symptomatic or rapidly enlarging, complete surgical resection, embolization, or hepatic artery ligation may be used for treatment.
- Hepatic adenomas are treated with complete surgical excision because these lesions have a small risk for:
  - Spontaneous rupture
  - Hemorrhage
  - Malignant transformation to hepatocellular carcinoma

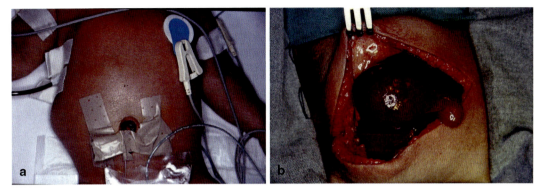

Fig. 61.6 Clinical (**a**) and intraoperative (**b**) photographs showing focal nodular hyperplasia of the liver which was resected

Hepatocellular Carcinoma

- Hepatocellular carcinoma is rare in children and accounts for 23 % of pediatric hepatic malignancies.
- Hepatocellular carcinoma typically presents in two incidence peaks:
  - The first is at age 0–4 years
  - The second is at age 10–14 years
- Predisposing conditions include:
  - Hepatic fibrosis and cirrhosis secondary to:
    - Metabolic liver disease
    - Viral hepatitis
    - Extrahepatic biliary atresia
    - Total parenteral nutrition
    - Chemotherapy-induced liver fibrosis
- Patients with hepatocellular carcinoma typically present with abdominal pain caused by the large size of the tumor.
- Associated weight loss, anemia, and fever may also be present.
- Hepatocellular carcinoma, when compared with hepatoblastoma, tends to have multiple lesions, more intravascular spread, and metastases.
- Liver function test findings are routinely elevated.
- Alpha-fetoprotein level is elevated in approximately half of the cases.
- Metastases usually occur in the lung and lymph nodes.
- More than 70 % of hepatocellular carcinomas are considered unresectable at the time of presentation and, unlike hepatoblastoma, respond poorly to chemotherapy.
- Combination chemotherapy has been used to treat patients with hepatocellular carcinoma but has been largely ineffective.
- Complete surgical resection or transplantation is often the only chance for cure.
- Newer therapeutic strategies have included chemoembolization, intra-arterial chemotherapy, and intraoperative cryotherapy.
- The overall survival rate of hepatocellular carcinoma remains poor, with a 41 % disease-free survival rate at 2 years and a 27 % disease-free survival rate at a longer follow-up interval.
- Children with initially resectable hepatocellular carcinoma have a much better prognosis than those who present with advanced or disseminated disease.

Fig. 61.7 CT scan showing multiple secondaries in a patient with Wilms tumor

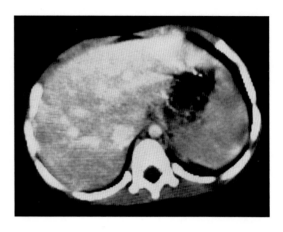

Hepatic Metastases

- Hepatic metastases are more common in children than primary tumors and may arise from various primary malignancies including:
  - Neuroblastoma
  - Wilms tumor (Fig. 61.7)
  - Rhabdomyosarcoma
  - Rhabdoid tumor
  - Non-Hodgkin lymphoma
  - Adrenal cortical carcinoma
- The role of surgical resection of these tumors is limited.
- Current criteria for resection of hepatic metastases include:
  - Control of the primary tumor
  - A solitary or limited number of metastases
  - A reasonable expectation of prolonged survival

Surgical considerations for hepatic tumors:

- Complete surgical resection is the treatment of choice of malignant hepatic tumors.
- Only 20% of the liver is necessary to maintain hepatic function; thus, postoperative insufficiency is rare.
- Start with adequate imaging studies to ensure resectability.
- Doppler ultrasonography and MRI provide valuable information regarding the vascular and biliary anatomy.
- The PRETEXT system was developed by the International Society of Pediatric Oncology on Childhood Liver Tumors (SIOPEL) group to identify suitable candidates for primary resection.
- Resection is typically performed through a bilateral subcostal incision, and, occasionally, a right thoracoabdominal approach is necessary for large lesions arising high in the right lobe.
- Intraoperative ultrasonography has been widely applied to determine the exact location of the tumor relative to the vessels.
- Once deemed resectable, the resection is marked out.
- Unresectability is usually determined by:
  - Involvement of hilar structures
  - Involvement of all hepatic veins

- Multicentricity
- Invasion of inferior vena cava or portal vein
- Centrally located tumors

- The most frequently performed procedure is a right hepatectomy (60%) because hepatoblastomas occur three times more often in the right lobe than in the left.
- Right hepatic lobectomy:
  - The gallbladder is dissected and cholecystectomy is performed.
  - The hilar plate is divided, exposing the bifurcation of the hepatic artery and portal vein.
  - The right hepatic artery and portal vein are ligated and divided.
  - The right hepatic vein is identified, ligated, and divided before any division of the hepatic parenchyma.
  - The hepatic parenchyma is divided using various measures.
  - In an extended right hepatectomy, the middle hepatic vein is ligated and segment 4 is resected. At completion, only segments 2 and 3 and the caudate lobe remain.
- Left hepatic lobectomy:
  - This begins the same way as right hepatic lobectomy, with cholecystectomy, division of the left hepatic artery and left branch of the portal vein.
  - The left and middle hepatic veins are identified after dissection through the sinus venosus.
  - The liver is then transected after vascular isolation of the resected segments.
  - An extended left hepatectomy includes removal of all or most of segments 5 and 8.
- Major intraoperative complications include:
  - Hemorrhage
  - Air embolism
  - Tumor embolus
  - Bile duct injury
- Postoperative complications include:
  - Hemorrhage
  - Bile leak
  - Abscess formation
  - Pulmonary complications
- Postoperative care consists of:
  - Adequate fluid replacement.
  - Intravenous albumin supplementation.
  - Vitamin K.
  - Clotting factors for the first 3–4 days.
  - The liver function test results generally normalize within the first 2 weeks, and hepatic insufficiency is rare.
- Postoperative monitoring consists of:
  - Frequent ultrasonography
  - Chest radiography
  - Serial alpha-fetoprotein level measurements

- Orthotopic liver transplantation:
  - This was first described in 1968 by Starzl.
  - Indications for liver transplantation:
    - The main indication for liver transplantation is nonmetastatic, unresectable lesions.
    - Hepatoblastoma now constitutes an indication for 3% of all pediatric liver transplantations.
    - Hepatocellular carcinoma.
    - Benign tumors such as diffuse hepatic hemangiomas.
  - The survival rate after liver transplantation in children with hepatoblastoma and hepatocellular carcinoma has been reported as 91% at 1 and 5 years and 82% at 14 years, respectively.
  - More generally, the 5-year survival rate for patients transplanted for hepatoblastoma is 70%.
- The survival rate following liver transplantation for hepatoblastoma and hepatocellular carcinoma with 1-, 5-, and 10-year survival of 79, 69, and 66% for hepatoblastoma, respectively, and 86, 63, and 58% for hepatocellular carcinoma, respectively. The primary cause of death for both groups was metastatic disease.
- Liver transplantation for hepatic hemangioma has a 1-, 5-, and 10-year patient survival rates of 93, 83, and 72%, respectively.
- Early failure of liver transplant (<30 days) is usually due to vascular complications or primary nonfunction.
- Late failure is usually a result of:
  - Infection
  - Posttransplant lymphoproliferative disease
  - Chronic rejection
  - Biliary complications
  - Recurrence of malignant disease

Recommended Reading

Austin MT, Leys CM, Feurer ID, Lovvorn HN III, O'Neill JA Jr, Pinson CW, Pietsch JB. Liver transplantation for childhood hepatic malignancy: a review of the United Network for Organ Sharing (UNOS) database. J Pediatr Surg. 2006;41(1):182–86.

Avila LF, Luis AL, Hernandez F, Garcia Miguel P, Jara P, Andres AM, Lopez Santamaria M, Tovar JA. Liver transplantation for malignant tumours in children. Eur J Pediatr Surg. 2006;16:411–4.

Isaacs H Jr. Fetal and neonatal hepatic tumors. J Pediatr Surg. 2007;42(11):1797–803.

Pham TH, Iqbal CW, Grams JM, Zarroug AE, Wall JC, Ishitani MB, Nagorney DM, Moir C. Outcomes of primary liver cancer in children: an appraisal of experience. J Pediatr Surg. 2007;42:834–9.

Srouji MN, Chatten J, Schulman WM, Ziegler MM, Koop CE. Mesenchymal hamartoma of the liver in infants. Cancer. 1978;42:2483–9.

Chapter 62
Renal Tumors: Wilms Tumor (Nephroblastoma)

Introduction

- Wilms tumor is a malignant tumor of the kidneys that typically occurs in children.
- Dr. Max Wilms, a German surgeon (1867–1918), was the first to describe this tumor.
- Most cases of Wilms tumor are seen in children between 3 and 3.5 years old.
- Most nephroblastomas are unilateral, being bilateral in <5% of cases.
- The overall prognosis of Wilms tumor following surgical excision is excellent. At present, survival rates of children with Wilms tumor are approximately 80–90%.

Epidemiology

- The majority (75%) of Wilms tumor occurs in otherwise normal healthy children; but in about 25% of the cases, Wilms tumor is associated with other genetic and developmental abnormalities:
- It occurs in approximately seven in a million children in the USA.
- Girls are slightly more likely to develop Wilms tumor than are boys.
- Black children have a slightly higher risk of developing Wilms tumor than do children of other races.
- Asian children appear to have a lower risk of developing Wilms tumor than do children of other races.
- A positive family history of Wilms tumor increases the risk of developing Wilms tumor in other members of the family.
- Wilms tumor occurs more frequently in children with certain abnormalities present at birth, including:
  - Aniridia
  - Hemihypertrophy
  - Undescended testes
  - Hypospadias

Clinical Features

- The usual presenting symptoms are (Fig. 62.1):
  - An abdominal swelling or mass

Fig. 62.1 Clinical photograph showing *left-sided* Wilms tumor

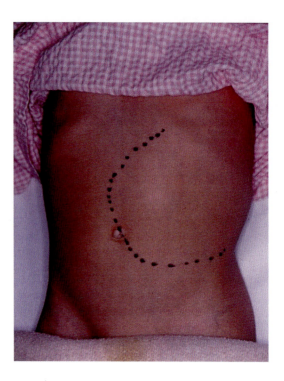

- Abdominal pain
- Fever
- Nausea and vomiting
- Hematuria
- High blood pressure

- The tumor can grow rapidly, which may result from bleeding into the tumor or from actual tumor growth.
- Hematuria:
  - May be seen in 10–15% of cases.
  - This is seen often after relatively minor trauma related to injury of an enlarged kidney involved by tumor.
  - Hematuria may be also a late presentation that is usually associated with tumor invasion of the calyces and is considered a bad prognostic sign.
- Hypertension:
  - Increased blood pressure may be present in 20% of cases.
  - Hypertension in Wilms's tumor results from pressure effect of the tumor on the renal vessels leading to increased secretion of rennin.
- Rarely, the tumor may produce erythropoietin leading to increased red blood cell production.
- Wilms tumor can occur as part of rare genetic syndromes, including:
  1. Wilms tumor, aniridia, genitourinary anomalies, and mental retardation (WAGR) syndrome. This syndrome includes:
     - Wilms tumor
     - Aniridia
     - Abnormalities of the genitals and urinary system
     - Mental retardation

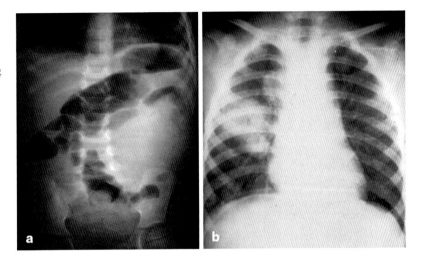

Fig. 62.2 Abdominal (**a**) and chest (**b**) X-rays in a patient with left-sided Wilms tumor. Note the soft tissue density pushing the bowel to the right and secondaries in the chest

2. Denys–Drash syndrome. This syndrome includes:
   - Wilms tumor
   - Kidney disease
   - Male pseudohermaphroditism
   - These patients mostly have bilateral or multiple tumors
3. Beckwith–Wiedemann syndrome. This syndrome includes:
   - Omphalocele
   - A large tongue (macroglossia)
   - Enlarged internal organs

Investigations

- These include a complete blood count, blood urea nitrogen (BUN), creatinine, abdominal X-ray, abdominal ultrasound, computed tomography (CT) scan of the chest and abdomen, and magnetic resonance imaging (MRI; Figs. 62.2, 62.3, 62.4, and 62.5).
- The aim is to evaluate the site, size, and extent of the tumor as well as the presence or absence of secondaries.
- This as well as the function of the affected and contralateral kidney.
- The presence or absence of synchronous tumors.
- It is of great importance to exclude extension of the tumor into the renal vein as well as the inferior vena cava.
- A plain abdominal radiograph often shows displacement of abdominal organs and occasionally the presence of calcification (<10%). The calcification usually is located on the edge of the tumor, whereas with a neuroblastoma, the calcification is speckled throughout.
- Abdominal ultrasound confirms that the kidney is the site of the tumor, determines whether the mass is a cystic or solid tumor, and indicates if the tumor extends into the renal veins and inferior vena cava. Doppler ultrasound is a valuable investigation in detecting tumor extension in the renal vein and inferior vena cava.
- CT scan defines the Wilms tumor site; identifies the presence of enlarged lymph nodes; evaluates the possible presence of a second Wilms tumor in the opposite kidney; assesses involvement of the tumor into the renal veins, inferior vena cava, and right atrium, and determines if the patient has intra-abdominal secondaries to the liver.

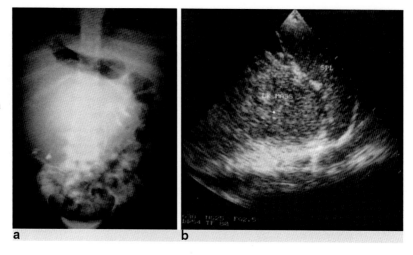

Fig. 62.3 An intravenous urography in a patient with right-sided Wilms tumor (**a**). Note the mass displacing and compressing the remaining calyces downward. Abdominal ultrasound in a patient with a *left*-sided Wilms tumor (**b**)

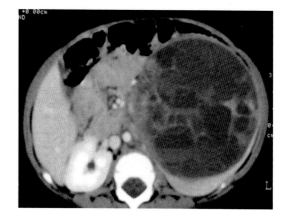

Fig. 62.4 Abdominal CT scan showing a large left-sided Wilms tumor. Note the thin rim of remaining kidney, which confirms that the tumor is arising from the kidney as opposed to neuroblastoma

- A chest CT is obtained to evaluate the presence of secondaries in the lungs.
- Small abnormalities seen on chest X-ray are suggestive of secondaries, but those seen on CT scan may need to be confirmed by biopsy.
- With the current radiological investigations, physical inspection of the opposite kidney by opening Gerota's fascia as suggested previously to check for synchronous tumor is no longer necessary.

Pathology

- Grossly, Wilms tumor is a large, solitary, and well-circumscribed mass with the remaining rim of normal kidney tissue. There is usually a well-defined membrane between them. On cut section, Wilms tumor is soft, homogenous, and tan-gray in color and may contain areas of hemorrhage and necrosis (Fig. 62.6).
- Pathologically, Wilms tumor is a malignant tumor composed of three elements (a triphasic nephroblastoma).
- These include metanephric blastema, mesenchymal stroma, and epithelium.

Pathology

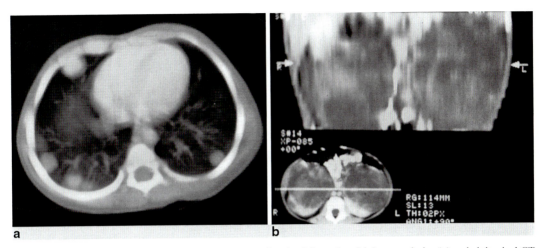

Fig. 62.5 Chest CT scan in a patient with Wilms tumor showing bilateral multiple secondaries (**a**) and abdominal CT scan showing bilateral Wilms tumor (**b**)

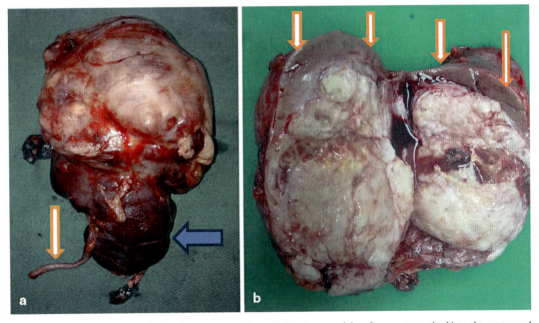

Fig. 62.6 a Clinical photograph showing a resected large Wilms tumor arising from upper pole. Note the ureter and lower pole. **b** Clinical photograph showing a bisected Wilms tumor. Note the small normal renal tissue at the *upper* pole of the kidney

- Characteristic of Wilms tumor is the presence of abortive tubules and glomeruli surrounded by a spindled cell stroma. The stroma may include striated muscle, cartilage, bone, fat, or fibrous tissue.
- The mesenchymal component may also include cells showing rhabdomyoid differentiation. The rhabdomyoid component may itself show features of malignancy (rhabdomyosarcomatous Wilms). This particular subtype shows poor response to chemotherapy.
- Pathologically, Wilms tumors are divided into two prognostic groups:

  1. Favorable: Contains well-developed components.

2. Unfavorable (Anaplastic): Contains anaplastic cells, which could be focal or diffuse. This is associated with higher frequencies of relapse and death.

- Most cases of Wilms tumor do not have mutations in any of the genes.
- A gene on the X chromosome, WTX, is inactivated in up to 30% of Wilms tumor cases.
- The gene WT1:
  - This is also called Wilms tumor-suppressor gene.
  - It has been found to make a protein that is found mostly in the fetal kidney and in tissues that give rise to the genitourinary system.
  - Inactivation of the gene may be responsible for the occurrence of Wilms tumor.
  - Mutations of the WT1 gene on chromosome 11 p 13 are observed in approximately 20% of Wilms tumors.
  - At least half of the Wilms tumors with mutations in WT1 also carry mutations in CTNNB1, the gene encoding the proto-oncogene beta-catenin.Staging (National Wilms Tumor Study—NWTS). Post-surgical staging.

Stage I (43% of patients):
For Stage I Wilms tumor, one or more of the following criteria must be met:

- Tumor is limited to the kidney and is completely excised.
- The surface of the renal capsule is intact.
- The tumor is not ruptured or biopsied (open or needle) prior to removal.
- No involvement of extrarenal or renal sinus lymph–vascular spaces.
- No residual tumor apparent beyond the margins of excision.
- Metastasis of tumor to lymph nodes not identified.

Stage II (23% of patients):
For Stage II Wilms tumor, one or more of the following criteria must be met:

- Tumor extends beyond the kidney but is completely excised
- No residual tumor apparent at or beyond the margins of excision
- Any of the following conditions may also exist:
  1. Tumor involvement of the blood vessels of the renal sinus and/or outside the renal parenchyma
  2. The tumor has been biopsied prior to removal or there is local spillage of tumor during surgery, confined to the flank
  3. Extensive tumor involvement of renal sinus soft tissue

Stage III (23% of patients):
For Stage III Wilms tumor, one or more of the following criteria must be met:

- Unresectable primary tumor
- Lymph node metastasis
- Tumor is present at surgical margins
- Tumor spillage involving peritoneal surfaces either before or during surgery, or transected tumor thrombus

Stage IV (10% of patients):

- Stage IV Wilms tumor is defined as the presence of hematogenous metastases (lung, liver, bone, or brain), or lymph node metastases outside the abdomenopelvic region.

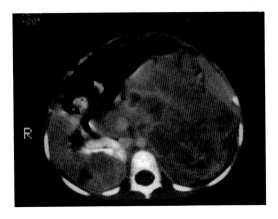

Fig. 62.7 Abdominal CT scan in a patient with bilateral Wilms tumor

Stage V (5 % of patients):

- Stage V Wilms tumor is defined as bilateral renal involvement at the time of initial diagnosis. Note: For patients with bilateral involvement, an attempt should be made to stage each side according to the above criteria (Stages I–III) on the basis of extent of disease prior to biopsy (Fig. 62.7).

Treatment

- The NWTS Group (NWTSG) and the International Society of Pediatric Oncology (SIOP) have identified several chemotherapeutic agents through clinical trials. When used together, these agents lead to a cure in most children with Wilms tumor. At present, survival rates of children with Wilms tumor are approximately 80–90 %.
- Stage I: Nephrectomy ± 18 weeks of chemotherapy depending on age of patient and weight of tumor, e.g., <2 years old and <550 g, only requires nephrectomy with observation.
- Stage II: Nephrectomy abdominal radiation + 24 weeks of chemotherapy.
- Stage III: Abdominal radiation + 24 weeks of chemotherapy + nephrectomy after tumor shrinkage.
- Stage IV: Nephrectomy + abdominal radiation + 24 weeks of chemotherapy + radiation of metastatic site as appropriate.
- Stage V: Individualized therapy based on tumor burden.
- The management of Wilms tumor in both kidneys must be individualized according to the extent of tumor present in both kidneys with a goal to preserving adequate kidney tissue to avoid kidney failure.

    - The initial procedure should be biopsies of both kidneys to establish the types in both kidneys.
    - Approximately 4 % of cases have different types between the two kidneys.
    - The patient is treated with chemotherapy and restudied by abdominal CT to evaluate tumor response and determine whether a surgical procedure would be beneficial.
    - If considerable tumor persists in both kidneys, additional chemotherapy is administered, and further surgery is delayed.
    - Radiation therapy is withheld if possible in these cases to reduce the risk of radiation injury to the remaining kidney tissue.
    - In some patients, the tumor persists in both kidneys, and resection of the tumor with preservation of functioning kidney tissue is not possible. The only remaining option for these rare patients ultimately is removal of both kidneys.

- Stages I–IV anaplasia:
  - Children with stage I anaplastic tumors can be managed with the same regimen given to stage I favorable histology patients.
  - Children with stage II through stage IV diffuse anaplasia, however, represent a higher-risk group.
  - These tumors are more resistant to the chemotherapy traditionally used in children with Wilms tumor (favorable histology), and require more aggressive regimens.

Prognosis

- Stage I: 98% 4-year survival; 85% 4-year survival, if anaplastic.
- Stage II: 96% 4-year survival; 70% 4-year survival, if anaplastic.
- Stage III: 95% 4-year survival; 56% 4-year survival, if anaplastic.
- Stage IV: 90% 4-year survival; 17% 4-year survival, if anaplastic.
- Stage V: The 4-year survival was 94% for those patients whose most advanced lesion was stage I or stage II; 76% for those whose most advanced lesion was stage III.
- Patients with synchronous bilateral tumors have a 70–80% survival rate whereas those with metachronous tumors have a 45–50% survival rate.
- Patients with anaplastic Wilms tumor have a worse prognosis compared with favorable histology Wilms tumor; the 4-year overall survival rates are 83, 83, 65 and 33% for stages I, II, III, and IV, respectively.

Clear Cell Sarcoma of the Kidney

- Clear cell sarcoma of the kidney (CCSK) is an uncommon renal neoplasm of childhood.
- It is characterized by:
  - Its propensity to metastasize to bone
  - Poor clinical outcome
  - The sarcomatous nonepithelial nature
- Bone is the most common site of metastases (15%), followed closely by lungs, abdomen, retroperitoneum, brain, and liver.
- Around 5% of patients have metastatic disease at presentation. Bone scan and brain CT scan or MRI are also part of the workup.
- CCSK may also recur many years after its initial diagnosis.
- CCSK represents <3% of pediatric renal tumors.
- Most patients are aged 1–4 years at diagnosis.
- Fifty percent of cases are diagnosed in children aged 2–3 years.
- A male predominance is observed.
- Histologically, CCSK shows three components, namely:
  1. Cord cells, which are small round-to-oval cells with deceptively bland cytologic features, including mitotic figures
  2. Septal cells, which are spindle-shaped cells along the fibrovascular septa (fibrovascular septa can be demonstrated more convincingly using reticulum stain)

- 3. An intercellular matrix composed of mucopolysaccharide, which ranges from minute indiscernible droplets to large pools imparting the clear appearance of clear cell sarcoma of the kidney.
- Several histologic variants of CCSK are recognized. The most common variant is the myxoid CCSK. The frequency of different CCSK variants is as follows:
  - Myxoid pattern (50%)
  - Sclerosing pattern (35%)
  - Cellular pattern (26%)
  - Epithelioid pattern (trabecular or acinar type) (13%)
  - Palisading (verocay-body) pattern (11%)
  - Spindle cell pattern (7%)
  - Storiform pattern (4%)
  - Anaplastic pattern (2.6%)
- Treatment of CCSK generally involves surgical excision coupled with radiation and chemotherapy.
- CCSK commonly responds poorly to treatment with vincristine and actinomycin alone, but the addition of doxorubicin to chemotherapy regimens has improved survival rates.
- The prognosis for CCSK, particularly for low-stage tumors, has improved with the addition of doxorubicin to chemotherapy regimens with a 66% reduction in overall mortality.
- Stage-dependent 6-year survival is:
  - 97% for stage I tumors
  - 75% for stage II tumors
  - 77% for stage III tumors
  - 50% for stage IV tumors
- Twenty-nine percent of patients with CCSK have lymph node metastases at the time of diagnosis, and bone metastasis is the most common form of relapse.
- Metastatic lesions have also been reported in the liver, brain, soft tissue sites, and lung with more unusual metastases to the skeletal muscles, testis, and salivary gland.
- Relapses of CCSK as many as 10 years after original diagnosis have been reported.

Malignant Rhabdoid Tumor of the Kidney

- Malignant rhabdoid tumor (MRT) is one of the most aggressive and lethal malignancies in children.
- MRT was initially described in 1978 as a rhabdomyosarcomatoid variant of a Wilms tumor because of its occurrence in the kidney and because of the resemblance of its cells to rhabdomyoblasts (Fig. 62.8).
- This tumor is now recognized as an entity separate from a Wilms tumor.
- The median age at presentation is 10.6 months, with a mean age of 15 months. Most patients are younger than 2 years at presentation.
- In contrast to a Wilms tumor, MRT is characterized by the early onset of local and distant metastases and resistance to chemotherapy.
- Whereas the overall survival rate for Wilms tumors exceeds 85%, the survival rate for MRT is only 20–25%.
- MRT is a rapidly progressive tumor, with most deaths occurring within 12 months of presentation. The most common sites of metastasis at presentation are the lungs, abdominal lymph nodes, liver, brain, and bone.

Fig. 62.8 Abdominal MRI in a patient with left-sided rhabdoid tumor of the kidney

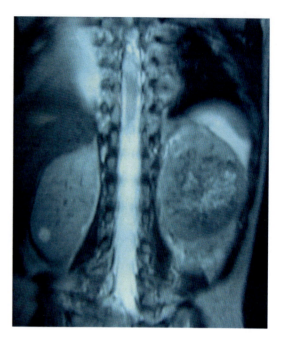

- Gross hematuria is a presenting feature in approximately 60% of patients with MRT. By contrast, only 20% of patients with Wilms tumor have gross hematuria.
- Fever is a presenting symptom in 50% of patients with a rhabdoid tumor of the kidney, compared with 25% of patients with a Wilms tumor.
- Hypertension is observed in up to 70% of patients.
- The rhabdoid tumor is seen commonly in children younger than 2 years of age and may occur in both kidneys as well as in areas outside of the kidney.
- This tumor has the worst prognosis of all renal tumors. Infants and children with rhabdoid tumors have aggressive disease, typically with much tumor spread, and frequently die early (within 1–2 years—90% tumor return rate and 86% mortality) despite intense multidrug chemotherapy.
- As many as 20% of patients with a rhabdoid tumor of the kidney have synchronous or metachronous central nervous system (CNS) lesions, including both metastases and second primary cancers.
- Mutations or deletions of the SMARCB1/INI1 gene play a role in the development of MRT.
- On microscopic examination, MRTs are characterized by sheets or solid trabeculae of large tumor cells with vesicular chromatin, nuclei with prominent cherry-red nucleoli, moderate amounts of eccentric eosinophilic cytoplasm, and a distinctive, globoid, hyaline pink intracytoplasmic inclusion.
- After the primary tumor is surgically removed (Fig. 62.9), chemotherapy is indicated as adjuvant MRT treatment.
- Chemotherapy for MRT was historically based on therapy for a Wilms tumor, which included vincristine, actinomycin, and doxorubicin with or without cyclophosphamide. With these agents, the estimated survival rate for patients with MRT was only 23%.
- Recent case reports have documented successful outcomes in patients with metastatic MRT treated with ifosfamide–carboplatin–etoposide (ICE) or ifosfamide–etoposide (IE) alternating with vincristine–doxorubicin–cyclophosphamide (VDC). On the basis of these reports, cyclophosphamide–carboplatin–etoposide (CCE) alternating with VDC is the main treatment now.
- Radiation therapy is a cornerstone of treatment for CNS MRT.
- High-dose chemotherapy with stem cell rescue is used to treat non-CNS MRT.

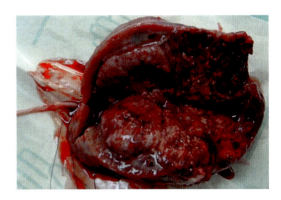

Fig. 62.9 Clinical photograph showing a resected rhabdoid tumor of the kidney

Mesoblastic Nephroma

- Mesoblastic nephroma is the most common renal tumor identified in the neonatal period and the most frequent benign renal tumor in childhood.
- It represents 3–10 % of all pediatric renal tumors.
- Mesoblastic nephroma is most commonly diagnosed in the first 3 months of life.
- Pathologically, the cut surface of the tumor specimen shows a yellow-tan tumor with a "whorled" appearance that is similar to a uterine leiomyoma (Fig. 62.10).
- There are two pathologic variants: classic and atypical or cellular.
- The classic form is characterized by rare mitoses and absence of necrosis. Entrapped tubules and/or glomeruli are usually seen at the periphery of the tumor.
- Atypical or cellular variant is characterized by:
    - A high mitotic index
    - Hypercellularity
    - An atypical growth pattern with necrosis, hemorrhage, and invasion of adjacent structures
- The cellular type accounts for 42–63 % of cases.
- Factors that increase the risk of recurrence and metastasis include:
    - Cellular variant
    - Older age at presentation
    - Positive surgical margins
- Metastases to distant organs such as the brain, bone, and lungs have been reported.
- Surgical resection of congenital mesoblastic nephroma is curative.

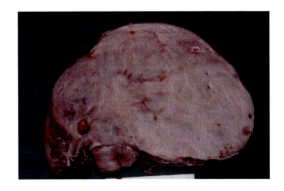

Fig. 62.10 Clinical photograph of a resected mesoblastic nephroma. Note the whorled appearance of the tumor

- Most cases of mesoblastic nephroma are clinically benign. However, there are reports of local recurrence in incompletely resected tumors and metastases to the brain, lung, heart, and bone.
- In such cases, patients may be treated with chemotherapy and/or radiation.
- When diagnosed in the first 7 months of life, the 5-year event-free survival rate is 94% and the overall survival rate is 96%.

Recommended Reading

Argani P, Perlman EJ, Breslow NE, Browning NG, Green DM, D'Angio GJ, Beckwith JB. Clear cell sarcoma of the kidney: a review of 351 cases from the National Wilms Tumor Study Group Pathology Center. Am J Surg Pathol. 2000;24(1):4–18.

England RJ, Haider N, Vujanic GM, Kelsey A, Stiller CA, Pritchard-Jones K, Powis M. Mesoblastic nephroma: a report of the United Kingdom Children's Cancer and Leukaemia Group (CCLG). Pediatr Blood Cancer. 2011;56(5):744–8.

Green DM. The treatment of stages I-IV favorable histology Wilms' tumor. J Clin Oncol. 2004;22:1366–72.

Hamilton TE, Ritchey ML, Haase GM, Argani P, Peterson SM, Anderson JR, et al. The management of synchronous bilateral Wilms tumor: a report from the National Wilms Tumor Study Group. Ann Surg. 2011;253(5):1004–10.

Tomlinson GE, Breslow NE, Dome J, Guthrie KA, Norkool P, Li S, Thomas PR, Perlman E, Beckwith JB, D'Angio GJ, Green DM. Rhabdoid tumor of the kidney in the National Wilms' Tumor Study: age at diagnosis as a prognostic factor. J Clin Oncol. 2005;23(30):7641–5.

Chapter 63
Teratoma

Introduction

- Teratoma is a word coined by Virchow in 1863 and it is derived from the Greek teras, meaning monster.
- Teratomas are tumors commonly composed of multiple cell types derived from all three germ layers. There are rare occasions when not all three germ layers are identifiable.
- The tissues of a teratoma, although normal in themselves, may be quite different from surrounding tissues and may be highly disparate; teratomas have been reported to contain hair, teeth, bone, and, very rarely, more complex organs such as eyes, torso, and hands, feet, or other limbs.
- The exact etiology of teratomas is not known but the most widely accepted theory suggests an origin from the primordial germ cells.
- Teratomas range from benign, well-differentiated (mature) cystic lesions to those that are solid and malignant (immature).
- Mature teratomas are highly variable in form and histology, and may be solid, cystic, or a combination of solid and cystic.
- Teratomas are thought to be present at birth (congenital), but small ones are often not discovered until much later in life.
- Teratomas arise from totipotential cells; these tumors typically are midline or paraxial.
- Excluding testicular teratomas, 75–80 % of teratomas occur in girls.
- The most common locations for teratomas are:
    1. Sacrococcygeal (57 %).
    2. Gonads (29 %): By far, the most common gonadal location is the ovary, although they also occur somewhat less frequently in the testes.
    3. Mediastinal (7 %).
    4. Retroperitoneal (4 %).
    5. Cervical (3 %).
    6. Intracranial (3 %).
    7. Rare sites include the stomach, intracranial, and mouth (Fig. 63.1).
- Fetus in fetu and fetiform teratoma are rare forms of mature teratoma that include one or more components resembling a malformed fetus. Both forms may contain or appear to contain complete organ systems, even major body parts such as torso or limbs. Fetus in fetu differs from fetiform teratoma in having an apparent spine and bilateral symmetry.
- A struma ovarii (literally, goitre of the ovary) is a rare form of mature teratoma that contains mostly thyroid tissue.

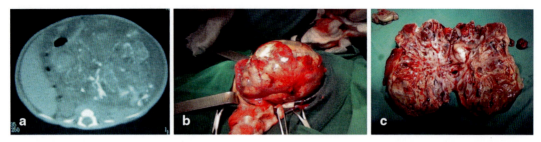

Fig. 63.1 a Abdominal CT scan in a newborn with a large gastric immature teratoma. Note the presence of calcifications. **b** Intraoperative photograph showing a large gastric teratoma. **c** a clinical photograph of a resected large immature gastric teratoma

- A dermoid cyst is a mature cystic teratoma containing hair (sometimes very abundant) and other structures characteristic of normal skin and other tissues derived from the ectoderm. The term is most often applied to teratoma on the skull sutures and in the ovaries of females.
- Teratomas commonly are classified using the Gonzalez-Crussi grading system:
  - 0 or mature (benign).
  - 1 or immature, probably benign.
  - 2 or immature, possibly malignant (cancerous).
  - 3 or frankly malignant. If frankly malignant, the tumor is a cancer for which additional cancer staging applies.
- Teratomas are also classified by their content:
  - A solid teratoma contains only tissues (perhaps including more complex structures).
  - A cystic teratoma contain only pockets of fluid or semi-fluid such as cerebrospinal fluid, sebum, or fat.
  - A mixed teratoma contains both solid and cystic parts.
  - Cystic teratomas usually are grade 0 and, conversely, grade 0 teratomas usually are cystic.

Sacrococcygeal Teratomas

- Sacrococcygeal teratomas are the most common tumors in newborns, occurring in 1 per 30,000–40,000 births.
- Sacrococcygeal teratomas occur more often in girls than in boys; ratios of 3:1 to 4:1 have been reported.
- Sacrococcygeal teratomas may be diagnosed antenatally during routine ultrasound, fetal anomaly scan, or when the mother presents with clinical symptoms such as inappropriate dates to gestational age or polyhydramnios.
- Those not diagnosed antenatally present in two patterns:
  - The most common pattern is in neonates, who present with a large, predominantly benign tumor protruding from the sacral area that is noted prenatally or at the time of delivery (Fig. 63.2).
  - Less commonly, the newborn may exhibit only asymmetry of the buttocks or present when aged 1 month to 4 years with a presacral tumor that may extend into the pelvis. Symptoms of bladder or bowel dysfunction may be present. The latter group is at a significantly higher risk for malignancy (Fig. 63.3).

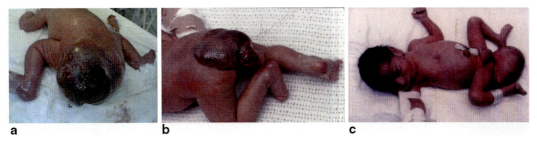

Fig. 63.2 a–c Clinical photographs of newborns with large sacrococcygeal teratoma

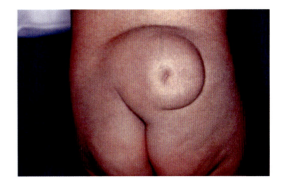

Fig. 63.3 A clinical photograph of a patient with sacrococcygeal teratoma. Note the deformity and asymmetry of the buttocks

- 15 % have associated congenital anomalies including:
  - Imperforated anus
  - Sacral bone defects
  - Duplication of uterus or vagina
  - Spina bifida
  - Myelomingocele
- Elevated serum alpha-fetoprotein (AFP) and beta-human chorionic gonadotropin (HCG) levels may be indicative of malignancy.
- Ultrasound examination may demonstrate cystic components and extension of the tumor into the pelvis or abdomen. Ultrasound may reveal mass displacement of the bladder and rectum, with compression of the ureters resulting in hydroureter or hydronephrosis.
- Computed tomography (CT) scanning and magnetic resonance imaging (MRI) of the abdomen and pelvis can further delineate sacrococcygeal tumor from normal anatomic features. May detect liver metastasis and retroperitoneal lymph node involvement in malignant cases (Figs. 63.4 and 63.5).

Altman's classification (Fig. 63.6):

- Type I (45.8 %): Tumors are predominantly external, attached to the coccyx, and may have a small presacral component.
- Type II (34 %): Tumors have both an external mass and significant presacral pelvic extension.
- Type III (8.6 %): Tumors are visible externally, but the predominant mass is pelvic and intra-abdominal.
- Type IV (9.6 %): Tumors are not visible externally but are entirely presacral (Fig. 63.7).

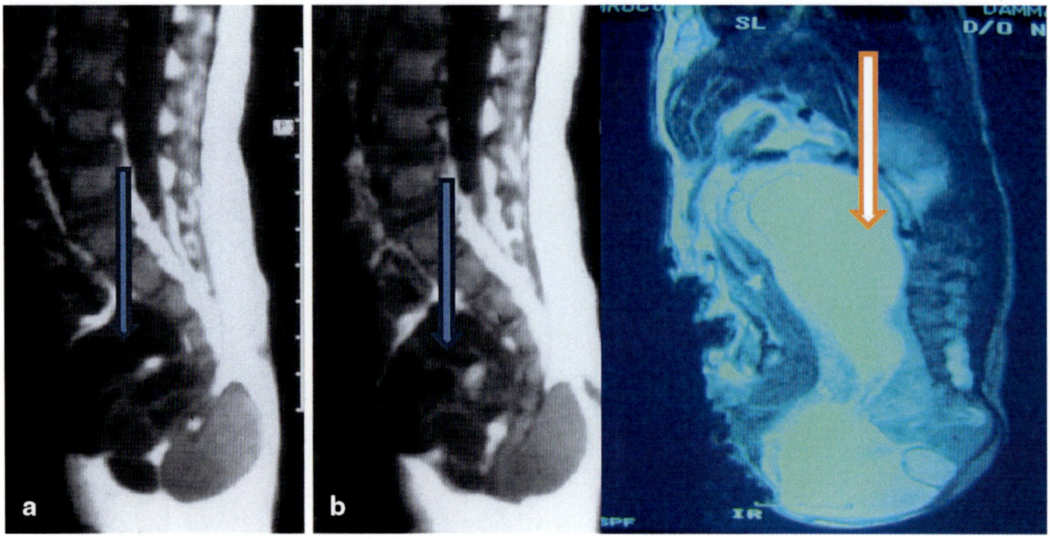

Fig. 63.4 a MRIs of a patient with sacrococcygeal teratoma. Note the intrapelvic extension of the tumor. **b** CT scan of a newborn with a very large sacrococcygeal teratoma. Note the large intra-abdominal extension of the tumor

Treatment

- Sacrococcygeal teratomas diagnosed prenatally should be monitored closely.
- In fetuses with larger tumors, cesarean delivery should be considered to prevent dystocia or tumor rupture.
- Because of the poor prognosis associated with development of hydrops prior to 30 weeks' gestation, these fetuses may benefit from in utero surgery.
- In most cases, sacrococcygeal teratomas should be resected electively in the first week of life, since long delays may be associated with a higher rate of malignancy.
- Most fetal teratomas can be managed by planned delivery and postnatal surgery.
- Holzgreve et al. have described an algorithm to approach the management of sacrococcygeal teratoma based on fetal lung maturity and the presence or absence of placentomegaly and/or hydrops fetalis. In the absence of placentomegaly and hydrops, the fetus should be followed by serial ultrasound until fetal pulmonary maturity is adequate for survival. The patient should then undergo elective early delivery by cesarean section to avoid trauma to the mass or dystocia.
- The occurrence of placentomegaly and/or hydrops fetalis appears to be a preterminal event indicating imminent fetal demise. Its occurrence in a fetus with adequate pulmonary maturity demands emergency cesarean section. Fetuses developing placentomegaly and/or fetal hydrops prior to adequate lung maturity are the most difficult management decisions. These fetuses may be candidates for transfusion or fetal surgical intervention.
- Complete excision should be done through a chevron-shaped buttock incision, with careful attention to the preservation of the muscles of the rectal sphincter.
- The coccyx always should be resected with the tumor, as failure to do so results in a 35–40 % recurrence rate with > 50 % being malignant (Fig. 63.8).
- Hemorrhage from the middle sacral vessels and hypogastric arteries is the most common complication.
- Prognosis of sacrococcygeal teratoma is improving due to prenatal detection, planned intrapartum management, and prompt surgical resection.

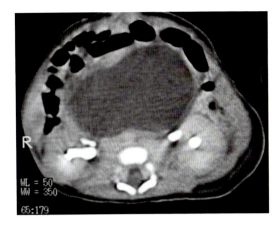

Fig. 63.5 CT scan of the abdomen showing a large intra-abdominal extension of the tumor

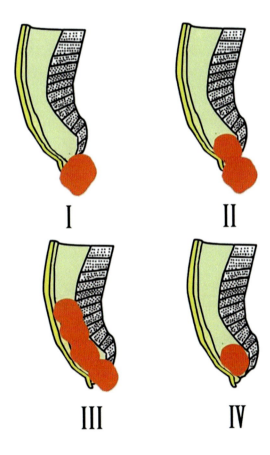

Fig. 63.6 Diagramatic representation of Altman's classification of sacrococcygeal teratoma

- In benign tumors, disease-free survival is >90%.
- Time of diagnoses is the key:
    - <2 months of age, only 7–10% are malignant.
    - Age 1 year, 37% malignant.
    - Age 2 years, 50% malignant.

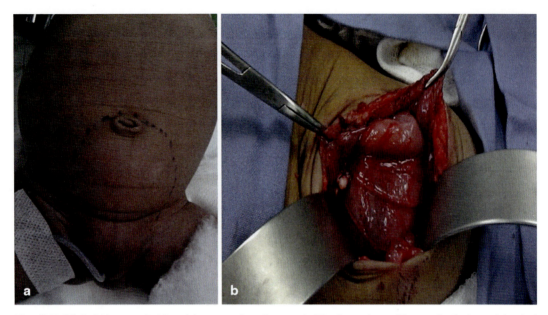

Fig. 63.7 Clinical photograph (**a**) and intraoperative photograph (**b**) of a patient with completely intra-abdominal sacrococcygeal teratoma (type IV)

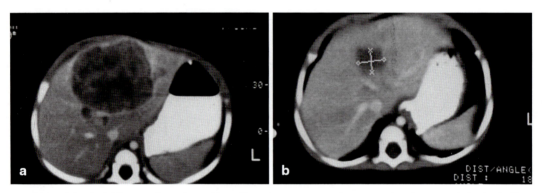

Fig. 63.8 Abdominal CT scan of a patient with malignant sacrococcygeal teratoma showing secondaries in the liver (**a**) and abdominal CT scan following chemotherapy (**b**). Note the response to chemotherapy

Ovarian Teratoma

- Teratoma is considered one of the germ cell tumors (teratomas, dysgerminoma, endodermal sinus tumor, choriocarcinoma, embryonal carcinoma, polyembryoma, and mixed germ cell tumors) which represent 15–20 % of all ovarian tumors.
- Ovarian teratomas are classified into three distinct types:
    - Mature teratomas
    - Immature teratomas
    - Monodermal teratomas

Immature Teratoma

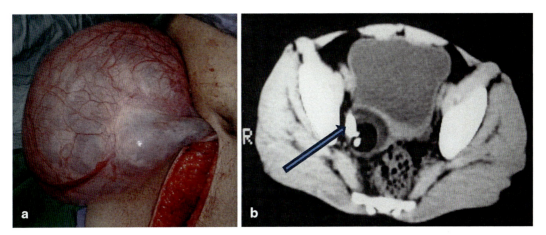

Fig. 63.9 Intraoperative photograph showing a large mature ovarian teratoma (**a**) and pelvic CT scan of a patient with ovarian teratomas (**b**). Note the calcification

Mature Teratoma

- Mature teratoma is one of the most common of all forms of ovarian germ cell tumor.
- Mature cystic teratomas account for 10–20 % of all ovarian neoplasms.
- This subtype is most likely to develop during the childbearing years.
- Mature teratoma is often called a dermoid cyst.
- The majority (98 %) of these tumors are benign, and around 2 % becomes malignant.
- Benign mature teratomas are bilateral in 10–15 % of cases.
- Mature teratomas are cystic tumors and consist of cysts lined by epidermis and adnexal structures.
- The cyst may be filled with hair, sebaceous material, and teeth. The cyst wall may contain differentiated tissues including bone, cartilage, muscle, thyroid follicles, lining of the gastrointestinal tract, respiratory tract, and other tissues (Fig. 63.9).

Immature Teratoma

- Immature teratoma is relatively rare.
- Immature teratoma is more frequently seen in children and young women, and tends to be very solid.
- Most of these tumors are malignant, grow quickly, and metastasize widely.
- Grossly, immature teratoma appear as large solid tumors with areas of necrosis and hemorrhage (Figs. 63.10 and 63.11).
- Microscopically, immature teratoma consists of embryonic cells from one to three germ cell layers. May contain immature elements differentiating to bone, cartilage, epithelium, muscle, nerve, and other tissues.
- Immature teratoma is classified as grade I–III depending on the extent of the immaturity of the various elements and the presence of neuroepithelium.

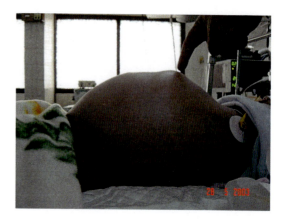

Fig. 63.10 Clinical photograph of a patient with a huge ovarian malignant teratoma

Monodermal Teratoma

- The cells in monodermal teratoma grow as a single germ cell layer and are mainly composed of one type of tissue, although there may be slight traces of other tissues found within the tumor itself.
- Examples include struma ovarii which consists of mature thyroid tissue and ovarian carcinoid.
- A monodermal teratoma may be malignant or benign and can occur in girls as well as adult women.

Staging of Malignant Teratoma

- Stage 1: The tumor is limited to the ovary (or both ovaries).
- Stage 2: The tumor has spread into the fallopian tube, uterus, or elsewhere in the pelvis.
- Stage 3: The tumor has spread to the regional lymph nodes or to the peritoneum.
- Stage 4: The tumor has spread to distant organs such as the lungs.

Gliomatosis peritonei: This is a rare condition characterized by the implantation of mature neural glial tissues on the surface of the visceral or parietal peritoneum. This is seen usually in patients with immature ovarian teratoma and rarely with mature ovarian teratoma.

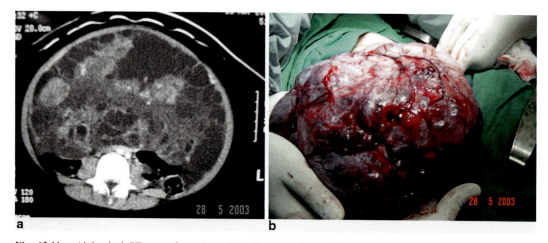

Fig. 63.11 a Abdominal CT scan of a patient with a huge ovarian malignant teratoma. **b** Intraoperative photograph showing a huge resected malignant ovarian teratoma

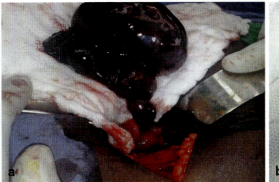 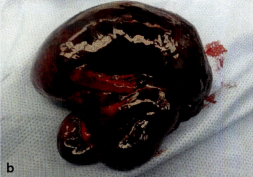

Fig. 63.12 a and **b** Clinical intraoperative photographs showing torsion of an ovarian teratoma that was resected

Struma ovarii:
This is an ovarian mature cystic teratoma composed entirely or predominantly of thyroid tissue and containing variable-sized follicles with colloid material. It accounts for 0.3–1 % of all ovarian tumors and for approximately 3 % of all mature cystic teratomas. About 5 % of these cases show symptoms or signs of thyrotoxicosis.

Complications

- Complications of ovarian teratomas include: torsion, rupture, infection, hemolytic anemia (autoimmune hemolytic anemia has been associated with mature cystic teratomas in rare cases, and in these reports, removal of the tumor resulted in complete resolution of symptoms), and malignant degeneration (Fig. 63.12).

Presentations

- Mature cystic teratomas of the ovary are often discovered as incidental findings on physical examination, during radiographic studies, or during abdominal surgery performed for other indications.
- Asymptomatic mature cystic teratomas of the ovaries have been reported in 6–65 % of cases.
- When symptoms are present, they may include: abdominal pain, abdominal mass or swelling, and abnormal uterine bleeding.
- The abdominal pain is usually constant and ranges from slight to moderate in intensity.
- Torsion and acute rupture commonly are associated with severe pain.
- Hormonal production is thought to account for cases of abnormal uterine bleeding.
- Bladder symptoms, gastrointestinal disturbances, and back pain are less frequent.
- Elevated serum AFP and beta-HCG levels may be indicative of malignancy.

Treatment

- Mature cystic teratomas of the ovaries may be removed by simple cystectomy rather than salpingo-oophorectomy. This can be done by laparotomy or laparoscopy.
- Treatment of malignant teratoma is oophorectomy, and if distant metastases are present, postoperative chemotherapy is necessary.

Testicular Teratoma

- The incidence of testicular tumors in men is 2.1–2.5 cases per 100,000 population.
- Germ cell tumors represent 95% of all testicular tumors after puberty, but pure benign teratomas of the testis are rare, accounting for only 3–5% of germ cell tumors.
- The incidence of all testicular tumors in prepubertal boys is 0.5–2 per 100,000, with mature teratomas accounting for 14–27% of these tumors.
- It is the second most common germ cell tumor in this population.
- Testicular teratomas most often present as a painless scrotal mass, except in the case of torsion.
- In most cases, the masses are firm or hard, nontender, and do not transilluminate.
- Testicular pain and scrotal swelling are occasionally reported with teratomas, but this is nonspecific and simply indicates torsion until proven otherwise.
- Hydrocele is frequently associated with teratoma in childhood.
- On examination, the testis is diffusely enlarged, rather than nodular, although a discreet nodule in the upper or lower pole sometimes can be appreciated. Testicular teratomas traditionally have been treated by simple or radical orchiectomy.
- More recently, conservative excision by enucleation also has been recommended for prepubertal teratomas of the testis.

Mediastinal Teratoma

- Benign teratomas of the mediastinum are rare, representing 8% of all tumors of this region.
- Mediastinal teratomas are often asymptomatic.
- Mediastinal teratomas are occasionally discovered incidentally on chest radiograph.
- When symptoms are present, they relate to mechanical effects including chest pain, cough, dyspnea, or symptoms related to recurrent pneumonitis.
- Many patients present with respiratory findings, and the pathognomonic finding of trichoptysis, or cough productive of hair or sebaceous material, may result if a communication develops between the mass and the tracheobronchial tree.
- Other serious presentations are superior vena cava syndrome or lipoid pneumonia.
- Open (sternotomy or lateral thoracotomy) or laparoscopic excision can be undertaken for these tumors. Due to the proximity of these tumors and adhesion to vital structures, excision of these tumors is sometimes difficult.

Intraperitoneal Teratoma

- These tumors are usually retroperitoneal in location.
- Retroperitoneal teratomas are rare and comprise 3.5–4% of all germ cell tumors in children.
- The majority of these tumors are benign.
- Retroperitoneal teratomas are usually seen in female infants under the age of 1 year.
- The majority present with an abdominal mass commonly on the left side which can attain a large size and rarely cause symptoms.
- The presence of calcification on plain x-ray should raise the possibility of a teratoma.

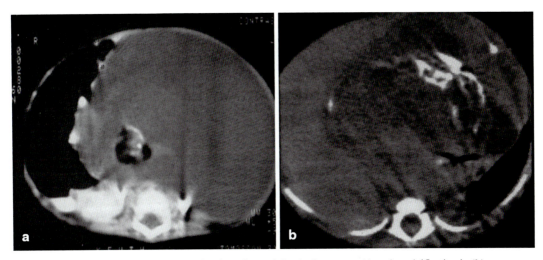

Fig. 63.13 a and **b** Abdominal CT scans showing a large abdominal teratoma. Note the calcification in (**b**)

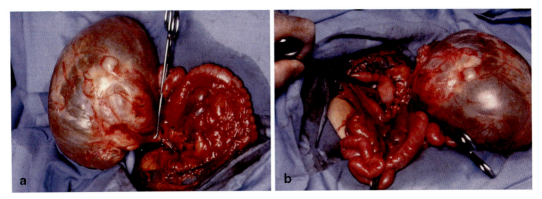

Fig. 63.14 a and **b** Clinical intraoperative photographs of a patient with a large abdominal teratoma. Note its relation to the blood vessels

- CT scan is valuable in delineating the extent of the tumor for proper planning and surgical excision (Fig. 63.13).
- In spite of the large size of these tumors, they are amenable to complete surgical resection.
- Careful attention to adjacent major blood vessels in the vicinity of the tumor is very important as these tumors tend to distort major blood vessels including the renal vessels (Fig. 63.14).

Cervical Teratoma

- Cervical teratomas are very rare tumors.
- In general, a cervical teratoma is a benign tumor, although there is a small possibility of malignancy.
- Although the majority of cervical teratomas are benign, they can cause significant morbidity and mortality.

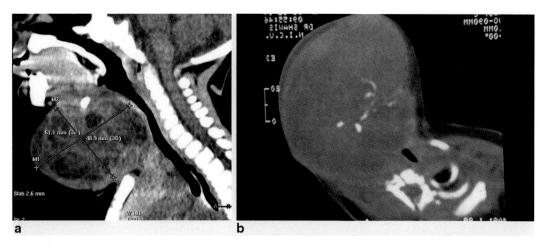

Fig. 63.15 a MRI of the neck showing a large cervical teratoma. Note its relation to the airways. **b** CT scan showing a large cervical teratoma. Note the calcification and its relation to the airways

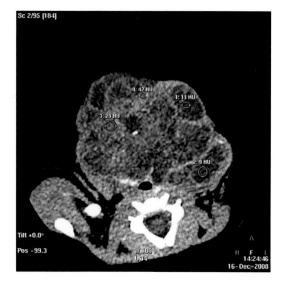

Fig. 63.16 CT scan of the neck showing a large cervical teratoma. Note its relation to the airways

- The antenatal diagnosis of large congenital cervical teratomas calls for early referral of these patients to specialized centers which allows for planned intervention by experienced personnel.
- Cervical teratomas tend to grow and attain a large size causing distortion of the normal anatomy with life-threatening upper airway obstruction.
- This makes postpartum intubation very difficult and sometimes impossible.
- Airway management at birth is critical in patients with large cervical teratoma. The delivery should be planned at a fetal therapy center prepared for high-risk deliveries as well as pediatric and fetal surgery (Figs. 63.15 and 63.16).
- Airway obstruction is life threatening and is associated with high mortality. One way to overcome this is the ex-utero intrapartum treatment (EXIT) procedure. This allows partial fetal delivery via cesarean section with the establishment of a safe fetal airway by intubation, bronchoscopy, or tracheostomy while fetal oxygenation is maintained through utero-placental circulation.

- Surgical removal of the tumor is performed often after the baby is stabilized. Care should be taken during excision to reduce the risk of nerve damage.
- Complete local excision of these tumors is the treatment of choice.
- This however may not be feasible always as these tumors may be extensive.
- To obviate postoperative morbidity and mortality, surgical excision of these large tumors needs to be planned also (staged surgical excision) which is also beneficial.
- A cervical teratoma may involve the thyroid and parathyroid glands. Therefore, these infants are at risk for developing hypoparathyroidism and hypothyroidism.

Recommended Reading

Altman RP, Randolph JG, Lilly JR. Sacrococcygeal teratoma: American Academy of Pediatrics Surgical Section Survey—1973. J Pediatr Surg. 1974;9:389.

Danzer E, Hubbard AM, Hedrick HL, Johnson MP, Wilson RD, Howell LJ, Flake AW, Adzick NS. Diagnosis and characterization of fetal sacrococcygeal teratoma with prenatal MRI. AJR Am J Roentgenol. 2006;187(4):W350–6.

Gabra HO, Jesudason EC, McDowell HP, Pizer BL, Losty PD. Sacrococcygeal teratoma- A 25-year experience in a UK regional center. J Pediatr Surg. 2006;41:1513–6.

Johnson N, Shah S, Shannon P, Campisi P, Windrim R. A challenging delivery by EXIT procedure of a fetus with a giant cervical teratoma. J Obstet Gynaecol Can. 2009;31:267–71.

Mann JR, Gray ES, Thornton C, Raafat F, Robinson K, Collins GS, et al. Mature and immature extracranial teratomas in children: the UK Children's Cancer Study Group Experience. J Clin Oncol. 2008;26(21):3590–7.

Tapper D, Lack EE. Teratomas in infancy and childhood. A 54-year experience at the Children's Hospital Medical Center. Ann Surg. 1983;198(3):398–410.

Chapter 64
Testicular Tumors

Introduction

- Testicular cancer is the most common cancer in males aged 20–39 years, and is rarely seen before the age of 15 years.
- Testicular tumors account for 1–2% of all pediatric tumors, with an incidence of 0.05–2 per 100,000 children.
- A bimodal age distribution is observed:
  - One peak occurs in the first 2 years of life.
  - The second occurs in young adulthood.
- Although testicular cancer can be derived from any cell type found in the testicles, more than 95% of testicular cancers are germ cell tumors.
- Most of the remaining 5% are sex cord-gonadal stromal tumors derived from Leydig cells or Sertoli cells.
- Of testicular tumors, 2–3% are bilateral.
- The two main categories of testicular tumors are:
  - Germ cell tumors (95%)
  - Sex cord-stromal tumors (5%)
- Germ cell tumors account for 60–77% of testicular tumors in children but account for 95% of testicular tumors in adults.
- Adult germ cell tumors with malignant potential, such as seminoma and embryonal carcinoma, are not seen in prepubertal patients.
- Teratomas, which are uniformly benign in children, are often malignant in adults.
- The most common germ cell tumors are:
  - Teratomas (62%).
  - Yolk-sac tumors (26%).
  - Prepubertal teratomas in children are uniformly benign.
- Gonadal stromal tumors are significantly less common than germ cell tumors and primarily include:
  - Juvenile granulosa-cell tumors
  - Leydig cell tumors
  - Sertoli cell tumors

- The vast majority (85%) of yolk-sac tumors in children present as clinical stage I disease, compared with 35% in adults.
- Alpha-fetoprotein (AFP) can be used as a reliable tumor marker because levels are increased in more than 90% of yolk-sac tumors.
- Epidermoid cysts are benign tumors of epithelial origin and account for 10–15% of cases.
- Seminomas and mixed germ cell tumors are extremely rare in prepubertal children.

Sertoli Cell Tumors

- Are the most common gonadal stromal tumors in prepubertal children.
- They tend to appear as painless masses in boys younger than 6 months.
- They produce no endocrinologic effects; however, 14% of patients present with gynecomastia.
- All reported cases in children younger than 5 years have been benign.
- Large-cell calcifying Sertoli cell tumor is a variant with large amounts of cytoplasm and calcification.
- One third of patients with this tumor have associated genetic abnormalities; however, these tumors are universally benign.

Leydig Cell Tumors

- These are the second most common gonadal stromal tumors in children.
- They are benign tumors.
- These tumors most often occur in boys aged 5–10 years.
- The synthesis of testosterone by these tumors may produce:
  - Precocious puberty
  - Gynecomastia
  - Elevated levels of 17-ketosteroids
- Leydig cell tumors must be differentiated from hyperplastic nodules that develop in boys with poorly controlled congenital adrenal hyperplasia (CAH).

Juvenile Granulosa Cell Tumors

- Account for approximately 3% of all neonatal testicular tumors.
- Commonly appear as cystic, painless testicular masses.
- They almost always appear in the first year of life, and most appear by age 6 months.
- They can be associated with:
  - Anomalies of the Y chromosome
  - Mosaicism
  - Ambiguous genitalia
- These tumors are hormonally inactive and benign.

Gonadoblastoma

- Occurs in association with disorders of sexual development (intersex).
- About 80% of cases involve phenotypic females with intra-abdominal testes or streak gonads.
- The gonadoblastoma gene is on the Y chromosome, and the tumor almost always develops in a child with a Y chromosome.
- The streak gonads in patients with mixed gonadal dysgenesis often develop gonadoblastomas.
- The incidence peaks at puberty, and early gonadectomy is recommended in patients at risk for gonadoblastoma.
- Metastatic spread of a gonadoblastoma occurs in 10% of patients.
- These tumors may have elevated serum levels of beta-human chorionic gonadotropin (beta-HCG).
  - Cystic dysplasia of the testis is a benign lesion that is often associated with ipsilateral renal agenesis or dysplasia. This association, along with a characteristic ultrasonographic appearance (i.e., hypoechoic lesions) permits preoperative diagnosis and possible treatment with testicular-sparing surgery.
  - Leukemia and lymphoma:
    - Are the most common secondary malignancies to affect the testis.
    - These tumors can present bilaterally.
    - Because the blood–testis barrier protects the intratesticular cells, the testis may be the site of residual tumor in children after chemotherapy.

Paratesticular Tumors

- Paratesticular structures can give rise to:
  - Benign tumors (lipoma, leiomyoma, hemangioma, or fibroma).
  - Malignant tumors; however, these are extremely rare.
    - Rhabdomyosarcoma is the most common malignant tumor (17%) and may arise from the distal spermatic cord and appear as a scrotal mass or hydrocele.
    - These tumors have a bimodal distribution and occur in boys aged 3–4 months and in teenagers.
    - Up to 70% of cases involve the retroperitoneal lymph nodes at presentation.
    - These tumors are highly aggressive and spread via the blood, lymphatics, or direct extension to the lungs, the cortical bone, or to the bone marrow in 20% of patients at the time of diagnosis.
    - Radical inguinal orchiectomy followed by retroperitoneal lymph node dissection is recommended for all children with retroperitoneal disease.
    - Patients with positive lymph nodes are treated with multimodal therapy (chemotherapy and radiation).

Clinical Features and Investigations

- The incidence of pediatric testicular tumors peaks in children aged 2–4 years.
- Most yolk-sac tumors occur in children younger than 2 years.
- About 85% of children with testicular tumors present with painless scrotal swelling.

- A few present with a hydrocele, scrotal pain, or a history of trauma.
- About 10–25% of patients with a malignant tumor present with a hydrocele.
- A hard mass may be palpable on physical examination. However, normal physical findings are not sufficient to exclude a tumor.
- Physical examination usually reveals a painless scrotal swelling with a hard mass or associated hydrocele.
- Some hormonally active tumors may appear in association with precocious puberty or gynecomastia
- Measure serum AFP level before treating a testicular mass.
    - AFP levels are elevated in 80% of patients with yolk-sac carcinomas and serve as a tumor marker.
    - The half-life of AFP is about 5 days, and levels should return to normal (<20 ng/mL) within 1 month after complete removal of the tumor.
    - Persistently elevated AFP levels after surgery suggest tumor metastases or recurrence.
- Serum testosterone levels may be elevated in Leydig cell tumors.
- Beta-HCG levels may be elevated in gonadoblastoma.
- Ultrasonography is helpful in evaluating the testicle and in distinguishing an extratesticular mass from an intratesticular mass.
- Chest radiography should be performed, as 20% of yolk-sac tumors occur with metastases to the lung.
- Patients with rhabdomyosarcomas require chest radiography, abdominal-pelvic CT scanning, bone scanning, and bone-marrow aspiration.
- About 90% of paratesticular rhabdomyosarcomas demonstrate a favorable embryonal pattern on histology.

Classification

- The testis is made up of:
    - Supporting cells (or stroma) that secrete testosterone (from Leydig cells).
    - 250–300 seminiferous tubules. These tubules are made up of:
        - Supporting or sertoli cells
        - Germ cells or spermatogonia
- Although testicular cancer can be derived from any cell type found in the testicles, more than 95% of testicular cancers are germ cell tumors. Most of the remaining 5% are sex cord-gonadal stromal tumors derived from Leydig cells or Sertoli cells.
- Testicular tumors are classified as:

    1. Primary neoplasms of testis
        a. Germ cell tumors (95%)
            - Seminoma (40%)
            - Spermatocytic seminoma
            - Nonseminomatous germ cell tumors:
                - Embryonal carcinoma (20–25%)
                - Teratoma (25–35%)
                - Choriocarcinoma (1%)
                - Yolk-sac tumors
        b. Nongerm cell tumors (5–10%)

2. Secondary neoplasms
  3. Paratesticular tumors

- Ninety-five percent of all testicular tumors originate from the germ cell and are hence called germ cell tumors. These tumors have the following subtypes:
  - Seminoma: This is a type of germ cell tumor that arise from the germinal epithelium of the seminiferous tubules with a possibility to metastasize. It accounts for 40% of the testicular tumors.
  - Spermatocytic seminoma: Is a subtype of seminoma. It hardly metastasizes.

- Nonseminomatous germ cell tumor comprises of a combination of any of following subtypes:
  - Embryonal carcinoma: It accounts for 20–25% of the tumors.
  - Teratoma: Teratoma of the testicle is the least aggressive form of cancer with a potential to relapse. It accounts for 25–35% of the testicular tumors.
  - Choriocarcinoma: Relatively rare (1% of testicular tumors) but most aggressive of the germ cell tumors. It spreads to the brain, lungs, and the liver quite early during the disease. Bleeding is common in patients with choriocarcinoma.
  - Yolk-sac tumors appear as large primary tumor.

- Testicular nongerm cell tumors: account for 5–10% of the testicular tumors. The various types are:
  - Specialized gonadal stromal tumors:
    ◦ Leydig cell tumors
    ◦ Sertoli cell tumors
    ◦ Other gonadal stromal tumors
    ◦ Gonadoblastoma
    ◦ Miscellaneous neoplasms
    ◦ Adenocarcinoma of the rete testis
    ◦ Mesenchymal neoplasms
    ◦ Carcinoid tumor
    ◦ Adrenal rest tumor

- The testis may also rarely be the site of a metastatic tumor from another organ.
- The testis may be the site of a lymphoma especially in a male above 60 years of age.
- Other structures that surround the testis, like its membranes and epididymis, can also, although rarely, produce benign or malignant tumors. These are called paratesticular tumors and an example is cystadenoma of epididymis or a mesothelioma.

Staging

- The testicular tumor is staged according to the tumor, node, metastasis (TNM) classification of malignant tumors. The size of the tumor in the testis is irrelevant to staging. Testicular cancer is staged as follows:
  - Stage I: The tumor remains localized to the testis.
  - Stage II: The tumor involves the testis and metastasis to retroperitoneal and/or para-aortic lymph nodes (lymph nodes below the diaphragm).
  - Stage III: The tumor involves the testis and metastasis beyond the retroperitoneal and para-aortic lymph nodes. Stage 3 is further subdivided into nonbulky stage 3 and bulky stage 3.
  - Stage IV: if there is liver and/or lung secondaries.

- The Intergroup Staging System for testicular germ cell tumors is as follows:
  - Stage I: The tumor is limited to the testis and completely resected (85% of children<4 years present with stage I disease (only 35% of adults present with stage I).
  - Stage II: The tumor is removed by transscrotal orchiectomy, involvement of scrotum or spermatic cord, persistently elevated tumor markers.
  - Stage III: There is retroperitoneal lymph node involvement (≤2 cm, no visceral or extra-abdominal involvement)
  - Stage IV: Distant metastases.

Treatment

- The treatment for yolk-sac tumors:
  - Inguinal orchiectomy and close surveillance. The tumor usually spreads to the lungs.
  - Current chemotherapeutic regimens for yolk-sac tumors are platinum-based protocols. Common agents include etoposide, bleomycin, and cisplatin.
  - Follow-up should include monthly tests of serum AFP levels, chest radiography every 2 months for 2 years, and CT scanning or MRI of the retroperitoneum every 3 months for the first year and then biannually.
  - Because spread to the retroperitoneal lymph nodes is uncommon, routine prophylactic dissection of the nodes is not performed.
  - Chemotherapy is administered in patients with radiographic evidence of metastatic disease or persistently elevated serum AFP levels.
  - The use of combination chemotherapy with cisplatin, etoposide, and bleomycin has been an effective treatment for metastatic disease, with a survival rate approaching 90%.
  - More than 99% of all patients with yolk-sac tumors are expected to survive.
  - Chemotherapy is recommended in all patients with yolk-sac tumors and stage II disease.
  - In boys with persistently elevated levels of tumor markers after chemotherapy, dissection of the retroperitoneal lymph node may be required.
  - Boys with stage III or IV germ cell tumors are treated with chemotherapy.
  - If elevated marker levels or retroperitoneal disease persists, biopsy or resection of residual tumor is performed.
- Prepubertal testicular teratomas, Leydig cell tumors, and Sertoli cell tumors are benign, and orchiectomy or testicular-sparing surgery with complete excision is curative.
- Stage II or higher teratocarcinomas require treatment with cisplatin, bleomycin, and vinblastine.
- Treatment of gonadoblastoma involves removal of the gonad. Streak gonads are routinely removed because of the risk of malignant degeneration.
- Seminoma is rare before puberty and is managed in a manner similar to that in the adult population.
- Juvenile granulosa-cell tumor is managed with inguinal orchiectomy and follow-up chest radiography for 1 year. Juvenile granulosa-cell tumors rarely metastasize.
- Paratesticular rhabdomyosarcoma:
  - Perform radical inguinal orchiectom.
  - If the scrotum is involved, hemiscrotectomy should be performed, with adjuvant chemotherapy.
  - All children with rhabdomyosarcoma require vincristine, adriamycin, and dactinomycin (VAC) chemotherapy or treatment with a combination of these drugs.
  - Patients with evidence of metastatic disease may require radiation therapy.

- Routine dissection of the retroperitoneal lymph nodes is recommended in all patients aged 10 years or older (regardless of the imaging results) and in patients younger than 10 years whose images show retroperitoneal disease.
- Children younger than 10 years have a survival rate of nearly 95%. Children older than 10 years have a worse prognosis and an increased risk for involvement of the retroperitoneal lymph nodes; therefore, an aggressive approach with dissection of the retroperitoneal lymph nodes is recommended.
- Routine dissection of the retroperitoneal lymph nodes is not performed to manage prepubertal testicular tumors. The incidence of metastases to the retroperitoneal lymph nodes is lower for these tumors than for postpubertal testicular tumors. However, the prognosis of children older than 10 years who have rhabdomyosarcoma is poor; modified retroperitoneal lymph node dissection is now recommended for these patients.

- The prognosis for patients with benign testicular lesions is excellent.
- Even for patients with metastatic yolk-sac tumor, survival with chemotherapy is approximately 90%.
- Patients with rhabdomyosarcoma have an overall survival rate of more than 70% when treated with multimodal chemotherapy. Poor prognostic indicators include:

  - Alveolar histology
  - Age older than 7 years
  - Unresectable retroperitoneal disease
  - Distant metastatic disease

Recommended Reading

Agarwal PK, Palmer JS. Testicular and paratesticular neoplasms in prepubertal males. J Urol. 2006;176:875–81.
Ciftci AO, Bingo"l-Kologlu M, Senocak ME, Tanyel FC, Buyukpamukcu M, Buyukpamukcu N. Testicular tumors in children. J Pediatr Surg. 2001;36:1796–801.
Green DM. Testicular tumors in infants and children. Semin Surg Oncol. 1986;2:156–62.
Horwich A, Shipley J, Huddart R. Testicular germ-cell cancer. Lancet. 2006;367:754–65.
Ross JH, Rybicki L, Kay R. Clinical behavior and a contemporary management algorithm for prepubertal testis tumors: a summary of the Prepubertal Testis Tumor Registry. J Urol. 2002;168:1675–8.
Sokoloff MH, Joyce GF, Wise M. Testis cancer. *J Urol*. 2007;177(6):2030–41.

Chapter 65
Thyroid Tumors

Introduction

- Thyroid carcinoma is relatively rare in children.
- Thyroid cancer, the most common pediatric endocrine neoplasm, represents 1–1.5 % of all pediatric malignancies and 5–5.7 % of head and neck malignant tumors.
- Only 5 % of all thyroid cancers occur in children and adolescents.
- Thyroid nodules occur in 4–7 % of the general adult population but in only 1–2 % of the pediatric population.
- Whereas 5 % of thyroid nodules in adults are malignant, in the pediatric population, the percentage of malignant thyroid nodules is 26.4 %. Pediatric thyroid nodules are four times more likely to be malignant than adult thyroid nodules.
- The incidence of thyroid carcinoma is 2–3 times more in girls than boys and commonly occurs between 7 and 12 years of age.
- Prior radiation to the neck in childhood is established as a causative factor in development of thyroid cancer. Radiation and chemotherapy for other pediatric malignancies also have been implicated in the etiology of thyroid malignancy. Children who undergo pretreatment radiation therapy prior to bone marrow transplant and children who undergo primary radiation treatments for Hodgkin lymphoma are at increased risk for thyroid cancer.
- Thyroglossal duct cysts carry an increased small risk of malignant transformation.
- Most childhood thyroid nodules are asymptomatic and are detected by parents or by physicians during routine examination.
- About 50 % of children with thyroid carcinoma present with nodular thyroid enlargement as the presenting symptom.
- Follicular adenoma is the most common cause of solitary thyroid nodules in the pediatric population; however, solitary nodules in children reportedly have a 20–73 % incidence of malignancy.
- A painless noninflammatory metastatic cervical mass is the presenting symptom in 40–60 % of patients.
- Malignant lesions are usually papillary and follicular carcinomas.

Classification

1. Papillary (72–75 %)
2. Follicular (18–20 %)
3. Medullary (5 %)
4. Anaplastic (1–2 %)

- Papillary thyroid cancer is by far the common thyroid malignancy in children.
- Medullary thyroid cancer (MTC):
  - Constitutes 5% of pediatric thyroid malignancies.
  - Is usually associated with multiple endocrine neoplasia type 2 (MEN2) in the pediatric population.
  - The inheritance pattern occurs either sporadically or as familial MTC without other associated endocrine abnormalities.
  - MTC (25% hereditary vs. 75% sporadic) are of C-cell (calcitonin-producing) origin.
  - MEN2 consists of MTC and pheochromocytoma and either hyperparathyroidism (2A) or mucosal neuromas (2B).
  - MTC associated with MEN2B is more virulent and may occur and metastasize early in infancy.
- Follicular adenoma is the most common cause of solitary nodules of the thyroid in the pediatric population.
- Adenomas are solitary, well circumscribed, and well encapsulated and are composed of glandular epithelium. Most are histologically follicular but are occasionally papillary.
- Most thyroid cancers (papillary, follicular, anaplastic) originate from follicular cells.
- Thyroid malignancies in children are usually well-differentiated papillary or papillary-follicular subtypes, but all histological types have been observed.
- Papillary carcinoma:
  - Comprise 72–75% of pediatric thyroid cancers.
  - Present as irregular, solid, or cystic masses that arise from follicular epithelium.
  - Most contain both papillary and follicular components.
  - Psammoma bodies are rounded calcified deposits found in approximately 50% of papillary carcinoma.
  - Papillary carcinoma has frequent lymphatic and pulmonary metastases.
- Follicular carcinoma:
  - Comprise 18–20% of pediatric thyroid cancers.
  - These are usually encapsulated and have highly cellular follicles and microfollicles with compact dark-staining nuclei of fairly uniform size, shape, and location.
  - Pathologic diagnosis can be made only when invasion of the capsule, adjacent glands, lymphatics, or blood vessels is seen.
  - Follicular carcinoma metastasizes intravascularly to the lungs, brain, and bones.
  - When a portion of the cells in the tumor are found to be oxyphilic (Hürthle cells), it is called a Hürthle cell tumor. These lesions tend to have a less favorable prognosis.
- MTC arises from the thyroid parafollicular or C cells, which secrete calcitonin and are derived from the neural crest. Calcifications are observed in 50% of these lesions.

Clinical Features

- Children commonly present with advanced disease.
- The neck masses are typically discovered incidentally by parents, patients, or physicians during routine physical examination.
- At presentation, 70% of patients have extensive regional nodal involvement, and 10–20% of patients have distant metastasis.

- The lungs are the most common sites of metastasis.
- Pediatric thyroid carcinoma occurs more frequently in adolescents, although it has been reported in the neonatal period.
- Thyroid carcinoma in pediatric patients usually manifests as an asymptomatic neck mass, with a reported incidence of cervical lymphadenopathy that ranges from 35 to 83%.
- 10–20% of patients present with distant metastasis (most commonly to the lungs) and 70% of patients present with extensive regional nodal involvement.
- Family history of thyroid cancer (especially in medullary cancer) is important.
  - Many young patients have a family history of thyroid cancer.
  - Of the MTC cases, 25% are hereditary, while more than 75% are sporadic.
  - A family history of MTC, pheochromocytoma, or hyperparathyroidism may indicate multiple endocrine neoplasia 2A (MEN2A) or multiple endocrine neoplasia 2B (MEN2B), both of which are inherited in an autosomal dominant fashion.
- Fixation of the mass to surrounding tissues and vocal cord paralysis (hoarseness of voice) suggest malignancy. This however is rare in the pediatric age group.

Diagnosis

- T3, T4, and thyroid-stimulating hormone (TSH) are usually normal.
- Antithyroid antibodies are helpful in diagnosing chronic lymphocytic thyroiditis.
- Thyroglobulin levels may be elevated in differentiated thyroid carcinoma and may help in postoperative monitoring.
- Calcitonin (medullary carcinoma) levels before and after pentagastrin stimulation.
- Screening for multiple endocrine neoplasia 2 (MEN2) is now possible with DNA analysis for specific mutations in the ret proto-oncogene.
- Serum carcinoembryonic antigen (CEA) should be measured in those with suspected MTC.
- Ultrasonography of neck.
- Thyroid scan: Thyroid scintigraphy has not proven worthwhile in distinguishing malignant from benign lesions. Classic hot nodules show uptake only in the nodule area of the thyroid and are associated with about a 6% incidence of malignancy. Solid lesions that are cold on scintigraphy are malignant in about 30% of children.
- Fine needle aspiration biopsy or excision biopsy:
  - Fine needle aspiration biopsy is standard in the diagnostic workup of adult thyroid nodules.
  - Several studies report efficacy in the pediatric population but others feel that it is often not practical in children younger than 10 years; and excisional biopsy under general anesthesia is recommended in this age group.
  - High diagnostic accuracy with experienced pathologists improves the selection of pediatric patients for surgery and is an adjunct to guide further management.
  - Ultrasonography can be a useful guide for percutaneous needle biopsy when the lesion is difficult to identify with palpation.
- Chest x-ray/CT chest to rule out metastasis,

Staging

The American Joint Committee on Cancer (AJCC) created the following staging system:

- T1: Tumor diameter 2 cm or smaller.
- T2: Primary tumor diameter > 2–4 cm.
- T3: Primary tumor diameter > 4 cm limited to the thyroid or with minimal extrathyroidal extension.
- T4a: Tumor of any size extending beyond the thyroid capsule to invade subcutaneous soft tissues, larynx, trachea, esophagus, or recurrent laryngeal nerve.
- T4b: Tumor invades prevertebral fascia or encases carotid artery or mediastinal vessels.
- TX: Primary tumor size unknown, but without extrathyroidal invasion.
- N0: No metastatic nodes.
- N1a: Metastases to level VI (pretracheal, paratracheal, and prelaryngeal/Delphian lymph nodes).
- N1b: Metastasis to unilateral, bilateral, contralateral cervical or superior mediastinal mode metastases.
- NX: Nodes not assessed at surgery.
- M0: No distant metastases.
- M1: Distant metastases.
- MX: Distant metastases not assessed.

Stage I (any T, any N, M0).
Stage II (any T, any N, M1).

Treatment

- Surgery is the mainstay of treatment for thyroid malignancy.
- Because of the unusual combination of an excellent prognosis and an advanced-stage disease at presentation, the initial extent of surgery is still controversial.
- Some recommend that the initial surgical approach should be conservative, while others advocate aggressive management with total thyroidectomy and radioactive iodine for all patients. The relative infrequency of thyroid malignancy makes this controversy difficult to resolve.
- Thyroid lobectomy is the initial procedure of choice for most solitary thyroid lesions. The need for total versus near-total or subtotal thyroidectomy is controversial.
- Proponents for near-total or subtotal thyroidectomy believe that these procedures decrease the incidence of complications such as recurrent laryngeal nerve injury and parathyroid devascularization, although the need to identify and preserve these structures remains. On the other hand, the remaining thyroid tissue may interfere with the use of radioactive iodine in the postoperative diagnostic scanning and in the treatment of microscopic regional and distant disease.
- Selective ipsilateral neck dissection in pediatric thyroid surgery is indicated for proven or suspected regional lymph node metastasis.
- A near-total thyroidectomy with radical lobectomy on the side of the primary lesion and subtotal removal of the contralateral lobe is recommended if the lesion is proven to be or suggestive of carcinoma.
- Radioiodine is usually recommended only for patients with extensive unresectable cervical nodal involvement, invasion of vital structures, or distant metastases.
- Total thyroidectomy and central neck dissection are indicated for biopsy-proven medullary carcinoma.
- Postoperative suppression of TSH with thyroid hormone may decrease recurrence and is more effective in papillary and papillary-follicular carcinomas.

Prognosis

Prognosis of differentiated carcinomas is very good; more than 90% survival has been reported.

Recommended Reading

Desjardins JG, Khan AH, Montupet P, et al. Management of thyroid nodules in children: a 20-year experience. J Pediatr Surg. 1987;22(8):736–9.

Halac I, Zimmerman D. Thyroid nodules and cancers in children. Endocrinol Metab Clin North Am. 2005;34(3):725–44.

Ridgway EC. Clinical review 30: clinician's evaluation of a solitary thyroid nodules. J Clin Endocrinol Metab. 1992;74(2):231–5.

Scholz S, Smith JR, Chaignaud B, Shamberger RC, Huang SA. Thyroid surgery at children's hospital Boston: a 35-year single-institution experience. J Pediatr Surg. 2011;46(3):437–42.

Chapter 66
Disorders of Sex Development

Introduction

- Disorders of sex development (DSD), sometimes referred to as disorders of sex differentiation, are congenital conditions characterized by chromosomal, gonadal, or anatomic sex developmental abnormalities.
- This definition has replaced the older terms, such as intersex and ambiguous genitalia.
- DSD consequently include anomalies of the sex chromosomes, the gonads, the reproductive ducts, and the external genitalia.
- Infants born with DSD represent a true medical and social emergency.
- Salt-wasting nephropathy occurs in 75% of infants born with congenital adrenal hyperplasia (CAH), the most common cause of DSD. If unrecognized, the resulting hypotension can cause vascular collapse and death. Male infants with this syndrome may be phenotypically normal, which may cause the diagnosis to be missed.
- Modern treatment of infants with DSD involves a team approach. This team involves:
  - Neonatologists
  - Geneticists/genetic counselor
  - Pediatric endocrinologists
  - Pediatric surgeons
  - Social worker
  - Obstetrician/pediatric urologist
  - Psychologist
- The goal is to provide appropriate medical support, gender assignment, appropriate surgical management, and counseling regarding care and therapy.
- Sex assignment (gender identity) is determined not only by the phenotypic appearance of the infant but also by other factors. These and other factors must be taken into consideration during the process of sex assignment:
  - Genetic sex (chromosomal sex)
  - Gonadal sex
  - Phenotypic sex
- Most of the spectrum of DSD anomalies are genetically caused, except one in which virilization of a 46, XX fetus is caused by maternal virilizing tumors or maternal ingestion of androgenic drugs.
- Most causes of DSD are due to an autosomal-recessive inheritance, such as CAH, 5-alpha-reductase deficiency, and defects in testosterone biosynthesis.

Table 66.1 Comparison of old and new classification of disorders of sex development

Previous	Proposed
Intersex	DSD
Male pseudohermaphrodite, undervirilization of a Y male, and undermasculinization of an XY male	46, XY DSD
Female pseudohermaphrodite, overvirilization of an XX female, and masculinization of an XX female	46, XX DSD
True hermaphrodite	Ovotesticular DSD
XX male or XX sex reversal	46, XX testicular DSD
XY sex reversal	46, XY complete gonadal dysgenesis

- X-linked recessive inheritance suggests androgen resistance (the androgen receptor gene is on the X chromosome).
- There are several types of DSDs and their effects on the external and internal reproductive organs vary greatly.
- DSD also vary in frequency, depending on their etiology.
- CAH is the most common cause of DSD in the newborn.
- Mixed gonadal dysgenesis (MGD) is the second most common cause of DSD.
- The overall incidence of DSD has been estimated at 1.7%.
- The incidence of DSD presenting with ambiguous genitalia at birth is estimated at 1.8 per 10,000 live births.
- The incidence of 46, XY DSD is estimated at 1 in 20,000 live male births.
- Fifty-two percent of patients with DSD have 46, XY DSD, 35% have 46, XX DSD, and 14% have a disorder of gonadal development.
- Partial androgen insensitivity syndrome, the most common cause of 46, XY DSD, is estimated to be about one-tenth as common as classic CAH.
- Overall, in 46, XY DSD patients, a definitive diagnosis is made in less than 50% of patients.
- This is in contrast to 46, XX DSD, where classic CAH, the most common cause, accounts for 95% of cases.
- A comparison between the old and the new classification of DSD is shown in Table 66.1.

Embryology

- Normal sexual differentiation and subsequent development depend on the genetic sex (XX or XY).
- Until 7 weeks of gestation, the fetus has undetermined sex with indifferent gonads (bipotential gonad) and internally developing both Wolffian and Müllerian ducts.
- Various genes expressed by the Y chromosome are responsible for the differentiation of the bipotential gonad to develop into testes.
- A 35-kilobase pair (kbp) gene (testis-determining factor, TDF) on the 11.3 subband of the distal short arm of the Y chromosome, an area termed as the sex-determining region of the Y chromosome (SRY), is responsible for initiating differentiation of the bipotential gonad and testes formation.
- The SRY also codes for a transcription factor that acts in the somatic cells of the genital ridge. This triggers a cascade of events that leads to the development of testicular Sertoli and Leydig cells.
- The SRY expression directs testicular morphogenesis, leading to the production of Müllerian-inhibiting substance (MIS) by the Sertoli cells and, later, testosterone by the Leydig cells.
- Surprisingly, more than half of the patients with XX ovotesticular DSD lack SRY, despite the presence of testicular differentiation. This suggests that this gene codes for a product that reacts with other genes on Y, X, and/or autosomes to complete testicular differentiation.

Embryology

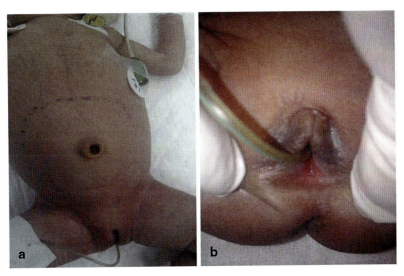

Fig. 66.1 a and **b** Clinical photographs of a newborn with vaginal atresia causing hydrocolpos

- In 46, XY males, the Sertoli cells of the testes are responsible for the production of MIS, which causes regression of the Müllerian ducts. The Leydig cells then produce testosterone which induces the primordial Wolffian (mesonephric) duct to develop into the epididymis, vas deferens, and seminal vesicle.
- MIS is produced by the Sertoli cells of the testis. It is a protein with a molecular weight of 15,000 d that is secreted by the testis beginning in the eighth fetal week. In a male fetus with normal testicular function, MIS represses Müllerian duct development (Fallopian tubes, uterus, and upper vagina).
- In the fetus with 46, XX, female gonadal development ensues.
- Ovarian differentiation from the bipotential gonad appears to rely on a mechanism that is triggered mostly, but not solely, by the absence of the SRY.
- Internal genitalia of the female fetus develop if there is no exposure to the *SRY* gene and its signaling molecules. The Wolffian duct (because of absence of SRY) regresses and the Müllerian duct (because of absence of MIS) then matures into the oviduct, uterus, cervix, and upper vagina.
- Hormone expression during the ninth week of gestation, from the testes or ovary, stimulates external genitalia development. By the 14th week of gestation, the external genitalia have been formed.
- The external genitalia of both sexes are identical during the first 7 weeks of gestation. Without the hormonal action of the androgens, testosterone, and dihydrotestosterone (DHT), external genitalia appear phenotypically female (Fig. 66.1)
- In the gonadal male:
  - Differentiation toward the male phenotype occurs over the next 8 weeks.
  - This is under the influence of testosterone, which is converted to 5-DHT by the action of 5-alpha reductase enzyme, present within the cytoplasm of cells of the external genitalia and the urogenital sinus.
  - DHT is bound to cytosol androgen receptors within the cytoplasm and is subsequently transported to the nucleus, where it leads to translation and transcription of genetic material.
  - This in turn leads to normal male external genital development from primordial parts, forming the scrotum from the genital swellings, forming the shaft of the penis from the folds, and forming the glans penis from the tubercle.

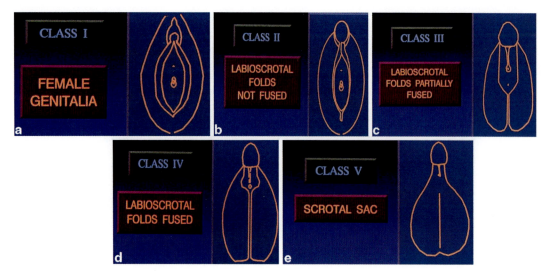

Fig. 66.2 a–e Diagrammatic representation of embryological differentiation of the external genitalia between males and females

- The prostate develops from the urogenital sinus.
- The timing of this testosterone-related developmental change begins at approximately 6 weeks of gestation, with a testosterone rise in response to a surge of luteinizing hormone (LH).
- Testosterone levels remain elevated until the 14th week.
- Most phenotypic differentiation occurs during this period.
- After the 14th week, fetal testosterone levels settle at a lower level, and are maintained more by maternal stimulation through human chorionic gonadotropin (HCG) than by LH.
- Testosterone's continued action during the latter phases of gestation is responsible for continued growth of the phallus, which is directly responsive to testosterone and to DHT (Fig. 66.2).
- Incomplete masculinization occurs:
- When testosterone fails to convert to DHT
- When DHT fails to act within the cytoplasm or nucleus of the cells of the external genitalia and urogenital sinus
- During the developmental process, there are multiple opportunities for errors in differentiation, all of which are possible causes of the DSD.
- In humans, genetic sex has traditionally been evaluated through establishing the karyotype of peripheral lymphocytes.
- The peripheral karyotypes of patients with ovotestes-DSD show marked variation:
    ○ Approximately 60% are 46, XX.
    ○ 15% are 46, XY.
    ○ 25% show various forms of mosaicism.
    ○ Less than 1% show 46, XX/46, XY chimerism or the existence of two or more cell lines, each of which has a different genetic origin.
- The existence of patients with 46, XX DSD, who have testicular tissue in the absence of a Y chromosome or SRY, clearly shows that other genetic components are involved. Other genes have been shown to play a role in testicular development. These include DAX1 on the X chromosome, S.1 on band 9q33, WT1 on band 11p13, SOX9 on bands 17q24-q25, and AMH on band 19q13.3. Fetal ovaries develop when the TDF gene (or genes) is absent.

Table 66.2 DSD classifications

Sex chromosome DSD	46, XY DSD	46, XX DSD
45, X (Turner syndrome and variants)	Disorders of testicular development: 1. Complete gonadal dysgenesis (Swyer syndrome) 2. Partial gonadal dysgenesis 3. Gonadal regression 4. Ovotesticular DSD	Disorders of gonadal (ovarian) development: 1. Ovotesticular DSD 2. Testicular DSD (e.g., SRY+, duplicate SOX9) 3. Gonadal dysgenesis
47, XXY (Klinefelter syndrome and variants)	Disorders in androgen synthesis or action: 1. Androgen biosynthesis defect (e.g., 17-hydroxysteroid dehydrogenase deficiency, 5αRD2 deficiency, StAR mutations) 2. Defect in androgen action (e.g., CAIS, PAIS) 3. Luteinizing hormone receptor defects (e.g., Leydig cell hypoplasia, aplasia) 4. Disorders of anti-Müllerian hormone (AMH) and AMH receptor (persistent Müllerian duct syndrome)	Androgen excess: 1. Fetal (e.g., 21-hydroxylase deficiency, 11-hydroxylase deficiency) 2. Fetoplacental (aromatase deficiency, P450 oxidoreductase [POR]) 3. Maternal (luteoma, exogenous, etc.)
45, X/46, XY (MGD, ovotesticular DSD)		Other (e.g., cloacal exstrophy, vaginal atresia, Müllerian, renal, cervicothoracic somite abnormalities [MURCS], other syndromes)
46, XX/46, XY (ovotesticular DSD)		

Classification

DSD classification is based on the new nomenclature as shown in Table 66.2.

- CAIS complete androgen insensitivity syndrome, PAIS *partial androgen insensitivity syndrome*
- Sex chromosome DSD:
    - 45, X (Turner syndrome and variants)
    - 47, XXY (Klinefelter syndrome and variants)
    - 45, X/46, XY (MGD, ovotesticular DSD)
    - 46, XX/46, XY (chimeric, ovotesticular DSD)
- 46, XY DSD: chromosomally male, but DSD results from:
    - Disorders of testicular development (complete and partial gonadal dysgenesis)
    - Disorders of androgen synthesis or action (complete and partial androgen insensitivity, disorders of AMH/anti-Müllerian receptor, androgen biosynthesis defect)
    - Syndromes associated with defects in genital development, including cloacal anomalies, vanishing testes syndrome, congenital hypogonadotropic hypogonadism, and severe hypospadias
- 46, XX DSD: chromosomally female, but DSD results from:
    - Disorders of ovarian development (ovotesticular DSD, testicular DSD, gonadal dysgenesis)
    - Disorders leading to androgen excess (fetal, e.g., CAH, fetoplacental, maternal)
    - Abnormalities of Müllerian ducts (Müllerian ducts dysgenesis or hypoplasia, vaginal atresia, cloacal exstrophy; Fig. 66.3).

Fig. 66.3 A clinical photograph of a patient with cloacal extrophy showing distorted anatomy of external genitalia

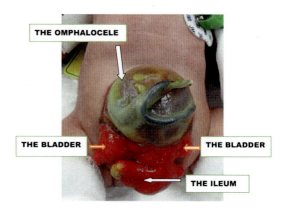

Etiology

- The etiology of DSD that is present at birth depends on the type of disorder (Fig. 66.4).
- Most causes of DSD are genetic.
- One exception is virilization of a 46, XX fetus due to maternal virilizing tumors or maternal ingestion of androgenic drugs.
- Genetic causes include:
  1. Sex chromosome DSD:
     - This presents as ambiguous genitalia due to meiotic or mitotic gain or loss of a chromosome, or due to chimerism.
     - 45X/46, XY MGD is due to postmeiotic errors, leading to loss of a Y chromosome in one cell lineage.
     - 46, XX/46, XY chimerism is due to the fusion of two zygotes.
  2. 46, XY DSD:
     - Gonadal dysgenesis may be due to mutations in one of several genes that are involved in testicular development.
     - Defects in SRY can cause ovotesticular DSD.
     - Disorders of androgen synthesis which include mutations in genes responsible for testosterone synthesis. These can be common to the adrenal gland and the testes, and thus cause deficiencies of glucocorticoids and/or mineralocorticoids or are just found in the testes and thus only lead to defects in testosterone biosynthesis. These include:
     - 17-hydroxylase deficiency and 20–22 lyase deficiency due to mutations in CYP17.
     - 3-hydroxysteroid dehydrogenase deficiency due to mutations in HSD3B2.
     - 5-alpha-reductase deficiency due to mutations in steroid 5-alpha-reductase (SRD5A2), which converts testosterone to DHT.
     - Steroidogenic acute regulatory (StAR) protein deficiency.
     - These are all autosomal-recessive conditions.
     - Partial androgen insensitivity syndrome is due to mutations in the androgen receptor on Xq11. This is an X-linked recessive condition.
     - Various genetic syndromes associated with defects in genital development, such as Smith–Lemli–Opitz syndrome
     - Congenital hypogonadotropic hypogonadism can be due to one of several gene defects.
  3. 46, XX DSD:
     - CAH.
     - CAH is due to 21-hydroxylase deficiency (CYP21A2 on chromosome 6p21.3).

Etiology

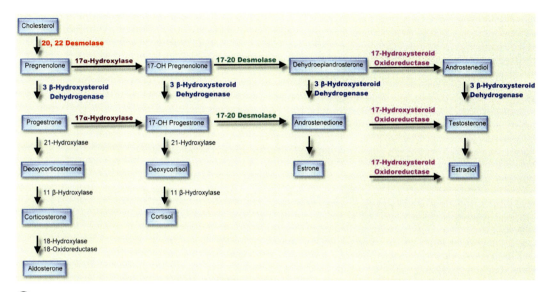

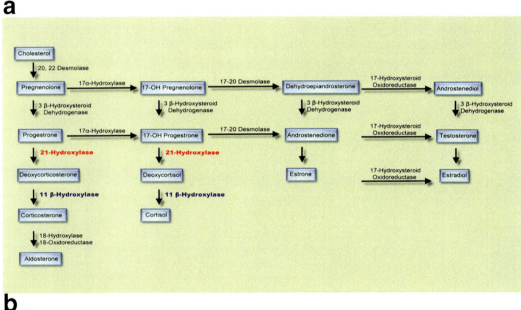

Fig. 66.4 a Diagrammatic representation of steroid biosynthesis. **b** The enzymes likely to be affected in congenital adrenal hyperplasia

- This is the cause in more than 95% of cases.
- This is an autosomal-recessive condition.
- Some of the other causes are 11-beta-hydroxylase deficiency (CYP11B1 on chromosome 8q21).
- 3-beta-hydroxysteroid dehydrogenase deficiency (HSD3B2 on chromosome 1p13.1).
- Gonadal dysgenesis can be due to translocation of an SRY gene onto an X chromosome or to duplication of the SOX9 region.

Pathophysiology

- MGD
  - Characterized by asymmetrical development of the gonads and internal genital ducts.
  - There is a dysgenetic testis and thus poorly developed Wolffian ducts on one side and a streak gonad (ovary) on the other side.
  - Variable degrees of external genital ambiguity are found.
  - The lack of a Y chromosome, and thus lack of the SRY gene, on one side presumably leads to the dysgenetic testis that produces some, but not enough, testosterone for normal male development.
  - The degree of virilization depends on the degree of functioning testes.
- In 46, XY DSD presenting as ambiguous genitalia, the degree of virilization depends on:
  - The amount of residual functioning testes.
  - The amount of testosterone synthesized.
  - The degree of androgen insensitivity.
- In 46, XX DSD with CAH due to 21-hydroxylase deficiency:
  - The degree of virilization depends on the residual activity of the 21-hydroxylase gene.
  - In the absence of any 21-hydroxylase activity, essentially all of the cortisol precursors are directed to androgen production leading to high androgen levels and severe virilization. These cases are associated with salt wasting.

Evaluation of a Newborn with DSD

- The diagnostic approach to a newborn with ambiguous genitalia involves a multidisciplinary team approach.
- This includes a pediatric endocrinologist, geneticist, pediatric surgeon, pediatric urologist, and a neonatologist.
- Sex assignment.
  - A sex is not assigned to the baby until the evaluation has been completed, but as soon as is feasible.
  - The child is referred to as "baby," not boy or girl.
  - The family should be encouraged to delay naming the baby until the sex has been assigned.
- The needs, background, culture, and expectations of the parents must be understood and respected.
- Parents should understand that children with a DSD can live normal lives and function well in society.
- Educating the parents regarding sexual development is also important, as this helps them understand and participate in the process.
- The most common disorder of DSD, CAH, results in virilization of a 46, XX female and thus is classified under the group of 46, XX DSD. It is important to distinguish CAH from other less common causes of DSD.
- Although different disorders may present with similar findings on physical examination, there are often aspects of the examination that are crucial and will help define the disorder and may help direct the necessary investigation.

Evaluation of a Newborn with DSD

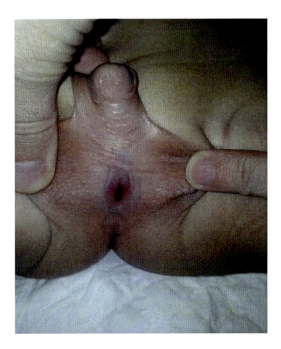

Fig. 66.5 A clinical photograph of a patient with severe hypospadias. This should be investigated to rule out associated DSD

- It is important to rule out a malformation syndrome in a patient with ambiguous genitalia.
- Gonadal and external genitalia examination:
  - Note the size and degree of differentiation of the phallus, since variations may represent clitoromegaly or hypospadias.
  - Phallus length:
    - A normal-term male penis is 3.5 ± 0.7 cm.
    - A length of less than 2.0 cm is considered abnormal.
    - A normal-term female clitoris is less than 1.0 cm.
    - Micropenis is thus defined as a stretch penile length of less than 2.0 cm in a term male infant, and clitoromegaly as a clitoris greater than 1.0 cm in a term female. In preterm infant males, the penile length is shorter.
  - Note the position of the urethral meatus (Fig. 66.5).
    - Hypospadias associated with separation of scrotal sacs or undescended testis suggests a DSD.
    - If the urethral opening is at the base of the phallus, it could be a urogenital sinus in a virilized female.
  - Labioscrotal folds may be separated or be fused at the midline, giving an appearance of a scrotum.
  - Newborns with 46, XX DSD due to CAH may have hyperpigmented labioscrotal folds.
  - Anogenital ratio:
    - This is the distance between the anus and posterior fourchette divided by the distance between the anus and base of the clitoris/phallus.
    - A ratio greater than 0.5 suggests virilization.
    - In a fully virilized male the ratio is 1.0.
  - Documentation of palpable gonads is important.
    - Although ovotestes have been reported to descend completely into the bottom of labioscrotal folds, in most patients, only testicular material descends fully.
    - If examination reveals palpable inguinal gonads, the diagnoses of a gonadal female, Turner syndrome, or pure gonadal dysgenesis can be eliminated.

- Impalpable gonads, even in an apparently fully virilized infant, should raise the possibility of a severely virilized 46, XX DSD patient with CAH.
- The presence of two gonads strongly favors the diagnosis of a 46, XY DSD.
- The presence of only one palpable gonad suggests the diagnosis of MGD, although it does not rule out a 46, XX ovotesticular DSD.
– Rectal examination may reveal the cervix and uterus, confirming internal Müllerian structures.

Evaluation of infants with ambiguous genitalia includes the following:

– Chromosomal analysis
– Endocrine screening
– Serum chemistries/electrolyte tests
– Androgen-receptor levels
– 5-alpha reductase type II levels

- A general approach to investigation includes karyotyping and palpation for gonads.
- Karyotyping should be ordered in all patients with suspected DSD.
- If the patient has no palpable gonads, a CAH screen should be ordered.
- If this is positive, an ultrasound and voiding cystourethrogram should be ordered to confirm the diagnosis.
- If there are palpable gonad(s) present, or CAH screen is negative, a biochemical profile, ultrasound, and gonadal inspection (with or without biopsy) should be ordered.
- Abdominal and pelvic ultrasound:

  – The adrenal glands may be enlarged in infants with CAH. They have a cribriform appearance.
  – A normal adrenal gland does not exclude a diagnosis of CAH.
  – A pelvic ultrasound is performed to determine whether Müllerian structures (uterus) are present.
  – In a neonate, findings of ambiguous genitalia, enlarged adrenal glands, and evidence of a uterus are pathognomonic for CAH.
  – Ultrasound may also help detect and locate undescended testes.

- Hormonal studies:

  – Hormonal tests should be performed in all patients and depend on the presence or absence of palpable gonads.

- No palpable gonads:

  – In the absence of palpable gonads, the most likely diagnosis is CAH secondary to 21-hydroxylase deficiency.
  – 17-hydroxyprogesterone (17-OHP) levels should be obtained and will be markedly elevated.
  – In CAH, electrolytes should be monitored closely, as salt wasting may take a few days to develop.
  – High plasma renin and elevated 17-OHP confirm salt wasting in CAH due to 21-hydroxylase deficiency.
  – If CAH is suspected and 17-OHP levels are not markedly elevated, adrenal precursors should be further evaluated to look for more rare causes of CAH, including 11-deoxycortisol and 11-deoxycorticosterone to rule out 11-beta-hydroxylase deficiency.

- Gonad(s) palpable:
- Testosterone and DHT:

  – A high testosterone to DHT ratio suggests a 5-alpha-reductase deficiency.
  – Partial androgen insensitivity syndrome is often a diagnosis of exclusion in a 46, XY patient. The testosterone may be elevated and, if so, facilitates the diagnosis.

Fig. 66.6 A genitogram showing a urinary bladder, vagina, and a common channel showing a urogenital sinus in a patient with congenital adrenal hyperplasia

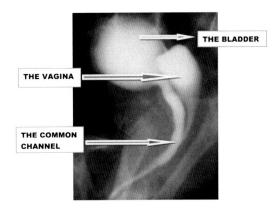

- LH and follicle-stimulating hormone (FSH):
  - These help evaluate the hypothalamic–pituitary–gonadal axis.
  - Low levels in the first week of life do not necessarily indicate hypogonadotropic hypogonadism and assessment at 2–4 months of life may be more informative when there is an increase in LH and FSH levels.
- ACTH (adrenocorticotrophic hormone) stimulation test:
  - This can identify a block in the testosterone biosynthesis pathway.
  - It may also reveal abnormalities of glucocorticoid and mineralocorticoid synthesis as in those with CAH.
- HCG stimulation test:
  - This helps assess the ability of the testes to respond to HCG and produce testosterone.
  - The ratio of testosterone to DHT after HCG stimulation is a sensitive way to detect 5-alpha-reductase deficiency.
  - The HCG stimulation test is also a good test to identify a block in the testosterone biosynthesis pathway and may be a better test than the ACTH stimulation test if a defect in glucocorticoid production is not suspected.
- MIS:
  - This can be obtained to assess testicular function in a child suspected to have 46, XY DSD and in the category of chromosomal DSD.
  - MIS levels are age and sex dependent.
- A MCUG (micturating cystourethrogram) is performed when there is a single opening at the base of the phallus to determine whether a urogenital sinus is present in a suspected virilized female.
- A Genitogram helps determine the reproductive system anatomy. Findings may indicate normal urethral anatomy, an enlarged utricle, a Müllerian remnant in a male, a common urogenital sinus, or an area of vaginal and urethral confluence in female neonates (Fig. 66.6)
- Computed tomography (CT) scan and magnetic resonance imaging (MRI) are usually not necessary but may help identify internal anatomy.
- Exploratory laparotomy/gonadal biopsy: Open exploration may help identify internal duct anatomy and allow gonadal tissue to be biopsied for histological evaluation. With the recent advances in minimal invasive surgery, many authors advocate laparoscopy for this purpose.
- Histological evaluation of gonadal biopsy specimens may identify ovarian tissue, testicular tissue, ovotestes, or streak gonads.

Management of Patients with DSD

- Medical and surgical therapy for patients with DSD depends on the underlying cause and is indicated for the conditions associated with ambiguous genitalia, including CAH. Supplemental hormone therapy may be given if gonadal function is compromised.
- In a virilized female, the surgical procedure is feminizing genitoplasty and includes vaginoplasty and clitoroplasty.
- Undervirilized males typically have hypospadias which require urethroplasty.
- Gender reassignment may be considered in patients with 46, XY males and inadequate external genitalia.

The More Common Causes of DSD

1. 46, XX DSD (formerly termed female pseudohermaphroditism)
   - CAH is the most frequent cause of DSD in the newborn. Excessive androstenedione production results in a gonadal female with a virilized phenotype.
   - The basic defect is an enzyme deficiency (commonly 21-hydroxylase deficiency) that prevents sufficient cortisol production.
   - Biofeedback via the pituitary gland causes accumulation of the precursor above the block.
   - CAH presents a spectrum of abnormalities, including the degree of phallic enlargement, the extent of urethral fold fusion, and the size and level of entry of the vagina into the urogenital sinus.
   - Although the degree of virilization seen in CAH can be extreme, internal Müllerian structures are consistently present.
   - In these children, endocrine stabilization must be individualized, a process that usually takes several weeks.
   - CAH may result from the following metabolic defects:
     - 21-Hydroxylase deficiency:
       - In 90% of patients with CAH, the block is at the 21-hydroxylation enzyme. This leads to a mineralocorticoid deficiency and a buildup of androgenic byproducts, which causes masculinization of a female fetus. The result is a female infant with varying degrees of virilization.
       - Biochemically, 75% of patients have salt-wasting nephropathy. This must be recognized to avoid vascular collapse.
       - The 21-hydroxylase defect is inherited as an autosomal recessive trait closely linked to the human leukocyte antigen (HLA) locus on chromosome 6.
       - The transmitted trait may have two varieties, which helps account for the clinical heterogenicity seen in patients with salt-wasting nephropathy.
       - Prenatal diagnosis is confirmed by noting an elevated amniotic fluid level of 17-OHP during the second trimester or by HLA typing of amniotic cells.
       - CAH is diagnosed more often following birth during evaluation of a 46, XX newborn with ambiguous genitalia.
       - The diagnosis is confirmed by an elevated serum level of 17-OHP.
       - 17-OHP levels may be markedly elevated also in the 11-hydroxylase form of CAH, as well as in the rare child with the 3-beta-hydroxysteroid dehydrogenase form of CAH.
     - 11-Hydroxylase deficiency:
       - CAH secondary to 11-hydroxylase deficiency leads to accumulation deoxycorticosterone (DOC) and 11-deoxycortisol.

- This leads to salt retention and hypertension because DOC is a potent mineralocorticoid.
            - This should be suspected in a 46, XX child with ambiguous genitalia in whom the 17-OHP level is elevated only mildly. The diagnosis can be confirmed by measurement of other steroid metabolites.
      ◦ 3-Beta-hydroxysteroid dehydrogenase deficiency:
            - CAH caused by 3-beta-hydroxysteroid dehydrogenase deficiency is rare.
            - This causes less severe virilization of a female infant than the virilization caused by 21-hydroxylase or 11-hydroxylase deficiency.
            - The buildup of pregneninolone, which is converted in the liver to testosterone, leads to virilization.
            - Patients can present with a salt-losing crisis caused by deficient mineralocorticoid production, similar to that occurring with 21-hydroxylase deficiency.
            - The diagnosis can be confirmed by identifying an elevated serum level of dehydroepiandrosterone or its sulfate metabolite.
            - 3-beta-hydroxysteroid dehydrogenase deficiency is the only common form of CAH that can also cause ambiguity in the genetic male. This ambiguity occurs because the enzyme defect is present in both the adrenal glands and the testes, leading to inadequate production of testosterone in utero.
      ◦ Maternal androgens
            - Although rare, female pseudohermaphroditism may be drug induced.
            - Virilization of a female fetus may occur if progestational agents or androgens are used during the first trimester of pregnancy.
            - After the first trimester, these drugs cause only phallic enlargement without labioscrotal fusion.
            - The incriminated drugs were formerly administered to avoid spontaneous miscarriages in patients who had a history of habitual abortion.
            - Extremely rare, various ovarian tumors (e.g., arrhenoblastomas, Krukenberg tumors, luteomas, lipoid tumors of the ovary, stromal cell tumors) have produced virilization of a female fetus.

2. Ovotesticular DSD (formerly termed true hermaphroditism)

    - Both ovarian and testicular tissues are present in ovotesticular DSD, an uncommon cause accounting for fewer than 10% of DSD cases.
    - The appearance of the genitalia varies widely but the tendency is toward masculinization.
    - The most common karyotype is 46, XX. Other karyotypes include 46, XY and 46, XX/46, XY as well as others.
    - A translocation of the gene coding for HY antigen from a Y chromosome to either an X chromosome or an autosome presumably explains the testicular material in a patient with a 46, XX karyotype.
    - The reason for patients with a 46, XY karyotype to have ovarian tissue is not known, since two X chromosomes are believed to be necessary to normal ovarian development. A possible explanation is the presence of unidentified XX cell lines in these patients.
    - Gonadal findings may be any combination of ovary, testis, or ovotestis.
      ◦ An ovotestis is the most common and is found in approximately two-thirds of patients.
      ◦ When an ovotestis is present, one-third of the patients exhibit bilateral ovotestes.
      ◦ A testicle, when present, is more likely to exist on the right (57.4%), and an ovary, when present, is more common on the left (62%).
      ◦ A palpable gonad is present in 61% of patients; of these, 60% are found to be an ovotestis.
      ◦ In 80% of patients with ovotestes, testicular and ovarian tissues are aligned in an end-to-end manner, emphasizing the need for a long longitudinal biopsy.

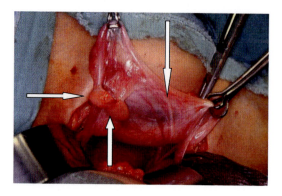

Fig. 66.7 Intraoperative photograph showing ovo-testes on one side in a patient with true hermaphrodite. Note the vas on one side

- In 20% of patients with ovotestes, testicular tissue is found in the hilar region of the gonad, reemphasizing the need for an adequate and deep biopsy.
- An ovary, when present, is found most commonly in the normal anatomic intra-abdominal position.
- The least common gonad in ovotesticular DSD is the testis; when present, a testis is found approximately two-thirds of the time in the scrotum, emphasizing that normal testicular tissue is most likely to descend fully.
- Ovotestes may present with either a fallopian tube or a vas deferens but usually not both (Fig. 66.7).
- If a fallopian tube has a fimbriated end, the end is closed in most patients, perhaps contributing to the usual lack of fertility.
- While rare, fertility has been reported.
- Gonadal tumors also are rare but have been reported in these patients.

3. 46, XY DSD (formerly termed male pseudohermaphroditism)

   a. Isolated deficiency of MIS (persistent Müllerian duct syndrome) (Fig. 66.8):
      - Isolated MIS deficiency is rare and results from a complete failure of the testes to produce MIS.
      - This usually does not present in the newborn period because the genitalia are those of a male with undescended testes.
      - The most common presentation is a phenotypic male with an inguinal hernia on one side and an impalpable contralateral gonad.
      - Herniorrhaphy reveals a uterus and fallopian tube in the hernia sac.
      - Since the testis produces normal levels of testosterone, a vas deferens presents bilaterally, usually running close to the uterus.
      - To avoid damage to the vas, care must be taken when excising Müllerian remnants. At times, the vas deferens ends blindly.
      - Appropriate surgical management includes:
        - Orchidopexy. This may necessitate division of the uterus to lengthen the vas.
        - A transverse testicular ectopia may be associated with this.
        - Removal of Müllerian remnants is unnecessary, since the remnants rarely produce symptoms and an extremely rare risk of subsequent malignancy.
      - 46, XY DSD occasionally occurs in families. Confined to males, inheritance may be either X-linked recessive or autosomal dominant.

Deficient testosterone biosynthesis:

- Testosterone is produced from cholesterol and this involves five enzymatic steps.
- Defects have been identified at each of these five steps.

The More Common Causes of DSD

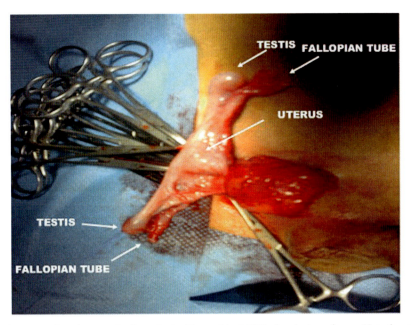

Fig. 66.8 An intraoperative photograph of a patient with persistent Müllerian duct syndrome. Note the uterus and fallopian tubes as well as the testes

- Of these five enzymes, three
  - 20-alpha hydroxylase
  - 3-beta-hydroxysteroid dehydrogenase
  - 17-alpha hydroxylase
- Are shared with the adrenal glands, and their deficiency leads to ambiguous genitalia and symptoms of CAH.
- The other two enzymes:
  - 17, 20 desmolase
  - 17-ketosteroid reductase
- Occur only as part of normal testosterone synthesis, and their defects leads to genital abnormalities, but are not associated with CAH.
- The diagnosis of these syndromes is possible by measuring the buildup of precursor products. This however is available in specialized centers only.
- During the newborn period, these patients present as 46, XY gonadal males with poor virilization and ambiguous genitalia.
- The genitalia respond to exogenously administered testosterone.
- Children with CAH manifestations also require treatment with steroid and mineralocorticoid replacement.
- Genetic counseling is desirable because 17-alpha hydroxylase and 3-beta-hydroxysteroid dehydrogenase deficiencies are transmitted as autosomal recessive traits.
- Additional rare causes for deficiencies in testosterone production include Leydig cell agenesis, Leydig cell hypoplasia, abnormal Leydig cell gonadotropin receptors, and delayed receptor maturation (Fig. 66.9).
  b. Complete androgen insensitivity syndrome (testicular feminization syndrome) (Fig. 66.10):
    - This results from failure of the end organ (external genitalia and prostate) in a 46, XY gonadal male fetus to respond to appropriately produced levels of DHT (dihydrotestesterone).

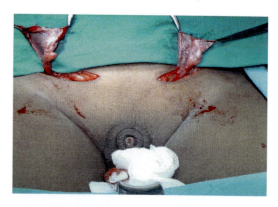

Fig. 66.9 An intraoperative photograph of a patient with bilateral atrophic testes

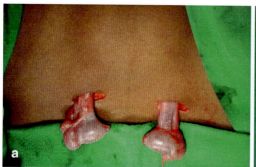
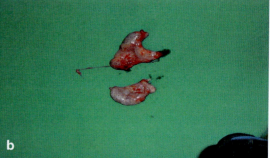

Fig. 66.10 a and b Intraoperative photographs showing intra-abdominal testes in a patient with testicular feminization syndrome. Both testes were excised

- The basic pathophysiology is based on assays of genital skin fibroblasts which defines two variants:
    - Receptor-negative: Some patients are receptor negative; their cytosol receptors cannot bind DHT.
    - Receptor-positive: Another variant is receptor positive in which receptors apparently permit DHT binding, but DHT does not lead to normal differentiation toward the male phenotype.
- Inheritance appears to be X-linked.
- Complete androgen insensitivity rarely presents in infancy with a shallow blind-ending vagina.
- Inguinal hernias are common in testicular feminization, and sometimes the diagnosis is made during inguinal herniorrhaphy when a gonad is present in the hernia and a fallopian tube cannot be seen.
- Failure to identify an internal Müllerian structure in a phenotypic female with an inguinal hernia should always raise the possibility of testicular feminization.
- If not detected this way, the diagnosis usually is not made until puberty, when the patient presents with amenorrhea.
- Despite a 46, XY karyotype and gonads with the typical appearance of testes, a feminine gender assignment is unquestionable because of the completely feminine phenotype.
- Confirmation of the diagnosis is crucial because the syndrome is associated with a significant incidence of gonadal malignancies.

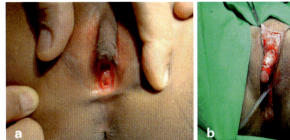

Fig. 66.11 a–c Intraoperative photographs of a patient with partial (incomplete androgen insensitivity syndrome). Note the vagina as well as the enlarged clitoris. Clitoroplasty was done

- The overall frequency of gonadal malignancies is approximately 6 %, with incidence rising to more than 30 % by age 50 years.
- Seminomas are the commonest malignant tumors.
- Other tumors include: Sertoli cell and Leydig cell tumors and tubular cell adenomas.
- The best timing for gonadectomy is still controversial. There are those who recommend gonadectomy after puberty. In contrast, others recommend early removal because morbidity is minimal in a young child.
- Pubertal changes are induced easily with hormone replacement, a requirement for all patients following gonadectomy.
- Although a vaginoplasty may be required later in life, many of these girls have an adequate vagina, requiring no vaginoplasty or possibly only vaginal dilation.

c. Partial androgen insensitivity syndrome (Fig. 66.11):
- An incomplete form of androgen insensitivity also occurs.
- These patients demonstrate a spectrum of external genitalia ranging from:
  - Very feminine (Lubs syndrome)
  - To increasingly masculine (Gilbert–Dreyfus syndrome).
  - To most masculine (Reifenstein syndrome)
- A diagnosis of incomplete androgen insensitivity is suggested by:
  - Elevated LH levels
  - Normal levels of plasma DHT
  - Normal 5-alpha-reductase activity in genital skin fibroblasts
- An early gonadectomy and feminizing genitoplasty are recommended in infancy.

d. 5-Alpha-reductase deficiency:
- This is seen in a 46, XY fetus with normal testes but lacks the enzyme 5-alpha reductase in the cells of the external genitalia and urogenital sinus.
- This leads to defect in the conversion of testosterone to DHT.
- The fetus is born with minimally virilized external genitalia (pseudovaginal perineoscrotal hypospadias).
- The fetus usually has a degree of phallic enlargement as a result of the direct action of testosterone.
- The striking feature in these patients is the extreme virilization at puberty. This is most likely caused by direct action of testosterone on the phallus. There will be increase in the penile size as well as the muscle mass and a masculine voice.
- The only characteristics that do not develop are those that depend on DHT (prostatic enlargement, facial hair, acne).
- There is a spectrum of 5-alpha-reductase deficiency which probably accounts for some of the variation in the phenotypes seen.

- Diagnosis of 5-alpha-reductase deficiency can be confirmed:
  - A patient with a 46, XY karyotype.
  - A high ratio of serum testosterone to DHT.
  - During the first 60 days of life, infants experience a surge of LH that obviates the need to carry out HCG stimulation, which may be useful to exaggerate the testosterone-to-DHT ratio characteristic of this syndrome.
  - The normal testosterone-to-DHT ratio is 8–16:1, while patients with 5-alpha-reductase deficiency characteristically have a ratio greater than 35:1.
  - Urinary metabolites of testosterone and DHT can be used to establish the diagnosis in a similar manner.
  - Cultured skin fibroblasts demonstrate decreased 5-alpha-reductase activity.
- Gender assignment in these patients has been debated because of the major virilization that occurs at puberty.
- Many recommend that all patients should be raised as males.
- Others say that only the most extremely virilized infant should receive a male gender assignment.
- Surgical results of a masculinizing operation in a mildly virilized infant are poor, and the burden to the child of growing up with inadequate genitalia hardly seems justified.
- Many authors recommend gonadectomy and feminizing genitoplasty in these patients.

e. Partial gonadal dysgenesis:
- Partial gonadal dysgenesis can be classified as either 46, XY DSD or sex chromosome DSD if there is mosaicism (45, X/46, XY).
- This represents a spectrum of DSD in which the gonads are abnormally developed.
- Typically, at least one gonad is either dysgenetic testis or a streak ovary.
- In MGD, a streak gonad is usually present on one side and a testis (usually dysgenetic) on the opposite side.
- Dysgenetic male pseudohermaphroditism (DMP): This is to describe patients with bilaterally dysgenetic testes and incomplete virilization of the internal sex ducts and external genitalia.
- A dysgenetic testis histologically demonstrates immature and hypoplastic testicular tubules in a stroma characteristic of ovarian tissue but that lack oocytes.
- Although the degree of virilization varies, all patients have a vagina and a uterus, and most have a fallopian tube, at least on the side of the streak gonad.
- Most patients with MGD have a mosaic karyotype, 45, X/46, XY.
- A characteristic of patients with a 45, X karyotype is short stature. Patients who have no internal Müllerian remnants usually have no 45, X component.
- There is a risk of gonadal malignancy when a Y chromosome is present in the karyotype.
- In MGD, 25% of gonads, including streak gonads, can be expected to undergo malignant change, most commonly to gonadoblastoma.
- In addition to gonadoblastomas, seminomas and embryonal cell carcinomas may develop.
- Early gonadectomy is recommended early in these patients.
- Gender assignment for patients with DMP and MGD remains controversial.
- There are those who recommend a male gender assignment to patients who are sufficiently virilized.
- Others prefer a feminine gender assignment for patients with MGD because a uterus and vagina always are present and one half of patients are markedly short and have a high incidence of inadequate external virilization.
- Estrogen support is required if these patients are raised as females.
- If the uterus remains in place, the unopposed estrogen can increase the incidence of endometrial carcinoma; thus, these patients must be cycled with a combination of estrogen and a progestational agent.

f. Pure gonadal dysgenesis:
   - These patients are phenotypically females.
   - They have bilateral streak gonads appearing as ovarian stroma without oocytes.
   - Usually this goes unrecognized in the newborn period.
   - These patients tend to present at puberty when they do not undergo normal pubertal changes.
   - Girls with Turner syndrome (45, XO) may be detected earlier by noting the characteristic associated with anomalies of short stature, webbing of the neck, and wide-spaced nipples.
   - Neither Turner syndrome (45, XO) nor the 46, XX type of pure gonadal dysgenesis appears to be associated with increased risk of gonadal malignancy.
   - Patients with 46, X pure gonadal dysgenesis on the other hand carry a significant potential for malignancy. Nearly one-third of patients develop a dysgerminoma or gonadoblastoma; therefore, gonadectomy should be done as soon as the diagnosis is confirmed.
   - Therapy in those with pure gonadal dysgenesis is primarily limited to appropriate estrogen and progesterone support.
   - Pure gonadal dysgenesis syndromes call for genetic counseling.
     - Turner syndrome appears sporadically, suggesting a postzygotic error.
     - The 46, XX type of pure gonadal dysgenesis appears to have an autosomal recessive transmission.
     - The 46, XY type is apparently an X-linked recessive trait.

Sex Assignment and Therapy

- Many factors must be considered during sex assignment, including:
  1. The phenotype
  2. The appearance of the genitalias
  3. The surgical options
  4. The need for future hormonal replacement therapy
  5. The potential for future fertility
  6. The culture and preferences of the family
  7. The effect of high levels of testosterone exposure on the brain development
- Sex assignment depends on the classification type (46, XX DSD, 46, XY DSD or chromosomal DSD).

  a. 46, XX chromosomes:

CAH

- These patients are usually assigned a female sex.
- Fertility is preserved.
- Surgical management, if necessary, is relatively straightforward.
- Glucocorticoids (usually hydrocortisone) are subscribed to replace cortisol, and, if there is associated salt wasting, fludrocortisone is given to replace aldosterone.
- Treatment is commenced as soon as the diagnosis is confirmed and is continued lifelong.
- Early surgical management is recommended.
  - Clitoroplasty
  - Vaginoplasty including separation of the vaginal opening from the urethral opening
  - Further genitoplasty in adolescence may be necessary

b. 46, XY chromosomes:
   1. Testosterone biosynthesis defects
      - Newborns are assigned a male sex, as fertility is preserved.
      - Patients with defects that are common to the adrenal gland and the testes have deficiencies of glucocorticoids and/or mineralocorticoids. Treatment with glucocorticoids and/or mineralocorticoids in these patients is commenced as soon as the diagnosis is confirmed and is continued indefinitely.
      - If hypospadias or chordee is present, it requires early surgical correction.
      - Testosterone replacement may be required at puberty, particularly if testosterone levels remain low.
   2. 5-alpha-reductase deficiency
      - Typically newborns are assigned a male sex.
      - Fertility is preserved.
      - If hypospadias or chordee is present, it requires surgical correction.
      - Virilization is usually adequate and these patients do not typically need hormonal replacement at puberty.
      - The rise in testosterone levels at the onset of puberty is sufficient to induce development of secondary sexual characteristics.
   3. Partial androgen resistance
      - Most of these patients are raised as males and fertility is preserved.
      - Some patients with severe partial androgen resistance may be raised as females, as adequate virilization at puberty may not be possible.
      - If the patient is raised as a male, early surgical correction of hypospadias or chordee is recommended.
      - Testosterone replacement may be required at puberty, particularly if testosterone levels remain low.
      - If the patient is raised as a female:
      - Early vaginoplasty (surgical separation of the urethral and vaginal openings) is recommended.
      - Clitoroplasty is indicated in cases of severe virilization.
      - Patients require gonadectomy before puberty to prevent virilization at puberty.
      - Estrogen is required at puberty to allow pubertal development.
      - Further genitoplasty in adolescence is usually necessary.
   4. Gonadal dysgenesis
      - Sex assignment is based on likelihood of fertility.
      - Other factors considered are:
      - The genital appearance
      - The size of the phallus
      - Presumed testicular function in puberty based on hormonal tests and gonadal development
      - If the patient is raised as a female:
      - Early vaginoplasty is recommended.
      - Clitoroplasty is indicated in cases of severe virilization.
      - Gonadectomy before puberty to prevent virilization at puberty.
      - Estrogen supplements at puberty to allow pubertal development.
      - Further genitoplasty in adolescence is usually necessary.
      - If the patient is raised as a male:
      - Early surgical correction of hypospadias or chordee is recommended.
      - Testosterone replacement may be required at puberty, particularly if testosterone levels remain low.

5. 45, X/46, XY mixed gonadal digenesis
    - Sex assignment is more complex.
    - If fertility is expected to be maintained, then the sex is best chosen to be consistent with fertility.
    - Other factors that must be considered are:
    - The genital appearance
    - The size of the phallus
    - The presumed testicular function in puberty based on hormonal tests and gonadal development
    - The risk of gonadal malignancy is highest in MGD in which there is a Y chromosomal and in those with an intra-abdominal testis.
    - In children assigned a male sex, hypospadias or chordee, if present, requires surgical correction.
    - A streak ovary, if present, should be removed.
    - Testosterone replacement may be required at puberty, particularly if testosterone levels remain low.
    - In children assigned a female sex:
    - Early vaginoplasty is recommended.
    - Clitoroplasty is indicated in cases of severe virilization.
    - Gonadectomy should be performed early in life to prevent malignancy.
    - This is best done before puberty to avoid any risk of virilization.
    - Estrogen will also be needed at puberty to allow pubertal development.
    - Further genitoplasty in adolescence is usually necessary.
    - Some patients have Müllerian structures (uterus) and need treatment with cyclic progesterone once breakthrough bleeding occurs.

Recommended Reading

Diamond M, Sigmundson HK. Management of intersexuality. Guidelines for dealing with persons with ambiguous genitalia. Arch Pediatr Adolesc Med. 1997;151(10):1046–50.

Nihoul-Fékété C, Thibaud E, Lortat-Jacob S, Josso N. Long-term surgical results and patient satisfaction with male pseudohermaphroditism or true hermaphroditism: a cohort of 63 patients. J Urol. 2006;175(5):1878–84.

Chapter 67
Persistent Müllerian Duct Syndrome

Introduction

- Persistent müllerian duct syndrome (PMDS) is characterized by the presence of a uterus, fallopian tubes, and upper vagina in an otherwise phenotypically and genotypically normal male (Fig. 67.1).
- Not uncommonly, it is seen in association with transverse testicular ectopia (TTE).
- PMDS, which is also called hernia uteri inguinal, is a rare congenital abnormality which results from a mutation in the gene encoding anti-müllerian hormone or by a mutation in the anti-müllerian hormone receptors.

Embryology

- Embryologically, the fetal testes secret two hormones.
- The Leydig cells secretes testosterone which is necessary for the development of the wolfian ducts into the epididymis, vas deferens, and seminal vesicles.
- The Sertoli cells on the other hand secrete the müllerian-inhibiting hormone which causes regression of the müllerian ducts that usually develop into the uterus, fallopian tubes, and upper third of the vagina.
- PMDS can be caused by deficiency or failure in the production of the müllerian-inhibiting hormone or abnormality in its receptors.
- As a result of this, the müllerian ducts fail to regress and develop into a uterus, fallopian tubes, and upper vagina in an otherwise normal male with testicular gonads and 46XY chromosomes.
- The presence of consanguinity in some of the reported cases as well as its occurrence in several pairs of brothers supports an autosomal male-restricted mode of inheritance. Others suggested an X-linked mode of inheritance.

Clinical Features

- Classically, PMDS is seen in an otherwise normal male with normal external genitalia who presents with unilateral or more commonly bilateral undescended testes and or inguinal hernia.
- It is also called hernia uteri inguinal because, at the time of hernia repair, uterus and fallopian tubes may be found in the hernia sac.

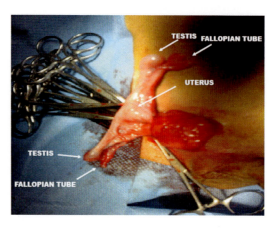

Fig. 67.1 Intraoperative photograph showing PMDS. Note the uterus, fallopian tubes, and testes

- There is an association between PMDS and hypospadias.
- Most cases of PMDS are diagnosed as a surprise at the time of surgery for an inguinal hernia or undescended testes.
- Rarely, the diagnosis is suspected preoperatively during evaluation of undescended testes.
- There is however a strong association between PMDS and TTE. PMDS is present in 30–50 % of all cases of TTE and in these cases cross-orchidopexy becomes a necessity.

Management

- The surgical management of PMDS is still controversial.
- Since these cases are discovered incidentally, a staged procedure is the most commonly accepted option.
- During the initial surgery, bilateral testicular biopsies are done followed by replacement of the uterus, fallopian tubes, and testes into the pelvis and herniotomy (Fig. 67.2).
- Once the diagnosis is confirmed, definitive surgery is planned.
- The confirmation of the diagnosis includes chromosomal analysis, hormonal assay including human chorionic gonadotropin (HCG) stimulation test, and the result of testicular biopsies.
- There is however still controversy whether to remove the müllerian remnants or not.
- There are those who advocate leaving the müllerian remnants to avoid injury to the vas deferens and testicular vessels at the time of their resection.
- On the other hand, there are those who strongly recommend their removal.
- Although very rare, there are reports of clear cell adenocarcinoma of the remnant uterus in PMDS.
- Add to this the fact that the remnant uterus can hypertrophy causing pain, and discomfort and removal of the uterus facilitates orchidopexy.
- The most commonly performed procedure is bilateral proximal salpingectomy, leaving the fimbriae with the epididymis, hysterectomy, and bilateral orchidopexy (Fig. 67.3).
- It is important to avoid injury to the vas deferens and vessels at the time of hysterectomy.
- One way to achieve this is to leave a pedicle of the myometrium and the fimbriae attached to the epididymis.
- Others advocated splitting the uterus in the midline bringing the testis with the vas deferens and attached uterine tissue into the scrotum.

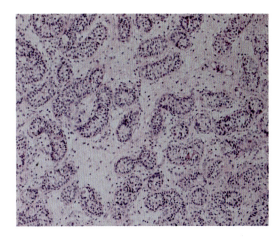

Fig. 67.2 Histological slide of testicular biopsy in a patient with PMDS

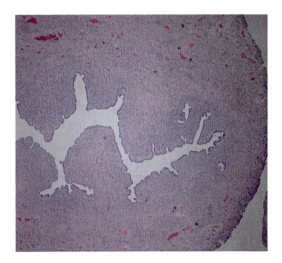

Fig. 67.3 Histological slide in a patient with PMDS showing a rudimentary uterus

- With the recent advances in minimal invasive surgery, laparoscopy is being increasingly used for both the diagnosis and the management of PMDS including testicular biopsy, orchidopexy, and herniotomy.

Follow-Up

- Follow-up of these patients is also important. There is a 5–15 % risk of testicular malignancy in these patients which is not different from that in patients with undescended testes.
- Most of these patients however are infertile because of azoospermia, low motility index, or ductal obstruction. It is also important to check the result of testicular biopsy. These usually show testicular tissue with variable degree of fibrosis, which may necessitate testosterone replacement at the time of puberty in those with hypoplastic or fibrotic testes.

Recommended Reading

Chertin B, Koulikov D, Alberton J. The use of laparoscopy in intersex patients. Pediatr Surg Int. 2006;22:405–8.

Crankson SJ, Bin Yahib S. Persistent mullerian duct syndrome in a child: surgical management. Ann Saudi Med. 2000;20:267–9.

Guerrier D, Tran D, Vanderwinden JM, Hideux S, Van Outryve L, Legeai L, et al. The persistent mullerian duct syndrome: a molecular approach. J Clin Endocrinol Metab. 1989;68:46–52.

Loeff DS, Imbeaud S, Reyes HM, Meller JL, Rosenthal IM. Surgical and genetic aspects of persistent mullerian duct syndrome. J Pediat Surg. 1994;29:65–6.

Chapter 68
Hypospadias

Introduction

- Hypospadias is a congenital abnormality of the urethra in which the urethral opening is located on the ventral aspect of the penis proximal to the tip of the glans penis.
- The site of the abnormal urethral opening is variable and may be located just proximal to the normal position of the external urethral meatus or as far down as the scrotum or perineum.
- Hypospadias occurs in approximately 1 in every 250 male births.
- The incidence of hypospadias is more in whites than in blacks, and it is seen more common in those of Jewish and Italian descent.
- Hypospadias is also known to run in families where several members of the same family are affected. The familial rate of hypospadias is about 7 %.
- There is increased rate of hypospadias in boys born prematurely and small for gestational age and boys with low birth weight.
- A higher incidence of hypospadias has been reported in those following in vitro fertilization.
- Clinically, hypospadias is associated with (Figs. 68.1 and 68.2)
    - A dorsal hood of foreskin.
    - An incomplete prepuce ventrally.
    - A glanular groove.
    - A proximally suited ectopic position.
    - Chordee (ventral shortening and curvature) is more likely with more proximal hypospadias.
    - Rarely, the foreskin may be complete and the hypospadias is discovered at the time of circumcision (Figs. 68.2, 68.3, and 68.4).

The treatment for hypospadias is surgical repair.

- More than 300 different types of repairs have been described in the medical literature.
- Hypospadias is generally repaired for functional and cosmetic reasons.
    - The more proximal the position of the urethral meatus, the more likely the urinary stream is to be deflected downward.
    - This is exacerbated by the presence of chordee.
    - Fertility may be affected as the abnormal deflection of ejaculate may preclude effective insemination.
    - Chordee can be associated with painful erections.
    - There is potential psychological stress of having abnormal genitalia.

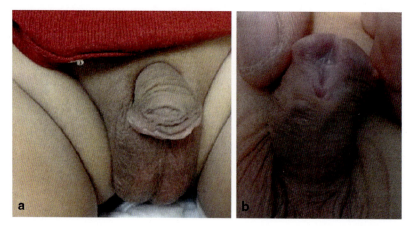

Fig. 68.1 a and **b** Clinical photographs showing a child with hypospadias. Note the dorsal hood of foreskin and a clinical photograph showing hypospadias. Note the ectopic urethral opening and the incomplete prepuce ventrally

Fig. 68.2 A clinical photograph showing hypospadias. Note the ectopic proximally located urethral opening as well as the widened glanular groove

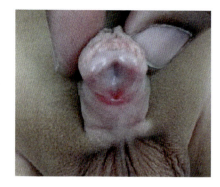

- The final outcome of hypospadias repair improved markedly as a result of several factors:
    - Modern anesthetic techniques
    - Fine instruments and better surgical techniques
    - Better sutures and dressing materials
    - Antibiotics

Embryology

- Hypospadias is a congenital defect that is thought to occur during urethral development, from 8 to 20 weeks' gestation.
- Testosterone is the main factor responsible for masculinization of the external genitalias.
- As the phallus grows, there is an open urethral groove which extends from the base to the level of the corona.
- The urethral folds than fuse in the midline forming a tubularized posterior and middle urethra.

Embryology

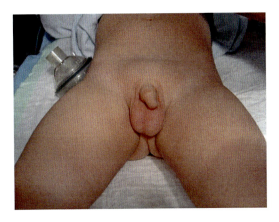

Fig. 68.3 A clinical photograph showing a normal intact prepuce with no evidence of hypospadias

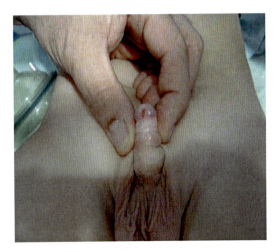

Fig. 68.4 A clinical photograph of the same patient in Fig. 68.3 showing hypospadias after retraction of the prepuce (Megameatus intact prepuce variant)

- The anterior urethra develops in a proximal direction, with an ectodermal core forming at the tip of the glans penis, which canalizes to join with the more proximal urethra at the level of the corona.
- The higher incidence of subcoronal hypospadias supports the vulnerable final step in this theory of development.
- Another theory suggests that the urethral folds fuse in the midline to form a seam of epithelium, which is then transformed into mesenchyme and subsequently canalizes by apoptosis or programmed cell resorption. This is also the case for the anterior urethra where the endoderm differentiates to ectoderm with subsequent canalization by apoptosis.
- The prepuce normally forms as a ridge of skin from the corona that grows circumferentially, fusing with the glans.
- Failure of fusion of the urethral folds in hypospadias impedes this process, and a dorsal hooded prepuce results.
- On rare occasions, a glanular cleft with intact prepuce may occur, which is termed the megameatus intact prepuce variant.
- Chordee is thought to result from the abnormal attenuated ventral urethra and associated tissues as well as the abortive spongiosal tissue and fascia distal to the urethral meatus which forms a tethering fibrous band.

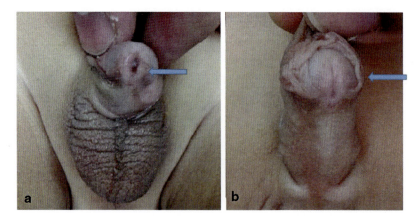

Fig. 68.5 A clinical photograph showing glanular hypospadias (**a**) and a photograph showing coronal hypospadias (**b**)

Fig. 68.6 A clinical photograph showing subcoronal hypospadias

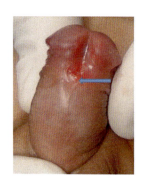

Classification

- In the past hypospadias was classified as follows:
    - First-degree hypospadias (50–75%): The urethral meatus opens on the underside of the glans penis.
    - Second-degree hypospadias (15–20%): The urethral meatus opens on the shaft of the penis.
    - Third-degree hypospadias (20–30%): The urethral meatus opens on the perineum.
- The more severe degrees of hypospadias are more likely to be associated with chordee.
- The recent classification of hypospadias was proposed by Barcat and modified by Duckett which is based on the site of the abnormal urethral meatus after correction of any associated chordee.
    - Anterior hypospadias (50%; Figs. 68.5 and 68.6)
        ◦ Glanular.
        ◦ Coronal.
        ◦ Subcoronal. The subcoronal position is the most common type.
    - Middle hypospadias (20%; Figs. 68.7 and 68.8):
        ◦ Distal penile
        ◦ Midshaft (Midpenile)
        ◦ Proximal penile

Etiology

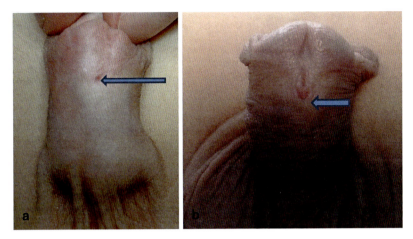

Fig. 68.7 **a** A clinical photograph showing distal penile hypospadias. Note the shallow glanular groove. **b** Clinical photograph showing a distal penile hypospadias. Note the deep glanular groove

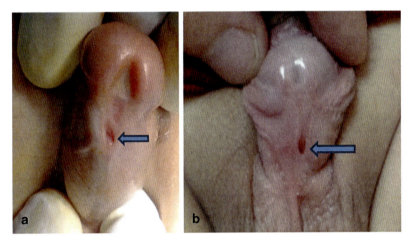

Fig. 68.8 Clinical photographs showing midpenile hypospadias (**a**) and proximal penile hypospadias (**b**)

- Posterior hypospadias (30%; Figs. 68.9 and 68.10):
  - Penoscrotal
  - Scrotal
  - Perineal

Etiology

- In most cases of hypospadias, the exact cause is not fully understood.
- Factors likely to increase the risk of hypospadias include:
  - Treatment with hormones such as progesterone during pregnancy.
  - Failure of the fetal testes to produce enough testosterone (transient deficiency of testosterone can occur during critical periods of fetal genital development, due to elevation of anti-müllerian hormone or more subtle degrees of pituitary-gonadal dysfunction).

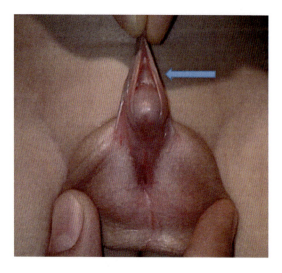

Fig. 68.9 A clinical photograph showing penoscrotal hypospadias

- Sixty-six percent of boys with mild hypospadias and 40 % with severe hypospadias were found to have a defect in testicular testosterone biosynthesis. Mutations in the 5-alpha reductase enzyme, which converts testosterone to the more potent dihydrotestosterone, have been associated with hypospadias.
- Failure of the body to respond to testosterone. A postnatal deficiency of, or reduced sensitivity to, androgens (testosterone and dihydrotestosterone).
- Genetic factors. There is about a 7 % familial recurrence risk of hypospadias.
- Maternal use of progestins and finasteride in the first two trimesters of pregnancy. Progesterone is a substrate for 5-alpha reductase and acts as a competitive inhibitor of the testosterone-to-dihydrotestosterone conversion.
- Maternal use of diethylstilbestrol.
- There also may be an increased risk of hypospadias in infant males born to women of an advanced age and increasing parity.
- There is an increased risk of hypospadias in males born following in vitro fertilization. This may be due to the mother's exposure to progesterone, or to progestin, administered during the in vitro fertilization.
- Environmental factors including pesticides on fruits and vegetables, endogenous plant estrogens, milk from lactating pregnant dairy cows, plastic lining in metal cans, and drugs.

Associated Anomalies

- Mild hypospadias most often occurs as an isolated anomaly.
- Those with more severe degrees of hypospadias will have additional anomalies:
  - Ten percent have at least one undescended testis.
  - Ten percent have an inguinal hernia.
  - An enlarged prostatic utricle is common in those with severe (scrotal or perineal) hypospadias. These predispose to urinary tract infections, pseudo-incontinence, or even stone formation.
  - Upper urinary tract anomalies are rarely associated with hypospadias and do not justify routine imaging in these patients.
  - Low-grade vesicoureteral reflux in those with severe hypospadias.
  - A karyotype and endocrine evaluation should be performed to detect intersex conditions or hormone deficiencies in those with severe degrees of hypospadias (Fig. 68.11).

Treatment

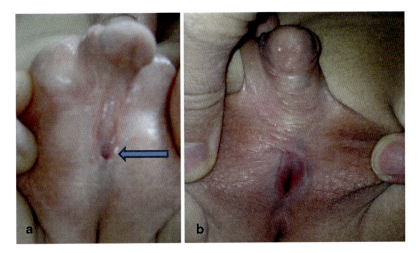

Fig. 68.10 Clinical photographs showing scrotal hypospadias. Note the associated severe chordee in **a** and perineal hypospadias in **b**. Note the site of the urethral opening and how close it is to the anal opening

Fig. 68.11 A micturating cystourethrogram showing bilateral reflux in a patient with hypospadias

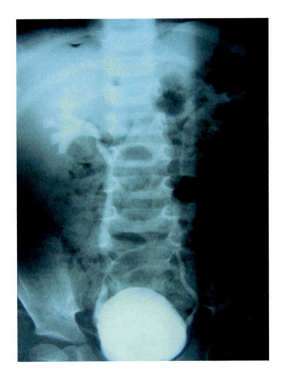

Treatment

- The treatment of hypospadias is surgical repair.
- The goals of treatment are (Fig. 68.12):
  - Orthoplasty: To create a straight penis.
  - Urethroplast: To create a urethra with its external meatus at the tip of the penis.
  - Glansplasty: To re-form the glans into a more natural conical configuration.
  - To achieve cosmetically acceptable penile skin coverage.

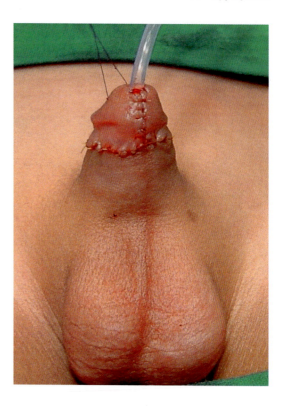

Fig. 68.12 A clinical photograph showing repair of hypospadias

- To create a normal-appearing scrotum.
- To construct a penis suitable for future sexual intercourse.
- To construct a penis that enable the patient to void while standing.
- To construct a penis that has an acceptable cosmetic appearance.

- Timing of surgery

  - Hypospadias is repaired around 4–18 months of age. This is beneficial from several points:
    - Better wound healing
    - Improved emotional and psychological effect
    - Less complication (urethrocutaneous fistula)
- Types of repair

  - Chordee must be corrected (Fig. 68.13):
    - Mild-to-moderate degrees of chordee are repaired either by excising the ventral fibrous tethering tissue or by dorsal plication of the tunica covering the corporal bodies.
    - Severe degrees of chordee require transection and excision of the tethered tissue which preclude the use of the urethral plate for urethroplasty and a type of graft may be necessary.
    - When local tissues are unavailable, buccal mucosa has been used for urethral grafting.
    - Preputial skin is often used for grafting and circumcision should be avoided prior to repair.
  - Treatment with testosterone injections or creams has been used to promote penile growth preoperatively for infants with small phallic size (Fig. 68.14).
  - There are many types of urethroplasties.
  - The tubularized incised plate (TIP) urethroplasty has become the procedure of choice to repair both distal and midshaft hypospadias without chordee.
  - The repair of hypospadias is generally planned as a single-stage procedure, but excessive chordee (especially if transection of the urethral plate is required) may be better approached in a staged repair.

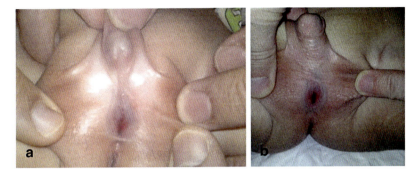

Fig. 68.13 Clinical photographs showing perineal hypospadias with chordee before (**a**) and after (**b**) release of chordee

Fig. 68.14 A clinical photograph showing hypospadias after treatment with long-acting testosterone. Note the hair growth as a side effect

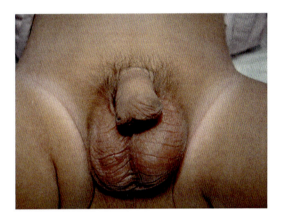

Postoperative Complications

- Early complications:
  - Penile edema
  - Penile hematoma
  - Postoperative bleeding
  - Infection
- Late complications:
  - Urethrocutaneous fistula (Figs. 68.15 and 68.16):
    - This is seen in < 10 % of hypospadias cases treated as a single-stage repair.
    - This may reach as high as 40 % in more complex cases.
    - Fistulas rarely close spontaneously and are repaired using a multilayered closure with local skin flaps 6 months after the initial repair.
    - After repair, fistulas recur in approximately 10 % of patients.
    - The use of protective covering layers between the urethroplasty and skin such as the single or double dartos flaps decrease the incidence of urethrocutaneous fistula (Fig. 68.17).
    - Temporary urethral stents also decrease the likelihood of fistula formation (Fig. 68.18).
  - Meatal stenosis:
    - Meatal stenosis can develop postoperatively.
    - This is treated by dilatation or meatoplasty.

Fig. 68.15 A clinical photograph showing two urethrocutaneous fistulas following repair of hypospadias. Note also the severe meatal stenosis at the tip of the penis

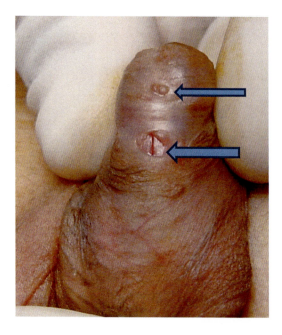

Fig. 68.16 A clinical photograph showing a urethrocutaneous fistula following repair of hypospadias with breakdown of the repair

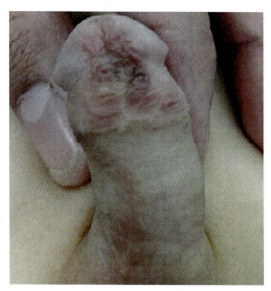

- Urethral strictures (Fig. 68.19):
    - May develop as a long-term complication.
    - These are generally repaired surgically.
- Urethral diverticula (Fig. 68.20):
    - This leads to ballooning of the urethra during urination.
    - A distal urethral stricture may cause outflow obstruction leading to a urethral diverticulum.
    - Diverticula can develop in the absence of distal urethral obstruction and are generally associated with graft- or flap-type hypospadias repairs.
    - This is treated by excision of the redundant urethral tissue.

Postoperative Complications

Fig. 68.17 A clinical photograph showing dissection of a dartos flap as a protective layer during the repair of hypospadias

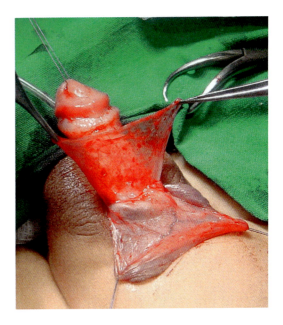

Fig. 68.18 A clinical photograph showing a urethral stent used to protect the repair of hypospadias

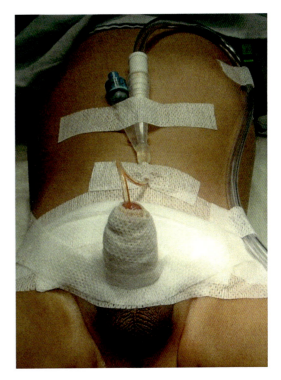

- Hairy urethra (Fig. 68.21):
    ◦ Hair-bearing skin is avoided in hypospadias reconstruction but was used in the past.
    ◦ When incorporated into the urethra, it can result in urinary tract infection or stone formation.
    ◦ This is treated using cystoscopy and laser or cautery.
    ◦ If severe, excision of hair-bearing skin and repeat hypospadias repair may be necessary.

Fig. 68.19 A urethrogram showing a urethral stricture following repair of hypospadias

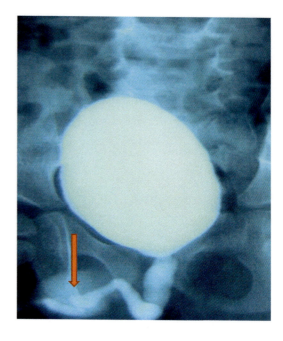

Fig. 68.20 A clinical photograph showing a urethral diverticulum following repair of hypospadias

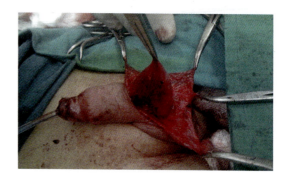

Fig. 68.21 A clinical photograph showing a hairy urethral. Note that skin was used in the creation of the urethra. This is a hair baring skin

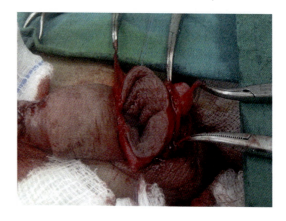

Recommended Reading

Baskin LS. Hypospadias and urethral development. J Urol. 2000;163(3):951–6.
Duckett JW. Successful hypospadias repair. Contemp Urol. 1992;4:42–55.
Duckett JW, Coplen D, Ewalt D. Buccal mucosal urethral replacement. J Urol. 1995;153(5):1660–3.
Gearhart JP, Jeffs RD. The use of parenteral testosterone therapy in genital reconstructive surgery. J Urol. 1987;138(4 Pt 2):1077–8.
Snodgrass WT. Tubularized incised plate hypospadias repair: indications, technique, and complications. Urology. 1999;54(1):6–11.
Snodgrass WT. The "learning curve" in hypospadias surgery. BJU Int. 2007;100(1):217.

Chapter 69
Pelviureteric Junction Obstruction

Introduction

- Pelviureteric junction obstruction (PUJ) is one of the most common congenital abnormalities of the urinary tract.
- It is defined as an obstruction at the junction of the renal pelvis and proximal ureter.
- Prior to the widespread use of prenatal ultrasonography, most cases of PUJ obstruction were not detected in the first year of life.
- Currently, the vast majority of PUJ obstructions (90 %) are detected with prenatal ultrasonography.
- The obstruction results in back pressure within the renal pelvis, which may lead to progressive renal damage and deterioration.
- The exact anatomy and function of the kidneys is crucial during the evaluation and treatment of these patients.
- PUJ obstruction is the most common cause of neonatally and antenatally diagnosed hydronephrosis.
- The frequency of unilateral PUJ obstruction is estimated to be 1 case in 5000–8000 live births.
- PUJ obstruction is more common on the left side than on the right. The left-to-right ratio is 5:2.
- PUJ obstruction is more common in males than in females. The male-to-female ratio is 3–4:1.
- PUJ obstruction occurs bilaterally in 6–10 % of cases (Fig. 69.1).
- Prior to the use of prenatal ultrasonography, most patients with PUJ obstruction presented with pain, hematuria, urinary tract infections, failure to thrive, or a palpable mass.
- With the increasing use and availability of prenatal ultrasonography, PUJ obstructions are being diagnosed earlier and more frequently.
- About 50–67 % of antenatally diagnosed hydronephrosis are due to PUJ obstruction.
- Initially, most patients with PUJ are treated conservatively and monitored closely.
- Surgical intervention is indicated in the event of significantly impaired renal drainage or poor renal growth.
- The treatment of PUJ obstruction has changed over the years and there are several corrective procedures including:
  - Laparoscopic pyeloplasty
  - Open pyeloplasty
  - Endopyelotomy
  - Endopyeloplasty
  - Robotic-assisted laparoscopic pyeloplasty

Fig. 69.1 Intravenous urogram (IVU) showing bilateral PUJ obstruction

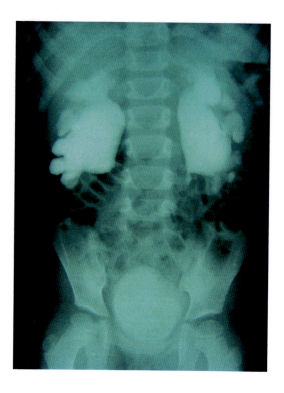

Etiology

- There are several possible etiologies for PUJ obstruction.
- These abnormalities all lead to impaired drainage of urine from the kidney into the ureter.
- As a result of this, there is increased intrapelvic pressure, which leads to elevated intrarenal back pressure, dilatation of the collecting system, and hydronephrosis.
- The etiologies of PUJ obstruction are classified into:
- Intrinsic causes:
  - Developmental anomalies of the PUJ leading to congenital stenosis.
  - Insertional anomalies in which the ureter inserts into the renal pelvis at a location that is not the most dependent. This prevents efficient drainage of the pelvis.
  - Functional abnormalities such as an aperistaltic section of smooth muscle.
  - Abnormal collagen architecture within the stenotic PUJ.
  - Asymmetry of ureteral wall musculature and ureteral hypoplasia. This may lead to abnormal peristalsis leading to defective emptying of the renal pelvis.
  - Mucosal folds and ureteral polyps that may be due to anatomical abnormalities. These obstruct the ureter at the PUJ in a ball–valve fashion during periods of diuresis.
  - Neural depletion and decreased neuronal markers and nerve growth factors within the smooth muscle layer of the pelviureteric junction.
- Extrinsic causes:
  - Due to causes exterior to the PUJ
  - Aberrant or accessory blood vessels (Aberrant polar vessels) (Fig. 69.2)
  - Scars and adhesions from previous surgery
  - Scarring and band formation from nephrolithiasis or urinary tract infection

Investigations

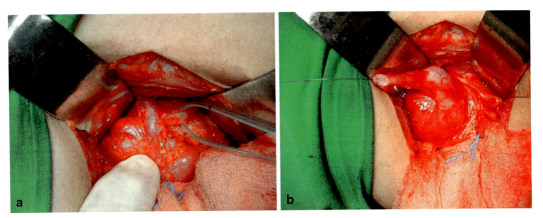

Fig. 69.2 Intraoperative photograph showing aberrant polar vessel causing hydronephrosis and intraoperative photograph showing the *upper* part of the ureter after its division. Note the normal ureter with no intrinsic cause of hydronephrosis

- Rotated and hypermobile kidney
- Vesicoureteral reflux leading to stenosis

• Additionally, PUJ obstruction is classified as primary and secondary.

- Primary PUJ obstruction is due to developmental anomalies of the PUJ.
- Secondary PUJ obstruction is due to other causes:
  ○ Previous surgical intervention on the kidney
  ○ Recurrent stone passage
  ○ Recurrent urinary tract infection
  ○ Vesicoureteral reflux
  ○ Rotated and hypermobile kidney (Fig. 69.3)
  ○ Failed repair of a primary PUJ obstruction

Clinical Features

- With the recent advancement in antenatal ultrasound, most cases of PUJ obstructions are diagnosed in utero.
- Older children may present with:
  - Urinary tract infection
  - A flank mass
  - Intermittent flank pain
  - Hematuria

Investigations

- All patients with possible PUJ obstruction should be evaluated with a complete blood count (CBC), coagulation profile, electrolytes, blood urea nitrogen (BUN) and creatinine, urine analysis, and culture. A plain abdominal X-ray may show a soft tissue density secondary to a hydronephrotic kidney (Fig. 69.4).

Fig. 69.3 IVU showing hydronephrotic pelvic kidney

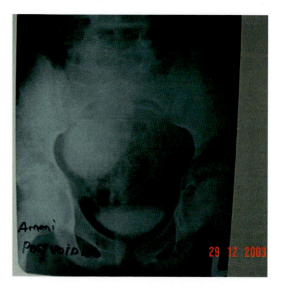

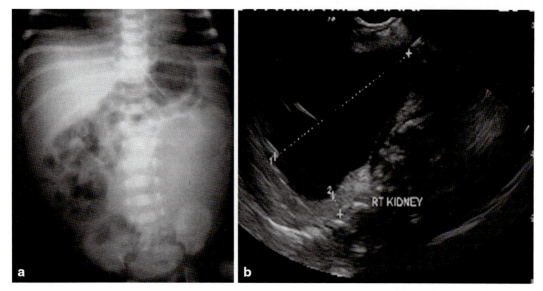

Fig. 69.4 A plain abdominal X-ray in a newborn with left hydronephrosis showing a soft tissue density on the *left* side and an abdominal ultrasound showing *right* hydronephrosis secondary to PUJ obstruction

- Renal ultrasonography (Fig. 69.4a).
- Micturating cystourethrography to rule out vesicoureteral reflux (Fig. 69.4b).
- Intravenous pyelogram (IVP) was used to evaluate patients with possible PUJ obstruction (Fig. 69.5).
- A renal isotope scan (mercaptotriglycylglycine [MAG-3], diethylenetriamine [DTPA], or dimercaptosuccinic acid [DMSA]):
  - Performed to quantify relative renal function and to define the extent of obstruction.
  - The differential renal function is important to decide the need for surgical intervention, especially in asymptomatic patients, and in selecting the appropriate treatment (pyeloplasty vs. nephrectomy).

Treatment

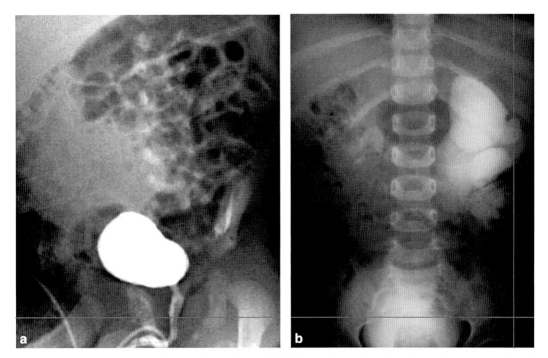

Fig. 69.5 A micturating cystourethrogram in a patient with PUJ obstruction, which showed no vesicoureteric reflux and IVP showing severe left PUJ obstruction

- Poorly functioning kidneys (< 10%) are often treated with nephrectomy.
- Renal isotope scans are also important to assess outcomes after surgical intervention.
- Abdominal computed tomography (CT) scan with three-dimensional reconstruction: this is helpful in establishing the anatomy of PUJ obstruction (Fig. 69.6).
- In children, retrograde ureteropyelography is sometimes performed to define the entire ureter just prior to surgical repair.
- Magnetic resonance urography (MRU)

Treatment

- The goals of treatment of PUJ obstruction are:
  - To improve renal drainage
  - To maintain or improve renal function
- Initially, most children with PUJ obstruction are treated conservatively and monitored closely.
- Conservative treatment is advocated:
  - If the obstruction is asymptomatic
  - If no evidence in deterioration of renal function exists
  - If patient is free from recurrent urinary tract infections or nephrolithiasis
- PUJ obstruction may resolve spontaneously in a substantial portion of children.
- Renal pelvic dilatation should be monitored with serial imaging to assess for changes in dilatation, renal parenchymal thickness and/or the presence of scarring, and function.

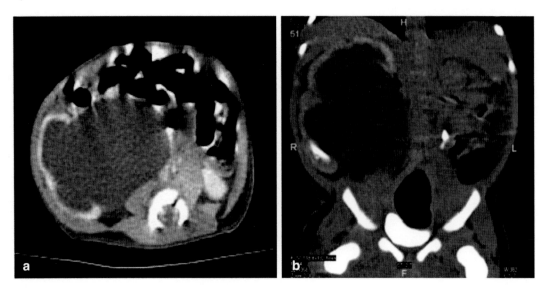

Fig. 69.6 CT-urography showing severe right hydronephrosis secondary to PUJ obstruction. Note the thin rim of renal tissue left as a result of the severe backpressure

- Typically, when imaging studies reveal an incomplete obstruction, the patient is monitored with routine renal ultrasonography and nuclear medicine renography every 3–6 months.
- In severe intrauterine PUJ obstruction, a temporary nephrostomy is indicated to decompress the kidney (Fig. 69.7).
- Surgical repair is indicated:
  - When there is a significant increase in the size of renal pelvis on serial imaging
  - When there is progressive deterioration of renal function
  - A renal pelvis size >5 cm in the maximum diameter signifies sever obstruction and is considered an indication for surgical intervention
  - A differential renal function <40%
  - A $t1/2$ s (The reaction half time ($t1/2$) of the clearance of the pharmaceutical tracer) >20 min
  - Ongoing renal parenchymal thinning
  - Intervention is also indicated in those with pain, hypertension, hematuria, secondary renal calculi, and recurrent urinary tract infection
- Open pyeloplasty is still considered the standard treatment for PUJ obstruction in infants and children.
- Laparoscopic pyeloplasty, with or without robotic assistance, is increasingly used and is becoming the treatment of choice in older children.
- An endopyelotomy refers to an endoscopic incision of the PUJ, performed to create a more funneled drainage system and to bring the ureteropelvic junction (UPJ) more dependent or caudad below areas of pathology.
- In children, the procedure of choice is an Anderson–Hynes dismembered pyeloplasty.
- The approach may be performed:
  - Through a flank incision
  - Through a dorsal lumbotomy incision
  - Through an anterior extraperitoneal incision
  - Via laparoscopy

Treatment

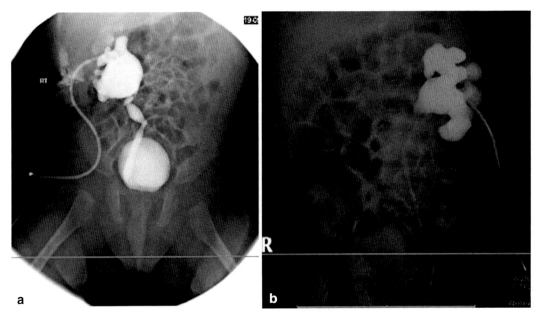

Fig. 69.7 Nephrostograms in patients with severe hydronephrosis. A percutaneous nephrostomy was inserted to decompress the kidney prior to surgery

- The use of a transanastomosis ureteral stent is still controversial.
- Postoperatively, a nephrostomy tube is occasionally left in place.
- A use of a transanastomotic ureteral stent that passes from the renal pelvis to the bladder is still controversial.
- Some surgeons leave a drain near the anastomosis; this is removed postoperatively when the output becomes minimal.
• The success rate of dismembered pyeloplasty for treating an obstructed UPJ exceeds 95 %.
• The Foley Y–V pyeloplasty is another alternative but cannot be used if transposition of a lower-pole vessel is needed.
• Laparoscopic pyeloplasty offers a minimally invasive treatment option for children with PUJ obstruction.
    - The success rates of laparoscopic pyeloplasty are comparable with those of open pyeloplasty.
    - Laparoscopy offers the advantages of decreased morbidity, shorter hospital stay, and quicker recovery.
    - Laparoscopic pyeloplasty is a technically demanding procedure that requires significant laparoscopic experience.
    - Robot-assisted laparoscopic pyeloplasty has become increasingly popular to treat PUJ obstruction.
• Postoperative complications from open surgical pyeloplasty include:
    - Urinary tract infection
    - Pyelonephritis
    - Urinary extravasation and leakage
    - Recurrent PUJ obstruction or stricture formation
• Endoscopic treatment alternatives to treat PUJ include an antegrade or retrograde endopyelotomy.
    - This is an endoscopic incision performed through the obstructing segment.

- The stricture should be short (<1.5 cm).
  - Endoluminal ultrasonography is particularly useful in evaluating an obstructed PUJ.
  - It allows for complete real-time evaluation with specific attention to the presence or proximity of blood vessels prior to an endoscopic incision.
  - It is also useful in defining the ureteral anatomy and in directing the incision technique in order to maximize the surgical outcome.
  - Endopyelotomy is contraindicated in the presence of a crossing posterior or lateral vessel.
  - An endopyelotomy incision is performed through the area of obstruction with a laser, electrocautery, or endoscopic scalpel.
  - The incision is most commonly performed posterolaterally.
  - Balloon dilation is performed after the incision is made to ensure completeness.
  - Ureteral stenting for 4–8 weeks after the endoscopic procedure.
  - The success rates with the percutaneous and ureteroscopic endopyelotomy are 80–90%.
- Spiral and vertical flaps pyeloplasties (e.g., Culp and DeWeerd, Scardino and Prince) are useful when a long-strictured segment of diseased ureter is present. The proximal ureter is re-created with redundant renal pelvis that is tubularized and anastomosed to the lower ureteric segment.
- Ureterocalicostomy:
  - Anastomosis of the ureter to a lower-pole renal calyx.
  - It is usually reserved for failed open pyeloplasty when no extrarenal pelvis and significant hilar scarring are present.
  - With this procedure, the ureter is sutured directly to a lower pole calyx.
- Endopyeloplasty:
  - It consists of horizontal suturing of a standard vertical endopyelotomy incision performed through a percutaneous tract via a 26 F nephroscope.
  - Indications for endopyeloplasty include:
    - Short-segment PUJ obstruction
    - Absence of crossing vessels
    - No prior PUJ surgery
  - Endopyeloplasty yields results comparable to those of endopyelotomy.
- Prophylactic antibiotics should be given postoperatively.
- Follow up with renal ultrasonography 1–3 months after surgery.
- Follow up with nuclear renal scan 3–6 months after surgery.
- Serial renal imaging is recommended for the first year after surgery and should be continued less frequently thereafter if results have normalized.
- Open and laparoscopic pyeloplasty yields long-term success rates that exceed 95%.
- The success rate for endopyelotomy approaches 80–90%.

Recommended Reading

Bernstein GT, Mandell J, Lebowitz RL, et al. Ureteropelvic junction obstruction in the neonate. J Urol. 1988;140:1216–21.

Helin I, Persson PH. Prenatal diagnosis of urinary tract abnormalities by ultrasound. Pediatrics. 1986;78(5):879–83.

Moon DA, El-Shazly MA, Chang CM, Gianduzzo TR, Eden CG. Laparoscopic pyeloplasty: evolution of a new gold standard. Urology. 2006;67(5):932–6.

Mufarrij PW, Woods M, Shah OD, Palese MA, Berger AD, Thomas R, et al. Robotic dismembered pyeloplasty: a 6-year, multi-institutional experience. J Urol. 2008;180(4):1391–6.
Patel V. Robotic-assisted laparoscopic dismembered pyeloplasty. Urology. 2005;66(1):45–9.
Schuessler WW, Grune MT, Tecuanhuey LV, Preminger GM. Laparoscopic dismembered pyeloplasty. J Urol. 1993;150(6):1795–9.

Chapter 70
Posterior Urethral Valve

Introduction

- A posterior urethral valve (PUV) is a congenital malformation of the posterior urethra leading to urinary outflow obstruction.
- It is an obstructing membrane in the posterior male urethra as a result of abnormal in utero development.
- This obstruction leads to back pressure with secondary effects on the bladder, ureters, and kidneys.
- PUV is the most common cause of lower urinary tract obstruction in male neonates.
- The incidence of PUV is 1 per 8000 to 1 per 25,000 live births.
- In the past, most children with PUV are diagnosed because of urinary tract infection (UTI) or progressive renal insufficiency and associated with a high mortality approaching 50%.
- Currently, most infants with PUV are diagnosed antenatally with ultrasound.
- Approximately 10% of patients with prenatal hydronephrosis detected by ultrasonography have PUV.
- In spite of this, some patients with PUV do present later in life.
- The most life-threatening problem in newborns with PUV is the potential pulmonary hypoplasia related to in utero renal dysfunction. This may be associated with oligohydramnios.
- At birth, these newborns may have pneumothoraxes which will complicate their management.
- PUV is a lifelong condition that requires continued medical management and close follow-up.
- Over the past 30 years, the prognosis of children with PUV has improved markedly.
- PUV continues to cause renal insufficiency and it is the cause in approximately 10–15% of children undergoing renal transplant.
- Approximately one third of patients born with PUV progress to end-stage renal disease.
- Elevated bladder pressures and recurrent UTIs further may compromise renal function.
- Approximately one third of patients with PUVs have problems with diurnal enuresis when older than 5 years.
- Improved dialysis and transplantation techniques have significantly improved not only the mortality rate for these children but also their quality of life.
- The management of PUV is complex and involves a team approach that includes:
    - A neonatologist
    - A general pediatrician
    - A pediatric urologist
    - A pediatric nephrologist.

Clinical Features

- The widespread use of antenatal ultrasonography has contributed markedly to the increased rate of antenatal diagnosis of PUVs.
- Neonates may present with severe pulmonary distress caused by lung underdevelopment due to oligohydramnios. Physical findings can include the following:
  - Poor fetal breathing movements
  - Small chest cavity
  - Ascites
  - Potter faces
  - Skin dimpling
  - Indentation of the knees and elbows due to compression within the uterus
- In older children, the diagnosis of PUV may be suspected in those with:
  - UTI
  - Diurnal enuresis in boys older than 5 years
  - Painful micturation
  - An abnormal urinary stream
  - An abdominal mass suggestive of urinary bladder or hydronephrosis
  - Renal failure
- Most patients with PUV have normal physical examination findings.
- Abnormal physical findings are the result of severe renal insufficiency.
- In older children, physical findings can include:
  - Poor growth.
  - Hypertension.
  - Lethargy.
  - An intermittent or weak urinary stream.
  - A large lower abdominal mass may represent a markedly distended urinary bladder.

Classification

- Type I:
  - Most common type.
  - It is due to anterior fusion of the plicae colliculi, mucosal fins extending from the bottom of the verumontanum distally along the prostatic, and membranous urethra.
- Type II:
  - Least common type.
  - It is due to vertical or longitudinal folds between the verumontanum and proximal prostatic urethra and bladder neck.
- Type III:
  - Less common variant.
  - It is due to a disc of tissue distal to verumontanum.
  - It is believed to originate from incomplete canalization between the anterior and posterior urethra.

Investigations

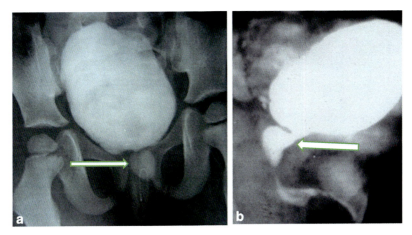

Fig. 70.1 a Micturating cystourethrogram showing dilated bladder with no vesicoureteric reflux. Note the dilated posterior urethra indicative of posterior urethral valve. **b** micturating cystourethrogram showing a dilated posterior urethra indicative of posterior urethral valve

- It is also thought to be a developmental anomaly of congenital urogenital remnants in the bulbar urethra.

Glassberg's Classification of Ureters

- Grade I: unobstructed with empty and full bladder
- Grade II: unobstructed with empty, but obstructed with full bladder
- Grade III: obstructed with full and empty bladder

Investigations

- Renal and bladder ultrasonography.
- All male children with antenatal diagnosis of hydronephrosis require voiding cystourethrography shortly after birth to confirm or exclude PUV.
- The diagnosis of PUV is made by voiding cystourethrography. (Figs. 70.1 and 70.2):
  - Visualization of the valve leaflets
  - A thickened trabeculated urinary bladder
  - A dilated or elongated posterior urethra
  - A hypertrophied bladder neck
  - The presence of diverticula, vesicoureteral reflux, and reflux into the ejaculatory ducts
  - Very thickened hypertrophied urinary bladder wall which may lead to secondary ureterovesical junction obstruction
- Renal scintigraphy
  - Tc-dimercaptosuccinic acid (DMSA) and mercaptoacetyltriglycine (MAG-3) renal scintigraphy provide information about relative renal function and areas of scarring or dysplasia.
  - MAG-3 renal scan with furosemide (Lasix) also provides information about renal drainage and possible obstruction.

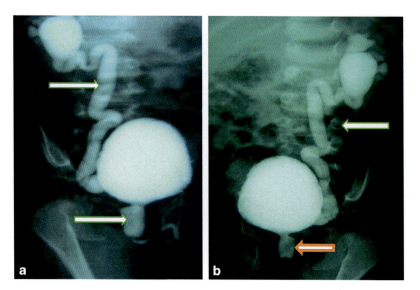

Fig. 70.2 a and **b** Micturating cystourethrogram showing dilated posterior urethra indicative of posterior urethral valve. Note the marked *right sided* and *left sided* vesicoureteric reflux

- Urodynamic evaluation:
  - Provides information about bladder storage and emptying.
  - The term "valve bladder" is used to describe patients with PUV and a fibrotic noncompliant bladder.
  - These patients are at risk of developing hydroureteronephrosis, progressive renal deterioration, recurrent infections, and urinary incontinence.
  - Patients with PUV require periodic urodynamic evaluation throughout childhood because bladder compliance may further deteriorate over time.
- Cystoscopy: serves both diagnostic and therapeutic functions.
  - Diagnostic cystoscopy:
    - Confirm the diagnosis
  - Therapeutic cystoscopy:
    - Transurethral incision of the PUV.
    - Multiple techniques have been described for ablating the valves.
    - Currently, valves are disrupted under direct vision by cystoscopy using an endoscopic loop, Bugbee electro cauterization, or laser fulguration.
    - In extremely small infants (<2000 g), a 2F Fogarty catheter may be passed either under fluoroscopic or under direct vision for valve disruption.
    - In some patients, the urethra may be too small and a temporary vesicostomy is performed.

Secondary effects of PUV:

- Vesicoureteral reflux (Fig. 70.3)
  - Vesicoureteral reflux is commonly associated with PUV and is present in as many as one third of patients.

Investigations

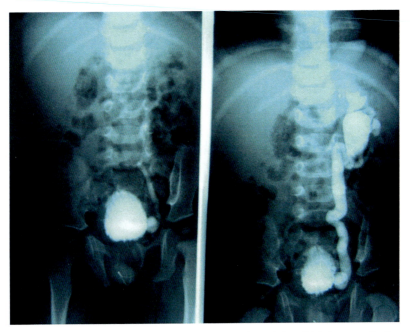

Fig. 70.3 Micturating cystourethrogram showing vesicoureteric reflux (*left*), which is severe in the second picture (*right*)

- When associated with PUV, reflux is generally secondary to elevated intravesical pressures.
- The treatment of vesicoureteral reflux in patients with PUV involves treatment of intravesical pressures using:
  1. Anticholinergics
  2. Timed voiding
  3. Double voiding
  4. Intermittent catheterization
  5. Bladder augmentation

- UTIs
  - Recurrent UTIs are common in patients with PUV. These are secondary to:
    1. Elevated intravesical pressures
    2. Increased post void residual urine volumes, leading to stasis of urine.
    3. Dilated upper urinary tracts, with or without vesicoureteral reflux.
  - UTI management is directed at:
    1. Lowering bladder pressures (anticholinergic medication)
    2. Lowering post void residual urine volume (via clean intermittent catheterization)
    3. Administering prophylactic antibiotics

- Urinary incontinence
  - The same factors that lead to vesicoureteral reflux and UTI also lead to urinary incontinence.
  - Correct management of bladder function depends on adequate bladder evaluation with urodynamic studies.

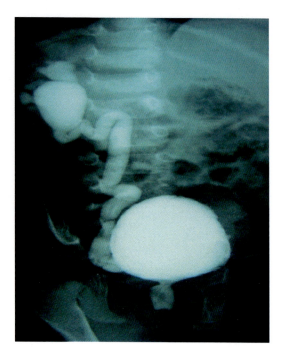

Fig. 70.4 Micturating cystourethrogram showing posterior urethral valve and marked reflux on the right side. There is marked hydronephrosis which act as a pop-off valve

- These include:
    1. Lowering bladder pressure.
    2. Improving bladder compliance.
    3. Minimizing post void residual urine volume.
    4. In some, bladder augmentation may be needed.

Pathophysiology

- An interesting group of patients are those with vesicoureteral reflux and renal dysplasia (VURD) syndrome.
    - In these patients, one kidney is hydronephrotic, nonfunctioning, and has high-grade vesicoureteral reflux.
    - The high-grade reflux is thought to act as a pop-off valve (Fig. 70.4), leading to reduced overall bladder pressures and preservation of contralateral renal function.
    - In the past, these patients were thought to have a better outcome due to preserved renal function in one kidney at the sacrifice of the other.
    - More recent data suggest that these patients may suffer long-term adverse renal function with hypertension, proteinuria, and renal failure.
- The obstructive urinary process leads to:
    - Increased collagen deposition and muscle hypertrophy can significantly thicken the bladder wall.
    - Hypertrophy and hyperplasia of the detrusor muscle and increases in connective tissue limit bladder compliance.

Management

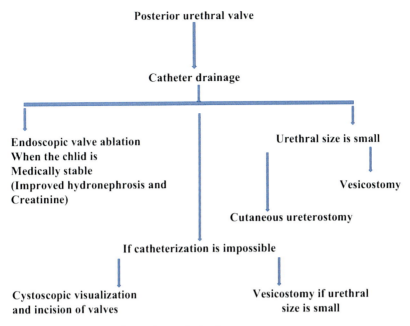

Fig. 70.5 Algorithm for management of posterior urethral valve

- Bladder emptying then occurs at high intravesical pressures, which, in turn, can be transmitted to the ureters and up into the renal collecting system.
- Patients with PUV may be susceptible to incontinence, infection, and progressive renal damage.
- As patients with PUV age, bladder decompensation may develop, resulting in detrusor failure and increased bladder capacity.
- Many boys with PUV will develop larger-than-expected bladder volumes in time possibly due to overproduction of urine caused by tubular dysfunction and an inability to concentrate urine (nephrogenic diabetes insipidus).
- Bladder function may change at puberty, resulting in high pressure, chronic retention and bladder dysfunction.
- The term "valve bladder" is used to describe patients with PUV and a fibrotic noncompliant bladder. These patients are at risk of developing:

  1. Hydroureteronephrosis
  2. Progressive renal deterioration
  3. Recurrent infections
  4. Urinary incontinence

- Patients with PUV require periodic urodynamic testing throughout childhood because bladder compliance may further deteriorate over time.

Management

- The goals of managing PUV consists of:
  - Relieving the obstruction and pressure on the urinary tract
  - Maintaining normal bladder and renal function

- The management consists of:
    - Catheter drainage of the bladder at birth (Fig. 70.5).
    - Close monitoring of serum electrolytes and renal function.
    - Antibiotics to prevent UTIs.
    - Those who do improve with catheter drainage undergo endoscopic ablation of the valves (transurethral ablation of the valves using the small resectoscopes).
    - If the patients are too small (under 2000 g), a vesicostomy is performed to alleviate the obstruction until the child is large enough for definitive treatment.
    - Fetal interventions:
        ○ Fetal surgery is a high-risk procedure reserved for cases with severe oligohydramnios, to try to limit the associated lung underdevelopment, or pulmonary hypoplasia.
        ○ These treatment options take the form of percutaneous fetal cystoscopy and valve ablation, vesicoamniotic shunting, and even open fetal surgery.
        ○ These highly complicated procedures are only undertaken when renal function is adequate and there is hope for benefit.
        ○ Fetal urine samples are often tested and the renal prognosis is considered good if the fetal urinary sample demonstrates Na <100 meq/l, Cl <90 meq/l, osmolality <200 mosm/l, and beta2 microglobulin <6 mg/L.
- In the newborn period, catheterization to drain the bladder may be difficult or even impossible because of the thickness of the valves or dilation of the posterior urethra with a hypertrophied bladder neck.
- Cystoscopic visualization with incision of the valves should be performed in the first few days of life once the child is metabolically stable.
- Approximately one-third of patients will require a second valve incision. Some authors recommend routine surveillance cystoscopy 1–2 months after initial incision to evaluate and treat any residual valvular obstruction.
- After the initial newborn period and successful bladder drainage, either by valve incision or by vesicostomy, long-term urologic care is needed.
- The medical management of PUV relates to the treatment of the secondary effects of the valves.
- Severe or prolonged urethral obstruction:
    - Leads to a fibrotic, poorly compliant bladder.
    - These bladders manifest poor compliance, leading to elevated storage pressures.
    - This, in turn, leads to increased risk of reflux, hydroureteronephrosis, and urinary incontinence.
    - Use of urodynamic testing to assess bladder compliance helps identify patients at risk.
    - Some patients may respond to anticholinergic medication, such as oxybutynin.
    - Institution of intermittent clean catheterization may aid some patients achieve continence by preventing the bladder from overfilling.
    - In patients who do not gain adequate bladder capacity and safe compliance despite optimal medical management, augmentation cystoplasty may be required.
- Vesicostomy: When urethral size precludes safe valve ablation, a vesicostomy can be created to provide bladder drainage.
- Cutaneous ureterostomies: Bilateral cutaneous ureterostomies (end stomal ureterostomy, loop ureterostomy, Y-ureterostomy) can be used to provide for urinary drainage.
- Secondary bladder surgery:
    1. Augmentation cystoplasty:
        - Augmentation can significantly improve patient lifestyle in those who have intractable incontinence due to poor compliance and bladder overactivity.
        - By lowering intravesical pressures, the upper urinary tract may also be protected.

- Indications for bladder augmentation include:
  - Inadequately low bladder storage volumes
  - High bladder pressures despite anticholinergic medication and clean intermittent catheterization
- The ileum is most commonly used; however, large bowel, stomach, and ureter are also used, depending on clinical conditions and surgeon preference.
- Augmentation should only be offered to patients willing to commit to lifelong intermittent catheterization.
- Potential complications include:
  - Bladder rupture (approximately 10% of patients)
  - Electrolyte disturbances, which may be worsened by the placement of intestinal mucosa in contact with urine, especially in those with a serum creatinine greater than 2 mg/dL
  - Mucus production, which can cause catheter blockage and may be a nidus for stone formation
- Malignant degeneration in augmented bladder have been reported.

2. Continent appendicovesicostomy (the Mitrofanoff procedure):

- This procedure involves placement of a nonrefluxing tubular conduit for catheterization between the bladder and skin to provide an alternative channel for catheterization.
- In children with PUV, intermittent catheterization through a sensate urethra can be difficult.
- Some patients may have a very dilated proximal urethra which may not be easily catheterizable.
- The appendix, ureter, and tubularized bowel can be used for the formation of this channel.

Medical Management

- The primary medications involved in bladder management are anticholinergic medications used to improve bladder compliance.
- Other medications include prophylactic antibiotics.
- Medications used in the management of renal insufficiency.
- Oxybutynin chloride (Ditropan): By inhibiting muscarinic action of acetylcholine on smooth muscle, it exerts an antispasmodic effect on bladder muscle.
- Hyoscyamine sulfate (Levbid, Levsin): Works by inhibiting postganglionic cholinergic receptors on smooth muscle cells.
- Tolterodine (Detrol): a new antimuscarinic drug with more selective receptor profile targeted for detrusor smooth muscle.
- Antibiotic prophylaxis, especially in the presence of vesicoureteral reflux.
- Appropriate antibiotics in children include:
  - Trimethoprim and sulfamethoxazole (Bactrim, Septra, Cotrim)
  - Trimethoprim (TMP)
  - Sulfamethoxazole (SMZ)
  - Nitrofurantoin
  - Amoxicillin

Prognosis

- Poor prognostic factors:
  - Echogenic kidneys, especially with multiple cysts, signify poor future renal function
  - Serum measurement of creatinine, which has been demonstrated to predict the likelihood of renal failure if above 1 mg/dL at 1 year of age
  - Delayed intervention
  - Reflux nephropathy
  - Growth retardation
  - Bilateral reflux at diagnosis
  - Presentation before 1 year of age (the earlier the diagnosis, the worse the prognosis)
  - Distal renal tubular acidosis
  - Incontinence by day at age 5 years
  - Hyperfiltration injury
  - Proteinuria in infancy

- Good prognostic factors:
  - Glomerular filtration rate at diagnosis
  - Ascites
  - Diverticula
  - Unilateral reflux or VURD syndrome

- If renal failure occurred early in life, it is most likely due to renal dysplasia.
- Renal failure that develops later in life is due to poor bladder function leading to further renal injury.
- Antibiotic prophylaxis is crucial to avoid UTIs.
- The urinary bladders of patients with PUV are divided into three groups:
  - Hyper-reflexic bladders: may respond to anticholinergic drugs.
  - Small noncompliant bladders: will need medical therapy, catheterization or even augmentation.
  - Myogenic bladders:
    - The bladder loses its contractile ability.
    - Catheterization is necessary for emptying.
    - The valve bladder may also lead to incontinence, with as many as 17–70% of children complaining of wetting at advanced ages.
    - The two main causes of this incontinence are bladder dysfunction and sphincter incompetence.
    - These children require management with timed/double voiding, anticholinergics, and clean intermittent catheterization.
    - In cases where conservative measures are not successful in protecting renal function, enterocystoplasty is required.
    - In addition, the kidneys in these children often have a concentration defect, producing large amounts of dilute urine.

- In the long term, many children with PUV develop end-stage renal disease and require renal transplantation.

Recommended Reading

Bajpai M, Dave S, Gupta DK. Factors affecting outcome in the management of posterior urethral valves. Pediatr Surg Int. 2001;17:11–5.

Denes ED, Barthold JS, Gonzalez R. Early prognostic value of serum creatinine levels in children with posterior urethral valves. J Urol. 1997;157:1441–3.

Glassberg KI. The valve bladder syndrome: 20 years later. J Urol. 2001;166:1406–14.

Karmarkar SJ. Long-term results of surgery for posterior urethral valves: a review. Pediatr Surg Int. 2001;17:8–10.

Lopez Pereira P, Martinez Urrutia MJ, Jaureguizar E. Initial and long-term management of posterior urethral valves. World J Urol. 2004;22:418–24.

Quintero RA, Shukla AR, Homsy YL, Bukkapatnam R. Successful in utero endoscopic ablation of posterior urethral valves: a new dimension in fetal urology. Urology. 2000;55:774.

Smith GH, Canning DA, Schulman SL, Snyder HM III, Duckett JW. The long-term outcome of posterior urethral valves treated with primary valve ablation and observation. J Urol. 1996;155:1730–4.

Yerkes EB, Cain MP, Padilla LM. In utero perinephric urinoma and urinary ascites with posterior urethral valves: a paradoxical pop-off valve? J Urol. 2001;166:2387–8.

Yohannes P, Hanna M. Current trends in the management of posterior urethral valves in the pediatric population. Urology. 2002;60:947–53.

Chapter 71
Vesicoureteral Reflux

Introduction

- Vesicoureteral reflux (VUR) is defined as retrograde flow of urine from the urinary bladder to the kidneys.
- Normally, there is a functional flap-valve mechanism at the ureterovesical junction, which is created by the oblique course of the ureter within the intramural portion of the urinary bladder wall.
- The normal valve mechanism of the ureterovesical junction is attributed to:
  - Oblique insertion of the intramural ureter
  - Adequate length of the intramural portion of the ureter
  - Strong detrusor muscle support
- The intravesical (intramural) length of the ureter is considered the most important factor.
- Defect in this mechanism leads to VUR.
- The extent of this retrograde regurgitation of urine from the urinary bladder up the ureter is variable.
- The exact incidence of VUR is not known but in healthy neonates, infants, and children the reported incidence is <1 %.
- The incidence of VUR, however, decreases as patient age increases.
- VUR is more prevalent in male newborns.
- VUR is five to six times more common in females older than 1 year than in males.
- VUR is known to be associated with repeated attacks of urinary tract infection (UTI) and if unrecognized lead to adverse effects on renal function (renal parenchymal scarring).
- Complications of VUR include:
  - Repeated attacks of UTI
  - Pyelonephritis
  - Hypertension
  - Progressive renal damage leading ultimately if bilateral to renal failure
- VUR is the fifth most common cause of chronic renal failure in children.
- Renal scarring secondary to VUR is one of the most common causes of childhood hypertension.
- Early diagnosis and treatment of VUR is important.
- To reduce the risk of UTI, prophylactic antibiotics are given as long as there is VUR.

Fig. 71.1 Micturating cystourethrogram (MCUG) showing VUR secondary to urethral stricture

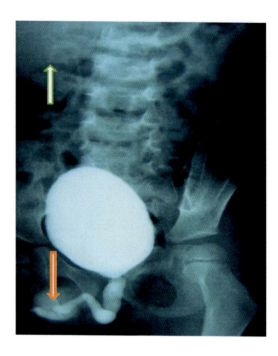

Etiology

- Normally, the ureter inserts into the trigone of the urinary bladder and courses obliquely through the intramural portion of the urinary bladder.
- The length of the intramural portion of the ureter is important to prevent reflux. Normally, the ratio of the intramural ureter to the diameter of the ureter is 5:1.
- As the bladder fills with urine and the bladder wall distends, the intramural portion of the ureter becomes compressed. This prevents retrograde flow of urine from the bladder back up to the ureter.
- Normally, this flap-valve mechanism prevents VUR.
- An abnormally short intramural ureteric segment results in a defective flap-valve mechanism and VUR.
- The exact cause of VUR is not known.
- There is, however, a definite genetic predisposition but the exact mode of inheritance remains unknown.
- There are several predisposing causes for VUR.
- Primary predisposing causes:
  - Short or absent intravesical (intramural) ureter
  - Absence of adequate detrusor backing
  - Lateral displacement of the ureteral orifice
  - Paraureteral diverticulum
- Secondary predisposing causes:
  - Cystitis or UTI
  - Chronic bladder outlet obstruction (Figs. 71.1 and 71.2)
  - Neurogenic bladder (e.g., myelomeningocele, spinal cord injury)
  - Detrusor instability and overactive urinary bladder

Classification

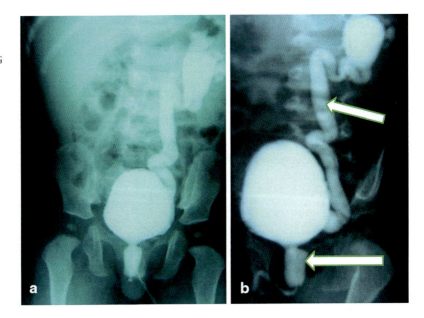

Fig. 71.2 a MCUG in a patient with posterior urethral valve showing unilateral VUR. b MCUG showing severe VUR in a child with posterior urethral valve. Note the dilated posterior urethra

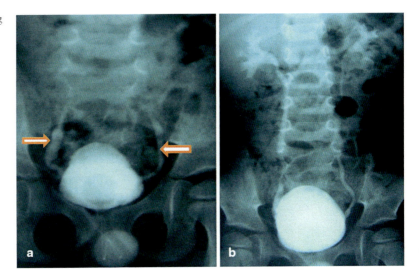

Fig. 71.3 MCUG showing bilateral grade I VUR in (a) and bilateral grade II and III VUR in (b)

Classification

The International Reflux Grading system classifies VUR into five grades, depending on the extent of retrograde filling and dilatation of the ureter and renal collecting system. This classification is based on the radiographic appearance during a voiding cystogram, as follows:

- Grade I: There is retrograde filling up into the ureter only. The renal pelvis and calyces appear normal (Fig. 71.3).
- Grade II: There is retrograde filling of the ureter, renal pelvis, and calyces. The renal pelvis and calyces appear normal.
- Grade III: There is retrograde filling of ureter and collecting system. The ureter and renal pelvis appear mildly dilated, and the calyces are mildly blunted.

Fig. 71.4 MCUG showing severe grade V VUR

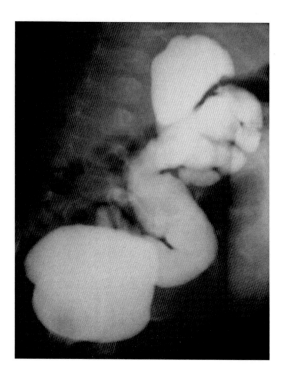

- Grade IV: There is retrograde filling of the ureter and collecting system. The ureter and renal pelvis appear moderately dilated, and the calyces are moderately blunted.
- Grade V: There is retrograde filling of the ureter and collecting system. The renal pelvis is severely dilated, the ureter appears tortuous, and the calyces are severely blunted (Fig. 71.4).

Pathophysiology

- VUR results from retrograde flow of urine from the urinary bladder up to the ureter and depending on the severity up into the renal collecting system.
- Unrecognized VUR may lead to long-term effects on the kidneys.
- This is more so in the presence of concomitant UTI.
- VUR leads to increased intrarenal reflux with increased intrarenal pressure and subsequent renal scarring and reflux nephropathy.
- This ultimately leads to impaired renal function, proteinuria, and hypertension.
- The presence of infection exacerbates the formation of renal fibrosis and scarring.
- VUR with intrarenal reflux of sterile urine that is not associated with increased intrapelvic pressures has not been shown to produce clinically significant renal scars.
- Sterile reflux however may also produce renal scarring when associated with high intravesical pressures.
- Pyelonephritic scarring may, over time, cause serious hypertension due to activation of the renin–angiotensin system.
- Renal scarring related to VUR is one of the most common causes of childhood hypertension.
- Hypertension develops in 10% of children with unilateral renal scars and in 18.5% in those with bilateral renal scars (Fig. 71.5).

Fig. 71.5 MCUG showing sever bilateral VUR

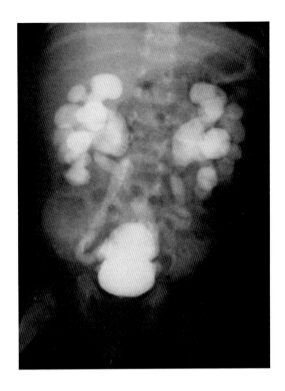

- Renal growth is also impaired in those with high grades VUR which if bilateral ultimately leads to impaired renal function and renal failure.
- Approximately 4% of children with VUR progress to end-stage renal failure.

Clinical Features

- VUR may be suspected prenatally on ultrasound demonstrating transient dilatation of the upper urinary tract in conjunction with bladder emptying.
- Approximately 10% of neonates diagnosed prenatally with dilatation of the upper urinary tract will be found to have VUR postnatally.
- In general, VUR may be asymptomatic and does not cause any specific signs or symptoms unless complicated by UTI.
- Older children may more clearly communicate signs and symptoms associated with a UTI (e.g., urgency, frequency, dysuria, incontinence), but, unless the UTI is associated with a fever, there is little reason to suspect VUR.

Investigations and Diagnosis

- Urine analysis and culture to rule out UTI.
- Blood urea, creatinine, and electrolytes.

- Abdominal and pelvic ultrasound.
  - To evaluate the presence and degree of hydronephrosis and ureter.
  - A dilated ureter in the presence of hydronephrosis may indicate VUR.
  - Hydronephrosis with an undilated ureter indicates pelviureteric junction obstruction.
  - To evaluate the bladder and bladder thickness.
  - To evaluate the lower urinary tract and bladder function.
- Micturating cystourethrogram.
  - Provides accurate grading of the degree of reflux.
  - Provides information regarding the urethra, voiding dysfunction and the presence or absence of posterior urethral valves.
- Nuclear renal scan.
  - DMSA
    - To visualize the renal cortex.
    - To evaluate renal function.
    - To evaluate the presence or absence of renal scars. Persistent photopenic defects on the DMSA scan represent renal scarring and irreversible renal damage.
- Nuclear cystography
  - May be more sensitive in revealing VUR.
  - It exposes the child to less radiation.
- Urodynamic
  - Valuable in patients with secondary VUR caused by lower urinary tract dysfunction.
- Cystoscopy
  - This is valuable:
    - When the anatomy of the urethra, bladder, or upper tracts is incompletely defined with radiographic evaluation.
    - When a ureterocele is suspected.

Treatment

- The goals of treating patients with VUR are:
  - To allow normal renal growth
  - To prevent UTI and pyelonephritis
  - To preserve renal function and prevent renal failure
- Indications for surgical management:
  - Relative Indications include:
    - Grades IV and V reflux
    - Persistent reflux despite medical therapy (beyond 3 years)
    - Breakthrough UTIs in patients who are receiving antibiotic prophylaxis
    - Lack of renal growth
    - Multiple drug allergies that preclude the use of antibiotic prophylaxis
    - Desire to terminate antibiotic prophylaxis (either by the physician or the patient/parents)
    - Medical noncompliance

- Absolute indications include:
  - Breakthrough pyelonephritis.
  - Progressive renal scarring in patients receiving antibiotic prophylaxis.
  - Associated ureterovesical junction abnormality
- Ureteral reimplantation is contraindicated as a first-line therapy in patients with secondary VUR resulting from an inappropriate increase in detrusor filling pressure.
- Three therapeutic options are available to treat children with VUR. They include:
  - Medical treatment
  - Surgical treatment
  - Surveillance
- The chance of spontaneous resolution of reflux is high in children younger than 5 years with grades I–III reflux and in children younger than 1 year with higher grades of reflux.
- Higher grades of reflux (grades IV and V) may resolve spontaneously as long as they remain infection free.
- Spontaneous resolution rates decrease as patient age increases and with higher grades of reflux.
- The medical management of VUR include:
  - Administering long-term prophylactic antibiotics.
  - Trimethoprim-sulfamethoxazole (Bactrim, Bactrim DS, Septra, Septra DS is an effective antibiotic used to treat uncomplicated UTIs and prevent recurrent infections.
  - In children <3 months, amoxicillin is preferred. Dosing in children >3 months is 1–2 mg/kg/d per os (PO) at bedtime (hs).
  - Correcting the underlying voiding dysfunction (if present).
  - Yearly follow-up radiographic studies (e.g., MCUG, nuclear cystography, DMSA scan).
  - Behavior modification protocol to ensure that the child empties his/her bladder completely at regular intervals (every 3 h), adequate hydration, and constipation prevention.
- Children with detrusor instability are treated with:
  - Anticholinergic medications.
    - Oxybutynin (Ditropan; 1–5 mg PO twice daily[bid]/thrice daily [tid]) inhibits action of acetylcholine on smooth muscle and has a direct antispasmodic effect on smooth muscles, which in turn causes bladder capacity to increase and uninhibited contractions to decrease.
    - Tolterodine tartrate (Detrol, Detrol LA) is a competitive muscarinic receptor antagonist used to treat overactive bladder. It has selectivity for urinary bladder.
- Surgical therapy includes:
  - Open surgical procedures
  - Endoscopic injection
- Surgical repair may be recommended in infants with persistent unilateral grades IV–V reflux or bilateral grades III–V reflux after a period of antibiotic therapy should the parents prefer definitive therapy over watchful management while receiving antibiotic prophylaxis.
- In children aged 1–5 years, surgical repair is a reasonable alternative for grades IV and V reflux (Fig. 71.6).
- In patients with bilateral grade V reflux, surgical repair is recommended.
- Surgery is recommended for children with persistent grades III–V reflux in whom antibiotic therapy has not kept them infection-free.

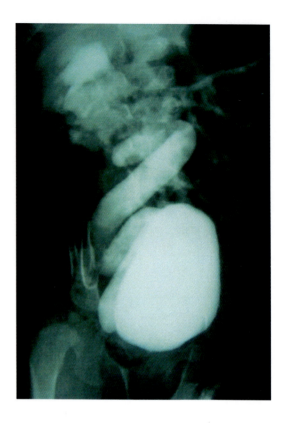

Fig. 71.6 MCUG showing severe VUR

- Endoscopic treatment may be recommended in children with grade III–IV who have not shown any improvement in the reflux grade, who do not wish to receive further antibiotics, or who have had UTI.
- In patients diagnosed with bilateral grades III–IV reflux at age 6–10 years, surgical repair is the preferred option, although continuous antibiotics is a reasonable alternative.
- Patients with grade V reflux should undergo surgical repair (Fig. 71.7).
- In patients with persistent grades I–II reflux after a period of antibiotic prophylaxis, consensus is lacking regarding the role of continued antibiotics versus surgery.
- However, surgery is an option for persistent reflux in children with grades III–IV reflux in whom initial antibiotic therapy has failed. They can undergo either open surgical or endoscopic treatment.
- Ureteral reimplantation:
  - Surgery (ureteral reimplantation or ureteroneocystostomy) is the definitive method of correcting primary VUR.
  - Surgical principles of successful reimplantation include:
    1. Creating a long submucosal tunnel to provide a 5:1 tunnel-to-diameter ratio
    2. Providing good detrusor muscle backing
    3. Avoiding ureteric kinking
    4. Creating a tunnel in the fixed area of the bladder
- Standard antireflux ureteral reimplantation procedures include:
  - The transtrigonal (Cohen)
  - The intravesical (Leadbetter–Politano)
  - The extravesical reimplantation (Lich–Gregoir)

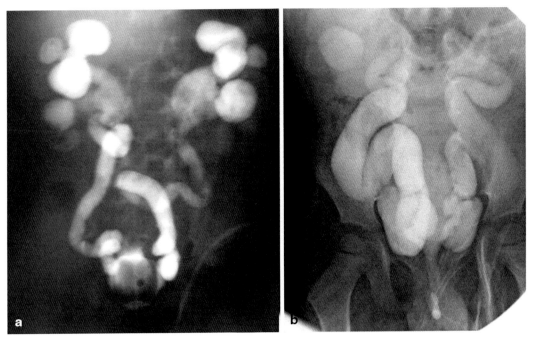

Fig. 71.7 MCUG images showing severe bilateral VUR (**a**) and severe grade V bilateral VUR (**b**)

- The Glenn-Anderson repair
- The extravesical detrusorrhaphy (Hodgson–Zaontz)
- Potential complications due to ureteral reimplantation of the ureters include (in < 1 %):
  - Bleeding in the retperitoneal space
  - Infections
  - Ureteral obstruction
  - Injury to adjacent organs
  - Persistent reflux
- Antireflux surgery does not completely prevent the frequency of recurrent nonfebrile UTIs (Fig. 71.8).
- Endoscopic treatment:
  - The principle of the procedure is to inject, under cystoscopic guidance, a biocompatible bulking agent underneath the intravesical portion of the ureter in a submucosal location.
  - The bulking agent elevates the ureteral orifice and distal ureter in such a way that the lumen is narrowed, preventing reflux of urine up the ureter but still allowing its antegrade flow.
  - Several bulking agents have been evaluated. These include:
    - Polytetrafluoroethylene (PTFE or Teflon).
    - Collagen.
    - Autologous fat.
    - Polydimethylsiloxane.
    - Silicone.
    - Chondrocytes.
    - A solution of dextranomer/hyaluronic acid (Deflux). This is the most commonly used agent.

Fig. 71.8 Post-reimplantation MCUG showing disappearance of VUR

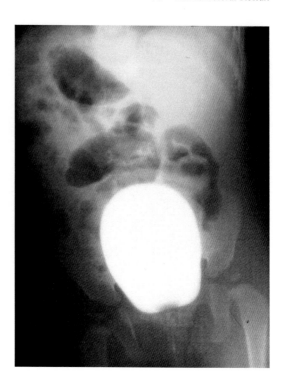

- The resolution rate of reflux per ureter for grades:
  - I and II is 78.5 %.
  - III is 72 %.
  - IV is 63 %.
  - V is 51 %.

- Laparoscopic and robotic reimplantation may be a possible alternative to open ureteral reimplantation.

Recommended Reading

Hayn MH, Smaldone MC, Ost MC, Docimo SG. Minimally invasive treatment of vesicoureteral reflux. Urol Clin North Am. 2008;35(3):477–88.

Hoberman A, Keren R. Antimicrobial prophylaxis for urinary tract infection in children. N Engl J Med. 2009;361(18):1804–6.

Park J, Retik AB. Surgery for vesicoureteral reflux. *Ped Urol.* 2001;4:421–29.

Roussey-Kesler G, Gadjos V, Idres N, Horen B, Ichay L, Leclair MD, et al. Antibiotic prophylaxis for the prevention of recurrent urinary tract infection in children with low grade vesicoureteral reflux: results from a prospective randomized study. J Urol. 2008;179(2):674–9.

Stenberg A, Hensle TW, Läckgren G. Vesicoureteral reflux: a new treatment algorithm. Curr Urol Rep. 2002;3(2):107–14.

Chapter 72
The Exstrophy–Epispadias Complex

Introduction

- The exstrophy–epispadias complex comprises a spectrum of congenital abnormalities that includes:
  - Classic bladder exstrophy
  - Epispadias
  - Cloacal exstrophy
  - Exstrophy variants
- Most of these patients have much more severe defects, involving a small and bifid phallus with bladder exstrophy or more severely, cloacal exstrophy.
- The prevalence of bladder exstrophy is 3.3 per 100,000 live births.
- The prevalence of male epispadias is 1 in 117,000 live births.
- The prevalence of female epispadias is 1 in 484,000 live births.
- The prevalence of cloacal exstrophy is 1 in 200,000–400,000 live births.
- Classic bladder exstrophy is more common in males (male to female ratio is 2.3:1 and as high as 6:1).
- No definitive risk factors or causative agents are known for exstrophy–epispadias complex.
- Offspring of patients with exstrophy–epispadias complex have a 1 in 70 risk (500 times that of the general population) of being affected. Nevertheless, familial occurrence is uncommon in large series.
- Growing evidence suggests an increased incidence of cloacal exstrophy and bladder exstrophy–epispadias in patients following in vitro fertilization pregnancies.
- A higher incidence of bladder exstrophy is also observed in infants of younger mothers and in those with relatively high parity.
- Maternal tobacco exposure is associated with more severe defects.

Embryology

- Embryologically, the primitive cloaca gets divided via the cloacal membrane into the urogenital sinus anteriorly and hindgut posteriorly.
- This occurs during the first trimester of pregnancy and coincides with the development of the anterior abdominal wall.
- Failure of mesenchyme to migrate between the ectodermal and endodermal layers of the lower abdominal wall muscles leads to instability of the cloacal membrane.

- Premature rupture of the cloacal membrane before its caudal translocation leads to this complex of anomalies.
- Rupture of the cloacal membrane after complete separation of the cloaca results in bladder exstrophy.
- Rupture of the cloacal membrane prior to the descent of the urorectal septum leads to cloacal exstrophy.
- Incomplete separation of the urinary tract, genital tract, and hindgut leads to cloacal malformation (persistent cloaca with no abdominal wall defect).

Clinical Features

- Most of these cases are diagnosed via antenatal ultrasound or fetal magnetic resonance imaging (MRI).
- Classic bladder exstrophy, exstrophy variants, epispadias, and cloacal exstrophy are obvious clinically.
- Unrecognized female epispadias or exstrophy variants may present as persistent childhood incontinence.
- In classic bladder exstrophy:
  - The bladder is open on the lower abdomen, with mucosa fully exposed.
  - The phallus in males is short and broad with upward (dorsal) chordee.
  - The urethral plate is open and extends the entire length of the phallus.
  - The bladder plate and urethral plate are in continuity, with the verumontanum and ejaculatory ducts visible within the prostatic urethral plate.
  - The anus is anteriorly displaced but with a normal sphincter mechanism.
  - The symphysis pubis is widely separated.
  - Inguinal hernias are common (>80% of males and >10% of females).
  - Reflux develops in approximately 40% of patients postoperatively.
  - In females:
    - The clitoris is bifid with divergent labia superiorly.
    - The open urethral plate is in continuity with the bladder plate.
    - The vagina is anteriorly displaced.
    - The anus is anteriorly displaced but with a normal sphincter mechanism.
  - Baseline ultrasound examination of the kidneys is recommended for all patients with bladder exstrophy because increased bladder pressure after bladder closure can lead to hydronephrosis and upper urinary tract deterioration.
  - Bilateral vesicoureteral reflux is present in nearly all patients with classic bladder exstrophy.
- In epispadias (Fig. 72.1):
  - The symphysis pubis is generally widened.
  - The rectus muscles are divergent distally.
  - In males:
    - The phallus is short and broad with upward chordee.
    - The urethral meatus is located on the dorsal penile shaft and can be limited to the glans penis or extends the whole length of the penis.
    - The glans penis lies open and flat.
  - In females:
    - The clitoris is bifid with divergent labia superiorly.

Clinical Features

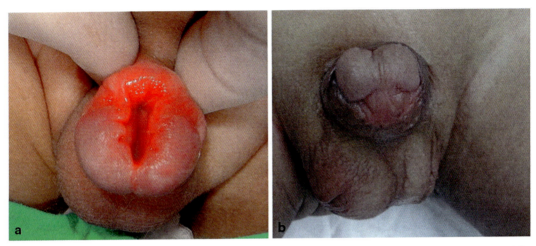

Fig. 72.1 Clinical photographs showing epispadias. Note the extent of the epispadias groove in (**a**) (glandular) and the dorsal chordee in (**b**)

- The dorsal aspect of the urethra is open distally.
- The urethra and bladder neck are patulous and may allow visualization of bladder.
- Bladder mucosa may prolapse through the bladder neck.

- In cloacal exstrophy (covered in detail in a separate chapter; Fig. 72.2):

  - Nearly all patients have an associated omphalocele.
  - The bladder is open and separated into two halves, with the exposed interior of the cecum between them.
  - The cecal plate contains openings to the remainder of the hindgut and to one or two appendices.
  - The terminal ileum may prolapse as a "trunk" of bowel onto the cecal plate.
  - The penis is generally small and bifid, with a hemi-glans located just caudal to each hemi-bladder.
  - Infrequently, the phallus may be intact in the midline.
  - In females, the clitoris is bifid and two vaginas are present.
  - The anus is absent.
  - Sixty-five percent of patients have a clubfoot or major deformity of a lower extremity.
  - Eighty percent of patients have vertebral anomalies.
  - Ninety-five percent of patients have myelodysplasia, which may include myelomeningocele, lipomeningocele, meningocele, or other forms of occult dysraphism.
  - These patients are at risk of neurologic deterioration, and they should be observed closely.
  - Early neurosurgical consultation is recommended if a radiographic abnormality of the spinal cord or canal is observed.

- In exstrophy variants:

  - The symphysis pubis is widely separated, and rectus muscles diverge distally.
  - The umbilicus is low in position or elongated.
  - A small superior bladder opening or a patch of isolated bladder mucosa may be present.
  - The intact bladder may be externally covered by only a thin membrane.
  - Isolated ectopic bowel segments have been reported.
  - Genitalia generally are intact, though epispadias can occur.
  - In the split-symphysis variants of exstrophy, the symphysis pubis is widely separated, and the rectus muscles are divergent.

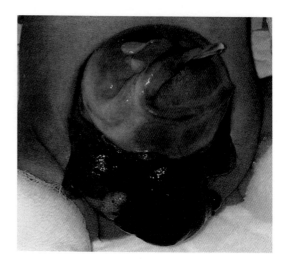

Fig. 72.2 A clinical photograph showing classic cloacal exstrophy. Note the omphalocele, the open urinary bladder, and the open trunk of bowel onto the cecal plate

Isolated Epispadias

Introduction

- Epispadias as an isolated malformation is very rare.
- It is an uncommon congenital malformation of the penis and more commonly seen as part of the epispadias–exstrophy malformation.
- Epispadias occurs more commonly in males than in females. The male to female ratio is 2.3:1.
- It occurs in around 1 in 50,000 to 1 in 120,000 male and 1 in 400,000 to 1 in 500,000 female live births.
- The extent of the defect can vary from a mild glandular defect to complete defects involving the whole length of the phallus.
- Evaluation of the bladder neck and proximal urethra is recommended in patients with epispadias in order to plan surgical management

Embryology

- Epispadias results from defective migration of the paired primordial genital tubercle that fuse on the midline to form the genital tubercle at the fifth week of embryologic development.
- Epispadias and exstrophy of the bladder are considered varying degrees of a single disorder.
- The extent of epispadias varies in severity depending on the time of the insult during embryologic development.

Classification

- Epispadias is classified into:
    - Glandular (Fig. 72.3)
    - Penile (Fig. 72.4a)

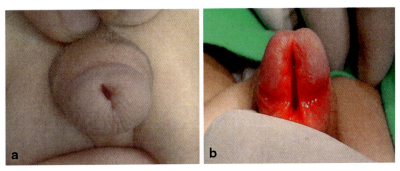

Fig. 72.3 a and **b** Clinical photographs showing mild glandular epispadias and full glandular epispadias

- Complete (penopubic; Fig. 72.4b)
- Epispadias associated with bladder exstrophy

- All forms of epispadias are associated with dorsal chordee. The extent of this is variable.
- In females, epispadias consists of bifid clitoris with diastases of the corpora cavernosa, flattening of the mons, and separation of the labia.
- Complete continence is expected in those with glandular and penile epispadias but in those with penopubic epispadias incontinence can be expected.
- The epispadias repair is performed commonly using the modified Cantwell–Ransley repair technique (Figs. 72.5, 72.6, 72.7, and 72.8).

Classic Bladder Exstrophy

Introduction

- Bladder exstrophy is rare with an incidence of 1 in 10,000 to 1 in 50,000 live births.
- The male to female ratio is 1.3:1.
- The risk of recurrence in a family is 1 in 100.
- Children born to parents with exstrophy have a 1 in 70 chance of having the defect.
- The diagnosis of bladder exstrophy can be made antenatally by a prenatal ultrasound and usually confirmed postnatally by the typical appearance of the lower abdomen which shows an open urinary bladder.
- The upper urinary tract is usually normal, but reflux develops in the vast majority of patients postoperatively.
- This will require later ureteroneocystostomy usually at the time of bladder neck repair.
- Inguinal hernias are noted in most patients due to the lack of obliquity of the inguinal canal. These are more common in males.
- Anal stenosis may be noted in some patients.
- Abnormalities of the pelvic muscles and bones are common.
- Of the patients with bladder exstrophy, 70–75 % are continent following modern reconstruction.

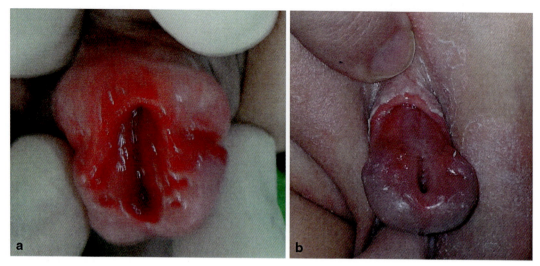

Fig. 72.4 Clinical photographs showing penile epispadias. **a** Note the opening of the urethra extending proximal to the glans penis. **b** shows complete epispadias. Note the open and flat glans penis

Fig. 72.5 Clinical photograph showing postoperative epispadias. Note the breakdown of the repair

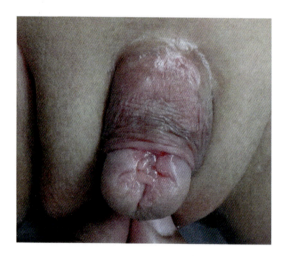

Management

- The management of bladder exstrophy must be done by an experienced team.
- The goals of surgical management are:
    - Preoperative stabilization of the patient
    - Initial closure of the bladder, posterior urethra, and abdominal wall aiming subsequently for urinary continence and preservation of renal function
    - Reapproximation of the symphysis pubis
    - Functional and cosmetically acceptable genitalia
- General preoperative supportive care.
- Keep the exposed urinary bladder covered by clean by plastic wrap.

Classic Bladder Exstrophy

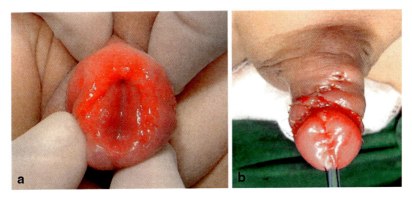

Fig. 72.6 Clinical photographs showing preoperative (**a**) and postoperative (**b**) glandular epispadias

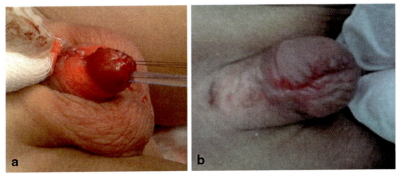

Fig. 72.7 A clinical photograph showing postoperative repair of glandular epispadias (**a**) and failed epispadias repair (**b**)

Fig. 72.8 Clinical photograph showing postoperative repair of failed epispadias

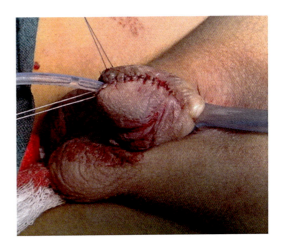

- Avoid moistened or impregnated gauze, which is irritating to the delicate bladder mucosa.
- Start antibiotic therapy which should continue through the early postoperative period.
- Daily prophylactic antibiotic therapy may be continued in the weeks after bladder closure.
- Approximately 30% of patients with bladder exstrophy have symptoms of latex allergy, and this must be taken in consideration.
- Staged functional closure for classic bladder exstrophy.
  - Initial bladder closure is attempted within in the first 48–72 h of life.
  - If repair is delayed, pelvic osteotomies are required to facilitate successful closure of the abdominal wall and to allow the bladder to lie within a closed and supportive pelvic ring.
  - Performance of anterior innominate osteotomy allows approximation of the pubic bones, closure of the symphysis pubis, and abdominal wall muscles without tension.
  - This is performed in conjunction with pediatric orthopedic surgeons.
  - Postoperatively, the patient is kept in modified Bryant traction for 3 weeks. Alternatively, spica casts, lower extremity wraps, and external pelvic fixators are used. This is to prevent separation of the pubic bones.
  - The urinary bladder is drained via a suprapubic tube or a urethral catheter and ureteral stents are also left in place.
  - At the end of the first stage procedure, the patient will be left with an epispadias.
  - Prophylactic antibiotics are continued postoperatively.
  - Epispadias repair with urethroplasty is performed at age 12–18 months. This allows enough increase in bladder outlet resistance to improve the bladder capacity as well as growth of the phallus.
  - The epispadias repair is performed using the modified Cantwell–Ransley repair technique.
  - Preoperative log-acting testosterone may be used to increase the penile length prior to epispadias repair.
  - Bladder neck reconstruction is performed at age 4 years. Ureteral reimplantation is usually performed at this time
  - Typically, a modified Young–Dees–Leadbetter repair is used. This allows continence and correction of vesicoureteral reflux.
  - The procedure is delayed until bladder capacity is adequate; better results are reported with a bladder capacity >85 ml.
- Complete primary repair for classic bladder exstrophy.
  - Primary bladder closure, urethroplasty, and genital reconstruction are performed in a single stage in newborns.
  - Hypospadias is a common outcome in males postoperatively and requires subsequent reconstruction (Fig. 72.9).
- Urinary diversion for classic bladder exstrophy may be performed in those with an extremely small bladder plate not suitable for functional closure.
- Postoperative complications include:
  - Bladder prolapse
  - Bladder outlet obstruction
  - Bladder calculi
  - Renal calculi
  - Wound dehiscence including urethra and bladder

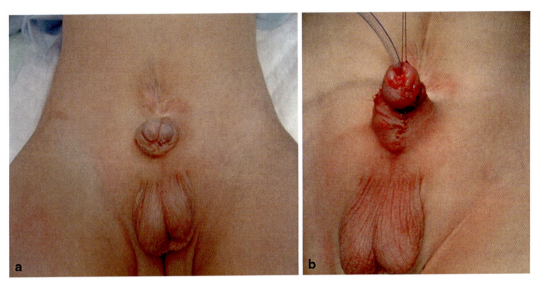

Fig. 72.9 a A clinical photograph showing hypospadias following primary repair of bladder exstrophy. **b** Clinical photograph showing postoperative repair of hypospadias that resulted following primary repair of bladder exstrophy

Recommended Reading

Bhatnagar V. Bladder exstrophy: an overview of the surgical management. J Indian Assoc Pediatr Surg. 2011;16(3):81–7.
Gearhart JP, Forschner DC, Jeffs RD, et al. A combined vertical and horizontal pelvic osteotomy approach for primary and secondary repair of bladder exstrophy. J Urol. 1996;155(2):689–93.
Grady RW, Mitchell ME. Complete primary repair of exstrophy. J Urol. 1999;162(4):1415–20.
Mitchell ME. Bladder exstrophy repair: complete primary repair of exstrophy. Urology. 2005;65(1):5–8.
Surer I, Baker LA, Jeffs RD, Gearhart JP. The modified Cantwell-Ransley repair for exstrophy and epispadias: 10-year experience. J Urol. 2000;164(3 Pt 2):1040–3.

Index

A

Abdominal distension, 139, 141
Abdominal wall defect, 253
Abdominal wall hernia, 15, 21
    in infants and children, 22, 25
Achalasia, 109
    clinical features of, 109
    diagnosis of, 110
        endoscopy, 110
    etiology of, 109
    incidence of, 109
    treatment of, 110–112
        Botulinum toxin injection, 111
        laparoscopic approach, 112
        operative, 112
        pharmacologic, 110
        pneumatic balloon dilatation, 111
Acute scrotum, 77
    causes of, 77, 85
    in children, 82
Ambiguous genitalia, 425
Angiographic occlusion, 75
Aniridia, 479, 480
Anomalous pancreaticobiliary junction, 286
Anorectal anomalies, 402
Anorectal malformations, 101, 203, 204, 401
    associated anomalies of, 401
    classification, 406
        high, 406
        intermediate, 406
        low, 406
    classification of, 406
    clinical features of, 402
    colostomy in, 409, 416
    diagnosis of, 407
    investigation techniques of, 403
    postoperative functional disorders of, 415
    prognosis of, 415
    tethered cord, 402
    treatment of, 406
Anti-müllerian hormone (AMH), 68, 541
Aplasia cutis congenital, 121
Ascent of testes, 67
Atresias, 150

B

Beckwith-Wiedemann syndrome (BWS), 431, 432
Benign,
    mesenchymal tumor, 57
    tumors, 461, 462
Biliary atresia, 291
    associated anomalies, 293
    classification of, 292, 293
    clinical features of, 293
    differential diagnosis of, 294
    etiology of, 291, 292
    postoperative care, 296, 297
        complication and outcome, 296, 297
    treatment of, 295, 296
Bilious vomiting, 139
    contrast studies of, 145
    examination of, 141
    history of, 140
    imaging studies of, 142
    investigation techniques of, 141
    treatment of, 147
Bochdalek hernia, 351, 352
Branchial clefts, 47
Branchial cysts, 47
    clinical features of, 49
    embryology of, 47
    investigation techniques of, 50
    pathology of, 47
    treatment of, 50
    types of, 48, 49
        first branchial cleft cysts, 48
        fourth branchial cleft cysts, 49
        second branchial cleft cysts, 48
        third branchial cleft cysts, 49
Bronchogenic cyst, 365
Bronchogenic cysts, 385
    clinical presentation of, 388
    embryology of, 385
    investigation techniques of, 389
    sites and pathology of, 386
    treatment of, 391
Bronchopulmonary sequestration *See* Pulmonary
    sequestration, 393

C
Calcitonin gene-related peptide (CGRP), 68
Caloric requirements, 6
Carbohydrates, 6
Cardiovascular anomalies, 249
Central nervous system, 249
Cervical teratoma *See under* Teratoma, 501
Choledochal cyst, 283
　classification of, 283
　clinical features of, 285
　diagnosis of, 285
　etiology of, 283
　treatment of, 286, 287, 289
Cholelithiasis, 277, 278
　complications in, 279
　etiology of, 278, 279
　treatment of, 280, 281
Cholesterol stones, 277
Chordee, 545, 547, 548, 552
Classic bladder exstrophy, 591, 592, 595
　clinical features of, 592
　management of, 596, 598
Cloacal exstrophy, 425, 591, 592
　associated anomalies, 427
　clinical features, 593
　clinical features and management of, 427–430
　embryology of, 425, 427
Cloacal malformation, 417
　associated anomalies of, 419
　classification of, 421
　clinical features of, 417
　investigation techniques of, 420
　management of, 421, 423
　　prognostic factors, 423
Colonic obstruction, 199
Common bile duct (CBD), 283, 284
Congenital,
　abnormality, 545, 559
　aplasia of the diaphragm, 345
　cystic adenomatoid malformation, 365
　cystic diseases of the lung, 365
　　bronchogenic cyst, 365
　　congenital cystic adenomatoid malformation, 365
　　congenital lobar emphysema, 365
　　pulmonary sequestration, 365
　diaphragmatic hernia, 329, 330, 333, 335–337, 343, 351
　　associated anomalies, 336
　　diagnosis of, 337
　　familial type, 333
　　long-term outcomes and prognosis of, 343
　　pathophysiology of, 330
　diverticulum, 181
　duodenal, 133
　　atresia, 133
　esophageal stenosis (CES), 105–107
　　classification of, 105
　　diagnosis of, 106
　　incidence of, 105
　　investigating techniques of, 107
　　symptoms of, 106
　　treatment of, 107
　lobar emphysema (CLE), 365–367, 369, 370, 372
　　associated malformations, 367
　　clinical features of, 367
　　diagnosis of, 367, 369, 370
　　pathogenesis of, 366, 367
　　treatment and outcome of, 370, 372
　lumbar hernias, 22
　　complications of, 22
　malformations, 29, 101, 569
　mass of the neck, 47
　paraesophageal hernia, 357–359, 361
　　classification of, 358
　　clinical features of, 359
　　etiology of, 357
　　treatment of, 359, 361
　pulmonary malformations, 393
　rectal atresia, 203–206
　　classification of, 203
　　clinical features of, 204
　　diagnosis of, 204
　　Dorairjan's classification of, 203
　　Gupta and Sharma's classification of, 203
　　treatment of, 205, 206
　segmental dilatation (CSD), 231, 233–235
　　diagnosis of, 234
Congenital abnormalities of the lung, 385
Congenital cystic adenomatoid malformation, 385
Congenital cystic adenomatoid malformation (CCAM), 373
　Adzick's classification of, 375
　　macrocystic CCAM, 375
　　microcystic CCAM, 375
　classification (based on cyst size), 373, 374
　　Type II CCAM, 374
　　Type III CCAM, 374
　differential diagnosis of, 377
　investigative techniques of, 377–380
　presentation of, 376
　treatment and outcomes of, 380–382
Congenital gastric outlet obstruction, 122
Congenital lobar emphysema, 385
Congenital pyloric atresia (CPA), 121
　anatomy of, 121
　clinical examination of, 123
　investigation techniques of, 123
　presentation of, 122
　prognosis of, 126
　treatment of, 124
Congenital:paraesophageal hernia:classification of:paraesophageal hernia, 359
Congenital:paraesophageal hernia:classification of:sliding hiatal hernia, 358
Continuous splenogonadal fusion *See under* Splenogonadal fusion, 273
Cooper's hernia, 22

Index

Cryptorchidism, 67, 71
  factors leading to, 69
  management of, 70
Cryptorchidism See also Undescended testes, 67
Cystic,
  dilatation biliary tract, 283
  fibrosis, 189
    etiology of, 189
  lesions, 491
Cystic Fibrosis Transmembrane conductance Regulator (CFTR), 189

D

Deep fibromatosis, 57, 60
Developmental abnormalities See Disorders of sex development (DSD), 519
Developmental pancreatic cysts, 309
Disorders of sex development (DSD), 519, 520
  classification, 523
    46, XX, 523
    46, XY, 523
    sex chromosome, 523
  common causes of, 530–537
  embryology of, 520–522
  etiology of, 524, 525
  evaluation of new born with, 526–529
  management of, 530
  pathophysiology of, 526
Disorders of sex differentiation See Disorders of sex development (DSD), 519
Down's syndrome See Trisomy 21, 133
Duodenal,
  atresia, 133
  stenosis, 133
Dysphagia, 109, 112

E

Echocardiogram, 91
Electrolytes, 1, 7
  outlines of, 2
Embolization, 43
Embryonic thyroglossal duct, 63
Epidermolysis bullosa (EB), 121
Epidermolysisbullosa (EB), 122
Epispadias, 592
  classification of, 594, 595
  clinical features of, 592, 593
  embryology of, 594
Esophageal,
  motility disorder, 109
  stricture, 98
Esophageal atresia (EA), 89, 105
  anatomy of, 89
  associated anomalies in, 92
  clinical features of, 90
  complications of, 98
  diagnosis of, 90, 91
    contrast-enhanced studies, 91
  embryology of, 89
  prognosis and outcome in, 95

  Spitz classification of, 99
  treatment of, 94
  Waterston classification of, 99
Esophagomyotomy, 112
Eventration of diaphragm, 345, 347, 351
  acquired type, 346
  congenital type, 345, 346
  diagnosis of, 348
  treatment of, 348
    surgical approaches, 348
Ewing sarcoma, 451
Exomphalos, 253, 256
Exstrophy, 429
  of bladder and intestine, 427
  of hemi bladders, 425, 428
  variants, 592, 593
    clinical features of, 593
Exstrophy See also Cloacal exstrophy, 429
Exstrophy-epispadias complex,
  congenital abnormalities in, 591
Extralobar sequestration See under Pulmonary sequestration, 395

F

Familial adenomatous polyposis (FAP), 315, 320, 321, 432
Fat, 6
Femoral hernias, 21
Fistula-in-ano, 241
  etiology of, 242
Fistulectomy,
  treatment of, 244
Fistulotomy, 244, 245
Foker technique, 95
Fowler-Stephens procedure, 71
Full-thickness intestinal necrosis, 209
Functional immaturity of the colon, 195

G

Gallstones, 277, 278
  hemolytic, 278
  idiopathic, 278
  non-hemolytic, 278
Gastric volvulus,
  classification (based on etiology), 128
    Type 1 (Idiopathic), 128
    Type 2 (Secondary or acquired), 128
  classification (based on presentation), 129, 130
    acute gastric volvulus, 129, 130
    chronic gastric volvulus, 129, 130
  classification (based on the site of volvulus), 130
    intra-abdominal gastric volvulus, 130
    intra-thoracic gastric volvulus, 130
  Singleton's classification of, 127
    mesentericoaxial, 127
    mixed (combined), 127
    organoaxial, 127
  treatment of, 130, 131
    anterior gastropexy, 130
    combined anterior and fundal gastropexy, 131

fundal gastropexy, 131
Gastroesophageal,
    junction (GEJ), 112, 357–359
    reflux, 357, 358, 361
Gastrointestinal anomalies, 92, 249
Gastroschisis, 247, 250
    associated anomalies, 249
    diagnosis of, 248
    etiology of, 247
    management and outcomes of, 249
Genitourinary,
    anomalies, 249
    defects, 401
Germ cell tumors, 461, 462, 505, 508, 509
    choriocarcinomas, 461
    dysgerminomas, 461
    non seminomatous, 508
    teratomas, 461
    yolk sac tumors, 461

H
Hamartomatous abnormality of the lung, 373
Hamartomatous polyposis syndromes, 315, 316, 319
Heller's myotomy See also Achalasia, 112
Hemangioma,
    characteristics of, 37
    complications in, 37
    prognosis of, 43
    treatment of, 39, 41–43
        interferon-alpha, 43
        laser therapy, 42
        sclerotherapy, 41
        surgical excision, 42
Hemihypertrophy, 479
Hepatic hemangioma, 45
Hepatoblastoma, 469, 470, 472, 475, 477, 478
    clinical feature of, 432
    etiology of, 431, 432
        Beckwith-Wiedmann syndrome, 431, 432
        familial adenomatous polyposis, 432
        hemihypertrophy, 432
        low birth weight, 432
    histological classification of, 437
    investigations, 432–434
    pathology, 435–437
    staging, 434, 435
    treatment and prognosis of, 438, 440
Hepatocellular carcinoma, 469, 474, 475, 478
    malignant tumors, 470
Hereditary multiple intestinal atresia (HMIA), 122
Hereditary-mixed polyposis syndrome (HMPS), 315, 326
Hirschprung's disease (HD), 219
    associated anomalies, 222, 223
    complications and outcome, 228, 229
    diagnosis of, 223
        abdominal x-ray, 223
    diagnosisof, 223–225
        anorectalmanometry, 224
        barium enema, 223
        rectal biopsy, 225
    enterocolitis in, 222
    etiology of, 220
    long-segment, 219, 227
    pathophysiology of, 219, 220
    short segment, 219
    symptoms and signs of, 220, 221
    treatment of, 225, 226
        laproscopic approach to, 226
    treatmentof, 225–227
        anorectal myomectomy, 227
        Duhamel procedure, 225
        Soave procedure, 226
        Swenson procedure, 225
        transanal pull-through, 226, 227
Hirschsprung disease, 201
Hodgkin's lymphoma, 443
    Ann Arbor staging classification, 444
    clinical features of, 445, 446
    diagnosis of, 446
    etiology of, 446
    lymphocyte depleted, 444
    lymphocytic predominance, 444
    mixed-cellularity, 444
    nodular sclerosing, 443
    treatment of, 447–450
H-type tracheoesophageal fistula, 101
    etiology of, 101
    investigation techniques in, 102
    presentation and diagnosis of, 101
    treatment of, 103
Human chorionic gonadotropin therapy, 70
    adverse effects of, 71
Hydroceles,
    characteristics of, 26
    definition of, 26
    of Canal Of Nuck, 27
    of cord, 27
    treatment of, 27
Hydrocolpos, 417, 418
    drainage of, 421
Hydronephrosis, 559, 560
    antenatally diagnosed, 559
Hypospadias, 479, 545
    anterior, 548
    embryology of, 546, 547
    etiology of, 549, 550
    middle, 548
    posterior, 549

I
Ileo-colic intussusception, 169
Imperforate anus, 401, 425, 427, 428
    without fistula, 401, 415
Incisional hernia, 24
Incomplete,
    fixation, 175
    prepuce, 545
    rotation, 173, 175

Indirect hernia, 181
Infantile fibromatosis, 57
   clinical features of, 58
   histopathology of, 58
Infantile hemangioma, 37
Infantile hypertrophic pyloric stenosis,
   incidence of, 115
   pathophysiology of, 116, 117
Infantile myofibromatosis, 57
   generalized form of, 59
   localized form of, 58
   multicentric form without visceral involvement, 59
   pathogenesis of, 57
   prognosis of, 61
   treatment of, 60
Infantile pyloric stenosis, 115, 116
   diagnosis of, 117
   epidemiology and etiology of, 115
   imaging techniques of, 117
   prognosis of, 118
   signs and symptoms, 116
   treatment of, 117
Infusion,
   guidelines of, 6
Inguinal canal, 67, 68, 70
Inguinal hernia,
   Amyand's hernia, 17
   Busse's hernia, 17
   classification of, 16
      irreducible hernia, 16
      reducible hernia, 16
   complications of, 17
   in infants, 17
   incarcerated, 17
   laparoscopic repair of, 19
      advantages of, 19
   Littre's hernia, 17
   obstructed, 16
   prevalence of, 15, 16
   Richter's hernia, 17
   strangulated, 17
   treatment of, 17
   types of, 15
      direct, 15
      indirect, 15
Inspissated meconium, 195
Intestinal,
   dilatation, 195
   fixation, 173
   malrotation, 173, 175, 177, 178
      clinical features of, 175
      embryology of, 173
      investigation techniques of, 177
      management of, 178
   neuronal dysplasia, 200
   nonrotation, 173
   obstruction, 149, 157, 161, 169
   polyps, 315, 316
      classification of, 316

Intracytoplasmic inclusions, 58
Intralobar sequestration *See* under Pulmonary
      sequestration, 395
Intravenous fluids, 1
Intussusception, 175
   diagnosis of, 169
   management of, 170
   signs and symptoms, 168
   treatment of, 172
      laparoscopy, 172
   types of, 167
   types of (based on etiology), 167
      idiopathic, 167
      secondary to a lead point, 167
   types of (based on site), 168
      enteroenteral, 168
      ileo-colic, 168
Ipsilateral testicular growth retardation, 75

J
Jejunoileal atresia, 149, 150, 156, 161, 162
   subtypes of, 155
      diagnosis of, 155
Jejunoileal stenosis, 149
Jejunoilealatresia,
   classification of, 150
   classificationof, 150
      atresias, 150
      stenosis, 150
   complications in, 153
   etiology of, 149
   subtypesof, 150–154
      clinical features of, 154
      pathophysiology of, 153
      Type I, 150
      Type II, 151
      Type IV, 152
      TypeIIIa, 151
      TypeIIIb, 152

K
Kasabach-Merritt syndrome, 39, 45

L
Laparoscopic,
   cholecystectomy, 280
      surgical complications of, 280
   myotomy, 113
Leydig cells, 505, 508
Lumbar hernias, 22
   types of, 22
Lymph nodes, 443, 445, 448
Lymphangiomas, 29
   characteristics of, 29
   classification of (based on microscopic
      characteristics), 30, 31
      capillary, 31
      cavernous, 31
      cystic, 31

hemangiolymphangioma, 31
classification of (based on size), 32
    macrocystic, 32
    microcystic, 32
    mixed, 32
Kennedy's classification of, 32, 33
    Lymphangioma circumscriptum, 33
sites of, 34
treatment of, 29, 34, 35

M
Macrocystic CCAM *See* under Congenital cystic adenomatoid malformation (CCAM), 375
Maintenance fluid, 2
Maldevelopment of the diaphragm, 345
Malignant neoplasms, 461
Maternal diabetes mellitus, 199, 200
Maydl's hernia, 17
Meckel's diverticulum, 181, 183, 185
    diagnosis of, 186
    embryology of, 182
    symptoms of, 183
    treatment of, 187
Meconium ileus, 189
    clinical presentation of, 190
    etiology of, 189
    investigation techniques in, 191
    treatment of, 191, 193
        long-term prognosis, 193
        nonoperative, 191
        post-operative management, 193
        surgical therapy, 193
    types of, 190
        complicated, 190
        simple, 190
Meconium plug syndrome, 195
    clinical features of, 196
    differential diagnosis of, 196
    etiology of, 195
    treatment of, 196, 197
        contrast enema, 197
        plain abdominal x-ray, 196
Medullary thyroid cancer (MTC), 514
    history of, 515
Megacystis microcolon intestinal hypoperistalsis syndrome (MMIHS), 237
    clinical features of, 239, 240
    etiology of, 237
    treatment of, 240
Microcystic CCAM *See* under Congenital cystic adenomatoid malformation (CCAM), 375
Morgagni's hernia, 351, 352
    associated anomalies, 353
    diagnosis of, 353, 354
    management of, 355
Multiple endocrine neoplasia (MEN), 514, 515
Musculoskeletal malformations, 249
Myotomy, 112

N
Necrotizing enterocolitis (NEC), 209
    clinical features of, 210
    clinical presentation of, 211
    diagnosis of, 212
    etiology of, 209, 210
    incidence of, 209
    radiographic signs of, 213
    surgical interventions in, 215
    treatment of, 214
Neonatal,
    distal small bowel obstruction, 189
    gastrointestinal disorders, 209
    hypoglycemia, 199
    intestinal obstruction, 139
        diagnosis of, 139
    neck mass, 53
    small left colon syndrome, 199–201
        clinical features of, 200
        etiology of, 199
        investigation techniques of, 201
        treatment of, 201
Nephroblastoma, 479, 482
Neuroblastoma, 451
    clinical features of, 452–454
    etiology of, 452
    investigations and diagnosis of, 454–456
    sites of origin, 452
    staging of, 456, 457
    treatment and outcome of, 457–459
Neuronal enteric plexus, 231
Neuronal nicotinic acetylcholine receptor (ηAChR), 237
Nissen's fundoplication, 357, 359
Non-Hodgkin lymphoma (NHL), 444, 448, 451
    staging, 444
    types of, 449
        aggressive, 449
        indolent, 449
Nutcracker phenomenon, 74
Nutrition requirements,
    for infants and children, 5

O
Obstructive cholangiopathy, 291
Omphalocele, 231, 247, 253, 254, 425, 427, 428, 430
    associated anomalies, 255
    etiology of, 253
    management and outcomes of, 256
    surgical management of, 257
Omphaloenteric duct anomalies, 182
Ovarian cyst, 465

P
Pampiniform plexus, 73
    diagnosis of, 74
Pancreatic cysts, 309
    clinical features of, 310

Index

embryology of, 310
pseudocysts, 309
true congenital pancreatic, 309
Pancreatic pseudocyst, 299, 302
  causes of, 303
  clinical features of, 303
  complications of, 304
    hemorrhage, 304
    infection, 304
    spontaneous rupture, 304
  surgical management of, 302
Pancreaticobiliary system, 299
Pancreatitis, 299
  acute, 300–302
    clinical features of, 300, 301
    diagnosis, 301, 302
  causes of, 299
  classification of, 299
  hereditary, 300
  surgical management of, 302, 303
Pantaloon hernia, 17
Papillary thyroid cancer, 514
Paraesophageal hernia, 351
Paraumbilical hernia, 21
Pediatric liver tumors,
  malignant tumors, 470
Pediatric primary liver tumor *See* Hepatoblastoma, 431
Pelviureteric junction obstruction (PUJ), 559, 564
  obstruction, 559–561, 566
    clinical features of, 561
    extrinsic causes, 560, 561
    intrinsic causes, 560
    short-segment, 566
Perianal abscess, 241–243
  clinical features of, 244
  etiology of, 242
Periodic acid–Schiff (PAS) test, 58
Peripheral percutaneous venous canulation, 9
Peripherally inserted central line (PICC), 9
Persistent cloacae, 417
Persistent müllerian duct syndrome (PMDS),
  clinical features of, 541, 542
  embryology of, 541
  management of, 542, 543
Pigment stones, 277
  black, 277
  brown, 278
Polyposis syndrome,
  inherited adenamatous, 316
  intestinal, 315
  noninherited, 316
Polysplenia syndrome, 293
Posterior fossa malformations, hemangiomas, arterial anomalies, cardiac defects, eye abnormalities, sternal cleft and supraumbilical raphe syndrome (PHACES), 39
Posterior sagittal anorectovaginourethroplasty (PSARVUP), 421

Posterior urethral valve, 569
  classification of, 570, 571
  clinical features of, 570
  management of, 575–577
    fetal interventions, 576
    secondary bladder surgery, 576, 577
  medical management of, 577
  pathophysiology of, 574, 575
  prognosis of, 578
  secondary effects of, 572–574
    urinary incontinence, 573, 574
    urinary tract infections, 573
    vesicoureteral reflux, 572, 573
Primitive neuroectodermal tumors, 451
Progressive obliterative cholangiopathy *See* Biliary atresia, 291
Protein, 6
Pulmonary hypertension, 330
  pathophysiology of, 335
Pulmonary hypoplasia, 330, 335, 337
  long-term outcomes and prognosis, 343
  pathophysiology of, 335
Pulmonary sequestration, 365, 385, 393
  classification of, 395, 396
    extralobar, 395, 396
    intralobar, 395
  diagnosis of, 396–398
    arteriography, 398
    chest computed tomography, 397
    chest radiography, 397
    magnetic resonance imaging, 398
    ultrasonography, 396, 397
  embryology of, 394, 395
  treatment of, 398
Pyeloplasty, 559, 562, 564, 565
  open surgical, 565, 566
Pyloric canal, 116, 117
Pyloromyotomy, 118
Pylorus, 115, 116
Pyocolpos, 417, 418

R
Ramstedt pyloromyotomy, 118
Rectal stenosis, 203, 206
Red blood cells (RBCs), 261, 263
Reed–Sternberg cells, 444
  multinucleated, 443
  pleomorphic, 444
Replacement solutions, 3
  outlines of, 3
Retractile testis, 67
Retrograde regurgitation of urine, 581
Rhabdomyosarcoma, 451

S
Sacrococcygeal teratomas *See under* Teratoma, 492
Salpingo-oophorectomy, 461, 465
Sclerosing agent, 35

Seminiferous tubule sclerosis, 75
Sertoli cells, 505, 508
Seton, 241
   use of, 245
Short bowel syndrome, 173
Sliding hernia, 17
Small and large bowel, 139
Spermatogenesis, 68
Spigelian hernia, 24
Spleen, 261
   embryology of, 261
   functions of, 261, 262
   pathological conditions of, 262–271
      accessory spleen, 264
      asplenia, 265
      congestive splenomegaly, 270
      hepatolienal fusion, 265
      massive splenic infraction, 268, 269
      massive splenomegaly, 263
      partial splenectomy, 270, 271
      polysplenia, 265, 266
      splenomegaly, 262, 263
      splenorenal fusion, 266
      splenosis, 264
      wandering spleen, 266, 267
Splenic cyst *See* under Spleen, 267
Splenogonadal fusion,
   clinical features of, 274
   diagnosis of, 275
   etiology of, 274
   types of, 273
      continuous, 273
      discontinuous, 273
Splenomegaly *See* under Spleen, 262
Sternocleidomastoid fibrosis, 54
Sternomastoid tumor of infancy, 53

T
Teratoma, 491, 492
   cervical, 501, 502
   immature, 497
   intracranial, 491
   intraperitoneal, 500, 501
   malignant (staging of), 499
      complications, 499
      presentations, 499
      treatment, 499
   mature, 497
   mediastinal, 500
   monodermal, 498
   ovarian, 496
   retroperitoneal, 500
   sacrococcygeal, 492, 493
   testicular, 500
   treatment, 494, 495
Testicular,
   cancer, 505, 508, 509
   germ cell tumors, 67
   torsion, 77–79, 81
      clinical features of, 79

   diagnosis of, 79
   etiology of, 77
   predisposing conditions to, 78
   treatment of, 81
   types of, 78
Thyroglossal cyst, 63
   clinical features of, 64
   complications of, 65
   infection sites of, 63
   treatment of, 64
Thyroglossal duct cysts, 63
Thyrohyoid membrane, 63
Thyroid cancer, 513, 514
   follicular carcinoma, 514
Thyroid gland, 64, 66
   embryology of, 63
Thyroid nodules, 513
   adult, 515
   childhood, 513
Torticollis, 53
   diagnosis of, 54
   etiology of, 53
   medical management of, 54, 55
      indications for, 54
      using surgical procedures, 55
   secondary effects of, 55
Total intestinal aganglionosis, 219, 220
Total parenteral nutrition (TPN), 6, 9
Trace elements, 7
Tracheoesophageal fistula (TEF), 89, 94, 101, 105
   anatomy of, 89
   clinical features of, 90
Transfusion,
   of blood and blood products, 4
Transverse testicular ectopia (TTE), 541, 542
Trisomy 21, 133
   features of, 133
   role in congenital duodenal obstruction, 134
Turner syndrome, 29, 33

U
Ultrasonography, 117
Umbilical hernia, 19
Undescended testes, 67, 479
   diagnosis of, 69
   effects of, 67
   embryology of, 67
   etiology of, 69
   prognosis of, 71
   role in testicular cancer, 72
   seminoma, 72
Ureterovesical junction, 571, 581, 587
Urinary tract infection (UTI), 581, 585, 588
   cystitis of, 582
   investigations and diagnosis, 585
   repeated attacks of, 581

V
Varicocele, 73
   classification of, 73

Index

clinical features of, 73
detection using venography, 75
diagnosis of, 74
etiology of, 74
histological studies on, 75
role in male fertility, 73
treatment of, 75
Varicocelectomy, 73, 75
    complications of, 75
Venography *See also* Venography, 75
Venous access, 9
    complications of, 13
    in infants and children, 11
    indicators for, 9
    percutaneous central, 9
Vertebral defects, Anorectal malformations, Tracheoesophageal fistula, Renal anomalies, Renal dysplasia (VATER), 93
Vesicoureteral reflux (VUR), 572–574, 577, 581
    classification of, 583, 584
        Grade I, 583
        Grade II, 583
        Grade III, 583
        Grade IV, 584
        Grade V, 584
    clinical features of, 585
    medical management of, 587
    pathophysiology of, 584
    predisposing causes for, 582
    treatment of, 586, 587
Vincristine, 43
Visceral myopathy, 237
Vitamins, 7

W

Water-soluble contrast enema, 201
Wilms tumor, 479–481, 484, 486–488
    anaplastic, 486
    epidemiology of, 479
    management of, 485
    pathology of, 482, 483

Y

Yolk sac tumor, 508, 509

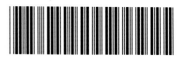